HEMOLYTIC ANEMIA
IN DISORDERS OF
RED CELL METABOLISM

TOPICS IN HEMATOLOGY

Series Editor: Maxwell M. Wintrobe, M.D.
University of Utah, Salt Lake City

THE RESPIRATORY FUNCTIONS OF BLOOD
  Lars Garby, M.D. and Jerry Meldon, M.D.

HEMOLYTIC ANEMIA IN DISORDERS OF RED CELL METABOLISM
  Ernest Beutler, M.D.

TRACE ELEMENTS AND IRON IN HUMAN METABOLISM
  Ananda S. Prasad, M.D.

HEMOLYTIC ANEMIA IN DISORDERS OF RED CELL METABOLISM

Ernest Beutler, M. D.

City of Hope National Medical Center
Duarte, California

PLENUM MEDICAL BOOK COMPANY • New York and London

Library of Congress Cataloging in Publication Data

Beutler, Ernest.
  Hemolytic anemia in disorders of red cell metabolism.

  (Topics in hematology)
  Includes index.
  1. Hemolytic anemia. 2. Erythrocyte disorders. I. Title. II. Series.
CR641.7.H4B48   616.1'52   78-2391
ISBN 978-1-4684-2459-1   ISBN 978-1-4684-2457-7 (eBook)
DOI 10.1007/978-1-4684-2457-7

© 1978 Plenum Publishing Corporation
Softcover reprint of the hardcover 1st edition 1978

227 West 17th Street, New York, N.Y. 10011

Plenum Medical Book Company is an imprint of Plenum Publishing Corporation

FOREWORD

I am prepared to predict that this monograph by Dr. Ernest Beutler will long serve as a model for monographs dealing with topics in medical science. I make this bold statement because we encounter in this work a degree of accuracy and authoritativeness well beyond that found in much of the medical literature. Too often, a monograph is simply a review of past reviews. The preparation of an exhaustive and completely accurate study such as the present one is a very laborious task; consequently, many authors make extensive use of the reviews of earlier writers assuming that the latter have checked and evaluated each previously published report. Unfortunately, however, this assumption of validity has not always been correct.

Dr. Beutler, who is a world authority on the subject about which he writes, was determined to make this book as correct and complete as possible, and, to this end, has checked all the original sources. Nowhere else will such an exhaustive bibliography be found. Moreover, he has also undertaken to reevaluate in the light of current knowledge material published in earlier days. This he is eminently able to do, and in some instances his investigations have resulted in new interpretations. The result is a volume that will be recognized as truly the last word on this important subject.

Maxwell M. Wintrobe

Salt Lake City

FOREWORD

PREFACE

Why another review of red cell enzyme defects associated with hemolytic anemia?

A good question, and one that I asked myself many times in planning and in writing this book. The fact that Professor Maxwell Wintrobe asked me to prepare this volume was the initial stimulus for the project. A request from Dr. Wintrobe is in itself very persuasive, but neither he nor I would have wanted this book to represent a mere reprise of what has been written before.

What, then, is new and what is different about this book?

First of all, most reviews of red cell enzyme deficiencies, particularly those dealing with G-6-PD, have relied on the accuracy of previous reviews for many of the data which they contained. This has had predictable, undesirable effects. Inadvertent errors, including some from my own early reviews, have been perpetuated in review after review. Moreover, the earlier data have never been carefully reevaluated in the light of current knowledge. Clearly, what was needed was a review of all of the original reports, regardless of obscurity of journal or strangeness of language. For example, the list of drugs to which G-6-PD-deficient persons are sensitive is published and republished, occasionally with the addition of new drugs. Seemingly, no drugs are ever deleted, for the original data seem never to be reevaluated. Persons with G-6-PD A− detected in population surveys are given cards which warn them not to take aspirin, Gantrisin, or chloroquine (none of which are hemolytic), but they are not counseled against the ingestion of hemolytic drugs such as Furadantin and Bactrim. Similar misinformation serves as a basis of "roundsmanship" as attending physicians display their knowledge of literature by warning house officers against the administration of drugs which are in reality innocuous to G-6-PD-deficient individuals. It seemed to me that a critical reappraisal of the drugs which produce hemolysis in G-6-PD deficiency was sorely needed. Many of the drugs on the list which is published, circulated, and republished were implicated before it was recognized that infection was a common precipitating cause of hemolysis in G-6-PD deficiency.

The inaccurate list of drugs which putatively produce hemolysis in G-6-PD deficiency is only one of many misconceptions which have been reiterated in the literature. Other common erroneous ideas examined in this book include the putative undesirability of the use of G-6-PD-deficient blood for transfusions, the etiologic role of glutathione reductase deficiency in a variety of diseases, and that of glutathione peroxidase, enolase, ATPase, and phosphogluconate dehydrogenase deficiency in hemolytic anemia.

There are data in this book which should be of value to the student of red cell abnormalities. A comprehensive review of the incidence of G-6-PD deficiency among various populations has not been published for many years. An up-to-date, carefully edited listing of properties of G-6-PD variants is also provided.

Although the biochemical details of the various types of enzyme abnormalities are of importance, and are given generous coverage in this book, I have tried to give primary emphasis to the clinical manifestations of the red cell enzyme defects. For example, a review of the effect of splenectomy in the various types of enzyme defects may guide the clinician who is charged with the responsibility for the care of one of these patients. In order to provide comprehensive coverage of some topics, it has been necessary to omit coverage of others. I have therefore reviewed only those red cell enzyme defects which are known to produce significant shortening of the red cell life span and those which have been alleged to do so. Various interesting and important red cell enzyme deficiencies are excluded. I have not attempted to discuss defects such as acatalasemia, galactose-1-phosphate uridyl transferase deficiency, galactokinase deficiency, adenosine deaminase deficiency, ITPase deficiency, phosphoglucomutase deficiency, UDP glucose-4-epimerase deficiency, lactate dehydrogenase deficiency, NADPH diaphorase deficiency, or acetylcholinesterase deficiency, because they are not associated with significant hemolytic consequences. Neither have important defects such as hereditary spherocytosis, elliptocytosis, or stomatocytosis been included; the enzymatic basis of these abnormalities is not known.

Preparation of this book, particularly with the necessity for consulting all of the primary references, was a difficult and time-consuming task which could not have been achieved without loyal assistance from both my staff and my family. Mrs. Janet Manning, Marianne Moss, and Sharyn Webb provided the secretarial assistance without which this work would have been impossible. Mr. John Carrigan, City of Hope librarian, aided me in a preliminary review of the literature concerning drug-induced hemolytic anemia and in making available to me obscure journals from obscure places. Mrs. Florinda Matsumoto aided me in the preparation of the table of G-6-PD variants. I am grateful to Dr. Akira Yoshida and Dr. Karl G. Blume for their critical reviews of the sections concerning G-6-PD and pyruvate kinase, respectively. My sons, Steve and Bruce, reviewed clinical reports on pyruvate kinase deficiency and data on incidence of G-6-PD deficiency, respectively. My wife, Bonnie, provided skillful editorial assistance and literary polish.

This work was supported, in part, by Grant HE 07449 from the National Heart, Lung, and Blood Institute.

Ernest Beutler

Duarte

CONTENTS

THE RED CELL

Evolution from single-celled organisms to complex metazoa requires the development of systems for the distribution of nutrients and oxygen to all cells of the body. The need to supply oxygen molecules reliably, consistently, and in large amounts has been met by different animals in different ways, but the most efficient system is one which has been adopted by all vertebrates. It consists of a specialized cell, the erythrocyte, filled with a protein uniquely suited to this task, hemoglobin.

By its very nature, specialization implies emphasis of certain attributes. Performance of its specialized function of oxygen transport required that the human erythrocyte evolve with the following characteristics: (1) the capacity to synthesize a high concentration of the respiratory pigment, hemoglobin; (2) the ability to maintain the integrity and function of the hemoglobin during its life span in the circulation; (3) a shape which allows efficient oxygen delivery to the tissues; and (4) the capacity to move rapidly through all areas of the body without loss of its contents. The development of these characteristics occurred at the expense of others; many of the metabolic functions normally carried out by most body cells, such as the citric acid cycle, have been sacrificed.

1.1. Red Cell Structure

The red cell has a structureless, relatively homogeneous interior bounded by a highly structured membrane at its interface with the plasma or other suspending medium. The interior of the cell consists of a highly concentrated aqueous solution of hemoglobin containing most of the glycolytic enzymes, nucleotides, 2,3-diphosphoglycerate, and other phosphorylated metabolic intermediates, glutathione, and electrolytes. The red cell, in contrast to the plasma, has a high potassium and low sodium content.

The red cell membrane is now generally regarded as a complex lipid bilayer. The outer and inner layers contain the hydrophilic phosphate groups of phospholipids, with the hydrophobic fatty acid chains pointing inward. The outer leaflet is particularly rich in phosphatidylcholine and sphingomyelin, while the inner leaflet contains more of the phosphatidyl-serine.[1] Cholesterol molecules are scattered throughout the outer leaflet so that it contains approximately one molecule of cholesterol for each molecule of phospholipid. The membrane is composed not only of lipids but also of a large number of different proteins. One of these, designated *spectrin,* seems to form a network lining the inner surface of the membrane.[2,3] An actin-like protein which may interact with spectrin has also been detected.[4] The glycoprotein, *glycophorin,* appears to pass through the entire lipid bilayer, being exposed both at the outer and inner aspects of the membrane. This substance has been studied in considerable detail, and its amino acid composition has also been studied.[5] A hydrophobic region is present in the central portion, the location of the membrane fatty acid chains; glycophorin is more hydrophilic at the outer and inner aspects of the membrane where it comes into contact with the plasma and with the red cell contents, respectively. Other proteins may also pass through the entire membrane, be exposed only at the outer or the inner portion, or lie entirely submerged within the lipid bilayer. Some enzymes, e.g., acetylcholinesterase, NADPase, ATPase, and glyceralde-hyde phosphate dehydrogenase (GAPD), appear to be firmly membrane bound.

The red cell membrane exhibits a highly selective permeability to various ions. Anions, such as chloride and bicarbonate, pass through the membrane extremely rapidly, and equilibrate according to the concentrations predicted by the Donnan membrane equilibrium. In contrast, the membrane is quite impermeable to cations, such as sodium and potassium.[6] A marked gradient exists between the concentration of potassium, which is approximately 90 mM within the cell and 4 mM in the plasma, and that of sodium, which is 8 mM within the cell and 140 mM in the plasma. Virtually no calcium gains access to the interior of the cell, but small quantities are present in the membrane. The amount of calcium in the membrane seems to be related to its flexibility.[7,8]

The resting human erythrocyte has a biconcave shape. It is clear that this shape is a function of the membrane rather than of the contents of the cell, since red cell ghosts are also biconcave. Furthermore, the location of various parts of the membrane with respect to the form of the cell does not appear to be fixed: a part of the membrane which is at the center of the biconcavity at one moment may be on the rim at another.[9] Under physiologic conditions the cell is rarely in an unstressed state. Continually buffeted by strong shear stresses in the circulation, its shape is distorted.

The normal human erythrocyte is remarkably deformable. It can be pulled into a long, fiber-like structure whose length is many times the diameter of the normal cell. It can assume dumbbell shapes to facilitate its passage through narrow apertures such as those of the spleen. It may fold over bifurcations in blood vessels, forming two greatly elongated teardrops until slipping down one channel or the other intact. It may twist and turn and flex to assume a great variety of other forms. The great deformability of the erythrocyte is not due to the membrane's capacity to stretch; in reality the membrane can tolerate very little stretch without rupturing. Rather, the red cell membrane offers very little resistance to bending. Since its surface area is considerably larger than that needed to enclose the contents, considerable distortion is possible without appreciable stretch. It is generally believed that loss of flexibility of the membrane may be a common denominator in the origin of many different types of hemolytic anemia.[10,11]

1.2. Red Cell Metabolism

The mature red cell of the human has been able to sacrifice many of the metabolic functions required for the existence of most other body cells. It has no nucleus or ribosomal apparatus, and hence cannot synthesize protein. It has lost its mitochondria, and therefore cannot metabolize pyruvate through the citric acid cycle. It cannot carry out *de novo* synthesis of nucleic acids or lipids. Yet the red cell is metabolically active, and loss of these functions has not compromised its ability to survive in the circulation or to carry out its major function of oxygen transport. Although it is sufficiently versatile to extract energy from a number of different substrates, its principal energy source normally is glucose. Deprived of glucose, the erythrocyte cannot function and survive. It cannot maintain the gradient of sodium and potassium which exists across the normal red cell membrane. Neither can it prevent the accumulation of calcium in the red cell membrane. Methemoglobin and oxidized glutathione accumulate, especially in the presence of oxidative stresses. The energy-deprived erythrocyte becomes echinocytic, then spherocytic, and ultimately undergoes osmotic lysis.

The red cell metabolizes glucose through two main routes, the Embden–Meyerhoff pathway, and the hexose monophosphate pathway (Table I). In the Embden–Meyerhoff pathway, glucose is catabolized to pyruvate or to lactate. A major portion of the energy derived from the glucose molecule is stored in the high energy phosphate of adenosine triphosphate (ATP). Reducing power is generated in the conversion of NAD^+ to NADH, the form of the coenzyme which reduces methemoglobin to he-

TABLE I
The Functions of the Two Main Pathways of Glucose Metabolism in the Erythrocyte

Functions of the Embden–Meyerhoff pathway	Functions of the hexose monophosphate pathway
(glucose-6-phosphate $\longrightarrow$ lactate)	(glucose-6-phosphate $\longrightarrow$ CO_2 + pentose, triose, etc.)
ADP $\longrightarrow$ ATP (pumps Na^+ and K^+)	
NAD$^+$ $\longrightarrow$ NADH (reduces methemoglobin)	NADP$^+$ $\longrightarrow$ NADPH (reduces GSSG and protein–SG disulfides)
1,3-DPG $\longrightarrow$ 2,3-DPG (regulates oxygen dissociation curve)	HEXOSE $\longrightarrow$ PENTOSE (provides substrate for nucleotide synthesis)

moglobin. 2,3-Diphosphoglycerate (2,3-DPG), an important modulator of hemoglobin oxygen affinity, is also synthesized in this pathway. The hexose monophosphate pathway (HMP) accounts only for approximately 10% of glucose metabolism in the resting cell. The rate of metabolism through the HMP is normally controlled by the availability of NADP$^+$. Under oxidative stress, therefore, when NADPH is oxidized to NADP$^+$, a much larger proportion of the total glucose metabolized may flow through this pathway. The principal function of the HMP is to maintain NADP$^+$ in its reduced form, NADPH. This coenzyme is required to maintain glutathione in the reduced form, a reaction which is important in protecting the erythrocyte from peroxidative damage. In reducing NADP$^+$ to NADPH the first carbon of glucose is oxidized to carbon dioxide, and a pentose is formed. This 5-carbon sugar may be used in the synthesis of nucleotides by the erythrocyte, or may undergo molecular rearrangements which result in further metabolism of the 3- and 6-carbon sugars formed in the Embden–Meyerhoff pathway. Thus, whereas ATP and 2,3-DPG are not formed in the hexose monophosphate pathway itself, glucose passing through the hexose monophosphate pathway may participate in the formation of these substances after the direct oxidative pathway has been traversed.

1.2.1.   Embden–Meyerhoff Pathway (Fig. 1)

Glucose enters the red cell rapidly through an unidentified carrier in the membrane.[12,13] Entry of glucose into erythrocytes is temperature sensitive[14] but not insulin dependent.[15] In contrast to that in most tissue cells, the glucose concentration within the red cell water is the same as that in plasma water. Entry of glucose into red cells never appears to be a limiting factor in its utilization.

The first step in the utilization of glucose is its phosphorylation by hexokinase. ATP serves as the phosphate donor, and magnesium is required. Some of the properties of human red cell hexokinase are summarized in Table II. Hexokinase deficiency is a rare cause of hereditary nonspherocytic hemolytic anemia (NSHA; see Chapter 4).

The product of the hexokinase reaction, glucose-6-phosphate, is in equilibrium with glucose-1-phosphate through phosphoglucomutase and glucose-1,6-diphosphate, and with fructose-6-phosphate through glucose phosphate isomerase (GPI; see Table II). It is the latter reaction which is

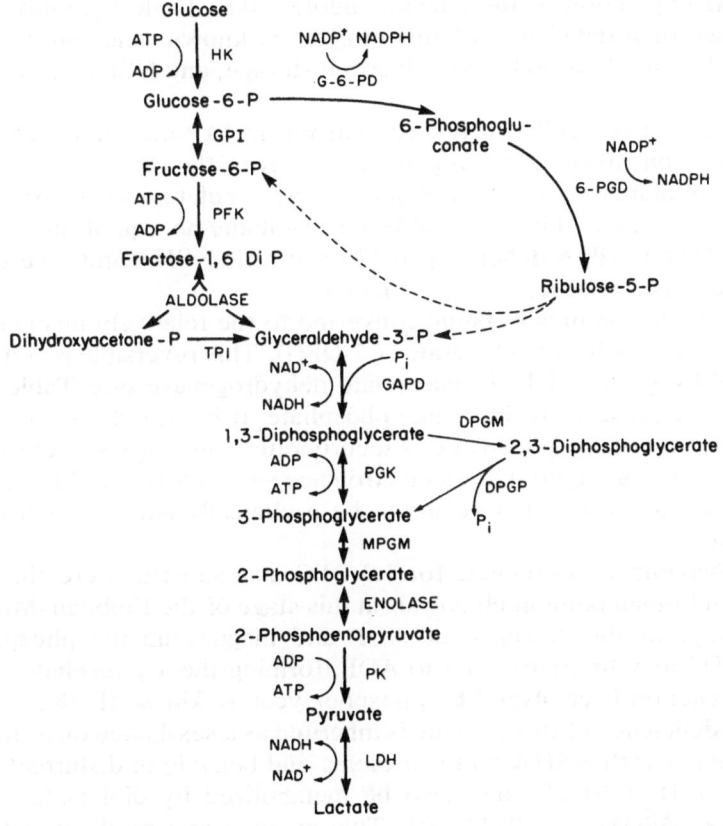

FIGURE 1.   Major pathways of red cell metabolism. The abbreviations are defined in the index.

metabolically of the greater importance since it is the second step in the Embden–Meyerhoff pathway. The "backward" GPI reaction is responsible for the "recycling" of glucose-6-phosphate which has entered the hexose monophosphate pathway. GPI deficiency is one of the more common of the known causes of NSHA (see Chapter 4).

The third step in the Embden–Meyerhoff pathway is the phosphorylation of fructose-6-phosphate to fructose-1,6-diphosphate (F-1,6-diP) in the reaction catalyzed by phosphofructokinase (PFK; see Table II). This reaction is essentially irreversible and is one of the most highly regulated steps in red cell glycolysis. A deficiency of the enzyme PFK leads to type VII (muscle) glycogen storage disease and may result in NSHA with or without myopathy (see Chapter 4).

Fructose-1,6-diphosphate is cleaved into two 3-carbon fragments, glyceraldehyde-3-phosphate (GAP) and dihydroxyacetone phosphate (DHAP) by action of the enzyme aldolase (see Table II). Only a single instance of a deficiency of this enzyme is known, and this has led to mental retardation, mild liver glycogen storage, and NSHA, as described in Chapter 4.

Normal red cells do not contain the DHAP-metabolizing enzyme, α-glycerophosphate dehydrogenase. However, the DHAP formed by the action of aldolase on F-1,6-diP does not accumulate because triose phosphate isomerase (TPI; see Table II) maintains an equilibrium between DHAP and GAP. A deficiency of TPI results in NSHA and severe neurologic disease, as described in Chapter 4.

GAP is continually being converted to the relatively unstable intermediate 1,3-diphosphoglycerate (1,3-DPG). This reversible reaction, catalyzed by glyceraldehyde phosphate dehydrogenase (see Table II), requires the presence of inorganic phosphate. It is the only metabolic step in which inorganic phosphate is incorporated into sugars in the erythrocyte. NAD^+ is required as an electron acceptor. Partial GAPD deficiency has been described, but seems to be a clinically benign condition (see Chapter 4).

Two enzymes compete for 1,3-DPG as a substrate, creating an important branch point in glycolysis at this stage of the Embden–Meyerhoff pathway. In the presence of ADP and magnesium the phosphate of 1,3-DPG may be transferred to ADP, forming the γ-phosphate of ATP. This reaction is catalyzed by phosphoglycerate kinase (PGK; see Table II). A deficiency of this enzyme is inherited as a sex-linked disorder and is associated with NSHA and neurologic and behavioral disturbances (see Chapter 4). 1,3-DPG may also be metabolized by diphosphoglycerate mutase (DPGM; see Table II). This enzyme apparently transfers the 1-phosphate of 1,3-DPG to the 2-carbon of 3-phosphoglyceric acid (3-PGA), to form a molecule of 2,3-DPG and one of 3-PGA. Hence, the overall result of the reaction is the conversion of a molecule of 1,3-DPG

TABLE II

Properties of Some Important Red Cell Enzymes

Enzyme (abbreviation)	E.C. number	Substrate	K_m (µM)	Product	Cofactor	Inhibitor	K_i (µM)	Activity mean ± SD 37°C (IU/g Hb)	Activity in young cells
Hexokinase (HK)	2.7.1.1	Glucose Fructose Mannose 2-Deoxyglucose Glucosamine ATP	48–80 10,000 600 1000 4500 570–1000[16]	Glucose-6-P 2-Deoxyglucose-6-P Glucosamine-6-P ADP	Mg^{2+}	2,3-DPG Glucose-6-P	1500[17] 35[18]	1.16 ± 0.17[19]	Markedly increased[20]
Glucose phosphate isomerase (GPI)	5.3.1.9	Fructose-6-P	50–80[21]	Glucose-6-P		2,3-DPG 6-PGA	940[21]	60.8 ± 11.1[19]	Normal[22]
Phosphofructokinase (PFK)	2.7.1.11	Fructose-6-P ATP	120[23] 120[23]	Fructose-1,6-diP ADP	Mg^{2+}	2,3-DPG ATP[23]	1500[17]	11.01 ± 2.23[19]	Normal or increased[22]
Aldolase	4.1.2.13	Fructose-1,6-diP	6250[24]	GAP DHAP		2,3-DPG	1500[17]	3.19 ± 0.86[19]	Markedly increased[20]
Triose phosphate isomerase (TPI)	5.3.1.1	DHAP	2250[25]	GAP				2111 ± 397[19]	Slightly increased[22]
Glyceraldehyde phosphate dehydrogenase (GAPD)	1.2.1.12	P_i GAP NAD^+	6600 21 143[26]	1,3-DPG NADH		2,3-DPG NADH	1400[17] 9.1[26]	226 ± 41.9[19]	Slight increase[22,27]
Phosphoglycerate kinase (PGK)	2.7.2.3	1,3-DPG ADP	1100[b] 370–1000[b,28]	3-PGA ATP	Mg^{2+}			320 ± 36.1[b,19]	Normal[22]
Diphosphoglyceromutase (DPGM)	2.7.5.4	1,3-DPG	0.53[29]	2,3-DPG	3-PGA	2,3-DPG	0.85[29]	4.78 ± 0.65[19]	

(continued)

TABLE II (continued)

Enzyme (abbreviation)	E.C. number	Substrate	K_m (μM)	Product	Cofactor	Inhibitor	K_i (μM)	Activity mean ± S D 37°C (IU⁻¹/g Hb)	Activity in young cells
phosphoglycerophosphatase	3.1.3.13	2,3-DPG	0.08–25[30]	3-PGH	P_i[30] Cl[30]	PEP ATP		0.003[30]	
monophosphoglyceromutase (PGM)	2.7.5.3	3-PGA	800[31]	2-PGA	2,3-DPG			19.3 ± 3.84[19]	Increased[22]
enolase	4.2.1.11	2-PGA	28[32]	PEP	Mg^{2+}			5.39 ± 0.83[19]	Normal or slight increase[22]
pyruvate kinase (PK)	2.7.1.40	ADP PEP	330[33] 46[33]	ATP Pyruvate	Mg^{2+} K^+			15.9 ± 1.99[19]	Markedly increased[22]
lactate dehydrogenase (LDH)	1.1.1.27	Pyruvate NADH	106[34] 15[34]	Lactate NAD^+	None			200 ± 26.5[19]	Slight increase[22]
mannose phosphate isomerase (PI)	5.3.1.8	Mannose-6-P		Fructose-6-P				0.064[35]	Increased[35]
galactokinase (GALK)	2.7.1.6	Galactose ATP	100–500+ 200–500[36]	Galactose-1-P ADP	Mg^{2+}			29.12 ± 5.97[19]	
galactose-1-phosphate uridyl transferase (GALT)	2.7.7.12	Galactose-1-P UDP glucose	150[37]	Glucose-1-P UDP galactose		UDP galactose	213[37]	28.4 ± 6.94[19]	
phosphoglucomutase (GM)	2.7.5.1	Glucose-1-P	270[38]	Glucose-6-P	Glucose-1,6-diP	2,3-DPG[17]	150[17]	5.5 ± 0.62[19]	

Enzyme	EC No.	Substrate	K_m (μM)	Product	K_m (μM)	Activity	
iokinase	2.7.1.28	Glyceraldehyde	11[39]	GAP		0.151 ± 0.011[39]	
		Dihydroxyacetone	0.5[39]	DHAP			
H exonate dehydrogenase	1.1.1.19	D-Glyceraldehyde	680[40]	Glycerol	0.08[40]		
		Glucose	396,000[40]	Sorbitol			
		NADPH		NAD+			
orbitol dehydrogenase	1.1.1.14	Sorbitol	1700[41]	Fructose			
		NAD+	200[41]	NADH			
cleoside phosphorylase (P)		Inosine	58[42]	Hypoxanthine	Ribose-1-P 550[42]		
		P_i	320[42]	Ribose-1-P			
ucose-6-phosphate dehydrogenase (-6-PD)	1.1.1.49	Glucose-6-P	40–60[43]	6-PGA	NADPH 9.1 ± 1.8[44]	8.3 ± 1.6[19]	Markedly increased [45,20,27,54]
		NADP+	1.3–2.6[43]	NADPH			
Phosphogluconate dehydrogenase (PGD)	1.1.1.43	6-PGA		R-5-P and CO_2		8.78 ± 0.78[19]	Increased [45,20]
		NADP+		NADPH			
lutathione reductase (R)	1.6.4.2	GSSG	25–42[46]	GSH		10.4 ± 1.5[19]	
		NADPH	11–13[46]	NADP+			
				FAD			
lutathione peroxidase (SHPx)	1.11.1.9	GSH	650[47]	GSSG		30.8 ± 4.7[19c]	
		Peroxide (R-O-O-H)	200[47]	Water			
				Alcohol (ROH + HOH)			

Micromoles substrate utilized per minute.
In the backward reaction.
For U.S.–European and U.S.–African. See Figure 20 for other groups.

to a molecule of 2,3-DPG. This reaction is particularly important since it represents the erythrocytes' only means for the net synthesis of 2,3-DPG. DPGM deficiency may be a very rare cause of NSHA (see Chapter 4). The proportion of 1,3-DPG metabolized by PGK, on the one hand, or DPGM, on the other, depends on the levels of a variety of substances within the erythrocyte. 2,3-DPG, for example, inhibits the DPGM reaction, thus retarding its own formation. Hydrogen ions also inhibit the DPGM reaction, thereby diverting 1,3-DPG to the PGK reaction. Increased amounts of ADP facilitate the conversion of 1,3-DPG to 3-PGA in the PGK reaction. 2,3-DPG is dephosphorylated to 3-PGA by the action of diphosphoglycerate phosphatase (DPGP; see Table II). This is the same product of 1,3-DPG metabolism which is formed in the PGK reaction.

Red cell 3-PGA is in equilibrium with 2-PGA through mediation of 2,3-DPG and the enzyme monophosphoglyceromutase (MPGM; see Table II). This enzyme apparently functions by transferring the 3-phosphate from 2,3-DPG to the 2 position of 3-PGA. The 2,3-DPG is thereby regenerated, but now 2-PGA is present instead of 3-PGA. Red cell 2-PGA is in equilibrium with phosphoenolpyruvate (PEP). This dehydration reaction is catalyzed by the enzyme enolase (see Table II).

Phosphoenolpyruvate donates its phosphate to ADP in the second ATP-synthesizing step of red cell glycolysis. This reaction is mediated by the enzyme pyruvate kinase (PK), the deficiency of which is one of the most important causes of NSHA (see Chapter 3).

The pyruvate formed in the PK reaction may either diffuse from the red cell or be converted within the cell to lactate by the enzyme lactate dehydrogenase. The fate of lactate depends on the intracellular NADH/ NAD$^+$ ratio and intracellular pH. When NADH is plentiful, and the pH low, pyruvate is reduced to lactate, which is also in equilibrium with plasma lactate.

1.2.2.   Hexose Monophosphate Pathway (Fig. 2)

Three enzymes compete for the glucose-6-phosphate formed in the hexokinase reaction: phosphoglucomutase, glucose phosphate isomerase, and glucose-6-phosphate dehydrogenase (Table II). The glucose-6-phosphate molecules metabolized by glucose-6-phosphate dehydrogenase (G-6-PD) are oxidized to 6-phosphogluconolactone and have thereby been diverted to the hexose monophosphate shunt. NADP$^+$ is reduced to NADPH in the G-6-PD reaction. It is the availability of NADP$^+$ which to a major extent regulates the diversion of glucose-6-phosphate into the HMP, and NADPH, a product of the reaction, is strongly inhibitory to G-6-PD. Deficiency of G-6-PD is the most common enzymatic abnor-

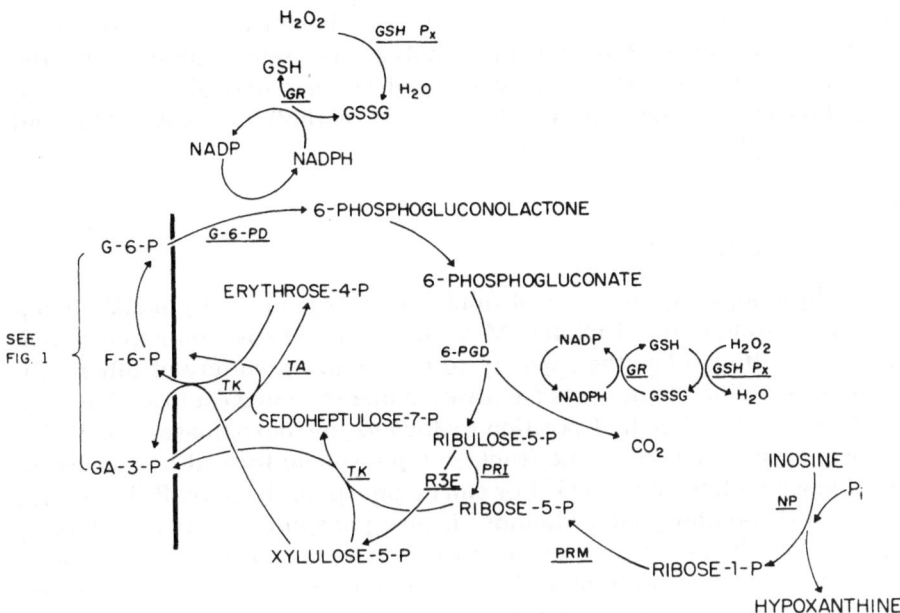

FIGURE 2.   The hexose monophosphate pathway of the erythrocyte. The abbreviations
are defined in the Index.

mality of red cells as is discussed in detail in Chapter 2. The
6-phosphogluconolactone formed in the G-6-PD reaction undergoes
spontaneous hydrolysis to 6-phosphogluconic acid and serves as a substrate for the second enzyme of the hexose monophosphate shunt,
6-phosphogluconate dehydrogenase (6-PGD; see Table II). 6-Phospho-
gluconate dehydrogenase deficiency produces little or no shortening of
red cell life span (see Chapter 4). In the 6-PGD reaction the 1-carbon from
the hexose is oxidized to carbon dioxide, and ribulose-5-phosphate is
formed. This pentose phosphate undergoes a series of isomerizations and
carbon transfers which are shown in Figure 2. Ribulose-5-phosphate is
maintained in equilibrium with ribose-5-phosphate and xylulose-
5-phosphate through two isomerases, phosphoribose isomerase[48] and ri-
bulosephosphate-3 epimerase.[49] The first two carbons are transferred
from a molecule of xylulose-5-phosphate to one of ribose-5-phosphate
through mediation of transketolase,[50,51] forming a 3-carbon and a 7-carbon
fragment.

The 7-carbon fragment, sedoheptulose-7-phosphate, reacts with gly-
ceraldehyde-3-phosphate, and through the action of transaldolase[51] the 10
carbon atoms are rearranged to form the 4-carbon sugar erythrose-
4-phosphate and the 6-carbon sugar fructose-6-phosphate. Erythrose-

4-phosphate, in turn, reacts with xylulose-5-phosphate to form fructose-6-phosphate and GAP in a reaction catalyzed by transketolase. Thus, the 5-carbon sugars in HMP are rearranged so that normal 3-carbon and 6-carbon intermediates of the Embden–Meyerhoff pathway, GAP and fructose-6-phosphate, are formed.

1.2.3. Other Pathways

Physiologically the red cell fulfills its energy needs by metabolizing glucose through the Embden–Meyerhoff and hexose monophosphate pathways. It also has the capacity to metabolize a variety of other substrates including the hexoses fructose, mannose, and galactose. Fructose is phosphorylated in the 6 position by the enzyme hexokinase, which also phosphorylates glucose. The fructose-6-phosphate formed is isomerized to glucose-6-phosphate by GPI or can be phosphorylated by PFK to form fructose-1,6-diphosphate. Mannose is also phosphorylated at the 6 position by hexokinase. However, the mannose-6-phosphate formed must be converted to fructose-6-phosphate by mannose phosphate isomerase[35] before it can be metabolized further by the erythrocyte. The significance of the presence of mannose-1,6-diphosphate in normal red cells[52] is not clear.

The metabolism of galactose by red cells follows a more complex pathway than that of fructose and mannose. Galactose is phosphorylated at the 1 position by galactokinase[36]:

$$\alpha\text{-galactose} + \text{ADP} \longrightarrow \alpha\text{-galactose-1-P} + \text{ADP}$$

Its conversion to glucose requires its exchange in the galactose-1-phosphate uridyl transferase reaction[53,54] with glucose-1-phosphate in uridine phosphoglucose (UDPG):

$$\alpha\text{-galactose-1-P} + \text{UDPG} \longrightarrow \alpha\text{-glucose-1-P} + \text{UDPGal}$$

The galactose-1-phosphate, now attached to uridine phosphate as uridine diphosphogalactose (UDPGal), is converted to glucose in the epimerase reaction:

$$\text{UDPGal} \rightleftharpoons \text{UDPG}$$

α-Glucose-1-phosphate is in equilibrium with α-glucose-6-phosphate through the phosphoglucomutase (PGM) reaction,[55] and in this way can enter the Embden–Meyerhoff pathway. If it is anomerized to β-glucose-6-phosphate, it can also be metabolized in the HMP. In addition, glucose-1-phosphate in the red cell may be incorporated into the small amount of glycogen that exists in erythrocytes.[56]

The erythrocyte can also metabolize trioses and, to a limited extent, pentoses. Dihydroxyacetone (DHA) is phosphorylated to DHAP in the triokinase[39] reaction:

$$DHA + ATP \longrightarrow DHAP + ADP$$

Triokinase also has the capacity to phosphorylate glyceraldehyde (GA) to glyceraldehyde-3-phosphate (GAP):

$$GA + ATP \longrightarrow GAP + ADP$$

Both DHAP and GAP are normal metabolites of the Embden–Meyerhoff pathway.

Xylitol, the 5-carbon polyol, reduces $NADP^+$ to NADPH in the xylitol dehydrogenase reaction and is oxidized to L-xylulose in the process.[57,58] Xylitol may also be oxidized through a NAD-linked enzyme[57] to form D-xylulose. Other metabolic transformations of carbohydrates may also occur in erythrocytes under appropriate conditions. For example, high concentrations of glucose and other aldoses, such as glyceraldehyde, are reduced to the corresponding polyol by the enzyme L-hexonate dehydrogenase which uses NADPH as a hydrogen donor.[40] In this reaction, glucose is reduced to sorbitol or glyceraldehyde to glycerol. Once formed, sorbitol may be reoxidized to fructose. In this reaction, catalyzed by sorbitol dehydrogenase,[41] NAD serves as the hydrogen acceptor. Thus, the L-hexonate dehydrogenase and sorbitol dehydrogenase reactions, working together, may act as a transhydrogenase, converting NADPH and NAD^+ to $NADP^+$ and NADH.

A "high K_m" pathway for the metabolism of galactose has been detected, but its steps have not been identified. Erythrocytes deficient in galactokinase or in galactose-1-phosphate uridyl transferase have the capacity to metabolize high concentrations of galactose;[59] it is apparent that the high K_m pathway bypasses these steps of galactose metabolism. Galactose metabolized through this pathway has the capacity to reduce NAD^+ to NADH.

The red cell is also able to derive energy from nucleosides, such as inosine. When inosine serves as substrate, phosphorolytic cleavage of the nucleoside catalyzed by nucleoside phosphorylase yields ribose-1-phosphate and the purine base hypoxanthine. The ribose-1-phosphate formed can be converted to ribose-5-phosphate through mediation of phosphoribomutase which, it has been claimed,[60] is distinct from phosphoglucomutase. The ribose-5-phosphate is a normal intermediate in the HMP (Fig. 2) and can thus serve as a source of high energy phosphate in the red cell, even when no ATP is available.

Erythrocytes contain enzymes that can catalyze certain interconversions of nucleosides and nucleotides. Adenylate kinase (AK) maintains an equilibrium between AMP, ADP, and ATP. Red cells also have the capacity to deaminate adenosine to inosine, through the action of the enzyme adenosine deaminase (ADA). This enzyme is of particular interest because a deficiency of ADA is often associated with combined immunodeficiency.[61,62] A genetically determined marked increase in the activity of ADA has also been observed (see Chapter 4). It produces nonspherocytic hemolytic anemia, probably by competing for the available adenosine with another enzyme, adenosine kinase,[63] which catalyzes the phosphorylation of adenosine to adenosine monophosphate. Cytosine deaminase (nucleoside deaminase) is distinct from ADA.[64] Its activity is markedly increased in the red cells of mice undergoing erythropoietic stress,[64,65] but an abnormality of this enzyme in human red cells has not been reported. Red cell nucleoside phosphorylase has the ability to provide phosphorylated sugars from inosine without expenditure of a high energy phosphate bond.[66,67] A deficiency of this enzyme has been associated with hereditary failure of T-cell immunity.[68,69] Guanosine monophosphate reductase is also reportedly present in erythrocytes.[70] Red cells contain an enzyme which dephosphorylates pyrimidine nucleotides.[71,72] A deficiency of this enzyme, pyrimidine 5-nucleotidase, results in NSHA characterized by marked basophilic stippling of erythrocytes. The enzyme is very sensitive to inhibition by lead, which may account for the basophilic stippling of red cells observed in hemolytic anemia associated with lead poisoning (see Chapter 4).

1.2.4. ATPase Activity and Ion Movements

Anions and water move rapidly through the red cell membrane. However, it presents a barrier to the movement of cations such as those of sodium, potassium, and calcium. It has been suggested that the membrane contains "pores" which are lined with positive charges and which repel positively charged ions.[73] Nonetheless, some leakage of cations across the membrane does occur, as sodium flows passively into the normal red cell at a rate of approximately 3 mmoles/liter/hr, and potassium leaves at approximately 2 mmoles/liter/hr.[73] If these passive movements were unopposed, equilibrium would ultimately be achieved between the electrolyte concentration inside and outside the cells. Since red cells contain a high concentration of proteins to which the membrane poses an absolute barrier, the colloid osmotic pressure exerted by the protein might be expected to result in an inflow of water and ultimately in lysis of the red cell. The achievement of such a destructive ionic equilibrium is prevented, however, by pumping systems which have the capacity to move ions "uphill" against an ionic gradient. These pumping systems derive their energy from ATP (see Table I). As they move ions, high energy phosphate is cleaved from ATP, producing ADP: the ion pumps of the membranes act as ATPases. Because these enzymes are membrane associated, and solubilized only with relatively harsh treatment, efforts to separate and characterize them have been far from satisfactory. One of these enzymes[74] appears to require both sodium and potassium for maximum activity and is completely inhibited by ouabain. This is presumably the ATPase which is involved in sodium and potassium pumping. Another activity, presumably of the enzyme associated with the pumping of calcium from the erythrocyte, appears to be strongly stimulated by Ca^{2+}.[75]

1.2.5. Methemoglobin Reduction

When oxygen dissociates from hemoglobin, it usually leaves the hemoglobin iron in the divalent ferrous state. On some occasions, however, the oxygen is expelled as the superoxide anion, removing one of the electrons from iron and leaving the hemoglobin in the methemoglobin state. The process of methemoglobin formation is greatly hastened by certain oxidant chemicals including aniline derivatives and nitrites. Although a number of physiologically present reducing agents, including glutathione (GSH) and ascorbic acid, have the capacity to reduce methemoglobin to hemoglobin, the reaction rates between methemoglobin and these compounds are negligible compared with that of the specific enzymatic mechanism for methemoglobin reduction which has evolved in erythrocytes.[76,77] This efficient system utilizes an NADH diaphorase which transfers an electron to cytochrome b_5. Reduced cytochrome b_5, in turn, reduces methemoglobin nonenzymatically. The NADH diaphorase-linked methemoglobin reduction system is the most important physiologic method for methemoglobin reduction; when a deficiency of this enzyme is present hereditary methemoglobinemia results.[76]

In the presence of certain dyes methemoglobin reduction may also take place through an NADPH-linked system. An NADPH diaphorase serves to transfer an electron from NADPH to an artificial carrier such as methylene blue or Nile blue. The reduced dye reacts nonenzymatically with methemoglobin, reducing it to hemoglobin.[78] In the absence of a linking dye NADPH diaphorase has no known function: its hereditary absence is unassociated with any clinical disorder.[79]

References

1. GORDESKY,S.E. AND MARINETTI,G.V., 1973, THE ASYMMETRIC ARRANGEMENT OF PHOSPHOLIPIDS IN THE HUMAN ERYTHROCYTE MEMBRANE. BIOCHEM BIOPHYS RES COMMUN 50:1027-1031

2. KIRKPATRICK,F.H., 1976, SPECTRIN: CURRENT UNDERSTANDING OF ITS PHYSICAL, BIOCHEMICAL, AND FUNCTIONAL PROPERTIES. LIFE SCI 19:1-18

3. SCHECHTER,N.M., SHARP,M., REYNOLDS,J.A. AND TANFORD,C., 1976, ERYTHROCYTE SPECTRIN. PURIFICATION IN DEOXYCHOLATE AND PRELIMINARY CHARACTERIZATION. BIOCHEMISTRY 15:1897-1904

4. TILNEY,L.G. AND DETMERS,P., 1975, ACTIN IN ERYTHROCYTE GHOSTS AND ITS ASSOCIATION WITH SPECTRIN. J CELL BIOL 66:508-520

5. SEGREST,J.P., KAHANE,I., JACKSON,R.L. AND MARCHESI,V.T., 1973, MAJOR GLYCOPROTEIN OF THE HUMAN ERYTHROCYTE MEMBRANE:EVIDENCE FOR AN AMPHIPATHIC MOLECULAR STRUCTURE. ARCH BIOCHEM BIOPHYS 155:167-183

6. PASSOW,H., 1964, ION AND WATER PERMEABILITY OF THE RED BLOOD CELL. THE RED BLOOD CELL BISHOP,C. AND SURGENOR,D.M. ED. 71-145, ACADEMIC PRESS, NEW YORK

7. KIRKPATRICK,F.H., HILLMAN,D.G. AND LA CELLE,P.L., 1975, A23187 AND RED CELLS: CHANGES IN DEFORMABILITY, K+,MG2+CA2+ AND ATP. EXPERIENTIA 31:653-654

8. PALEK,J., STEWART,G. AND LIONETTI,F.J., 1974, THE DEPENDENCE OF SHAPE OF HUMAN ERYTHROCYTE GHOSTS ON CALCIUM, MAGNESIUM, AND ADENOSINE TRIPHOSPHATE. BLOOD 44:583-597

9. BULL,B., 1972, RED CELL BIOCONCAVITY AND DEFORMABILITY. A MACROMODEL BASED ON FLOW CHAMBER OBSERVATIONS. NOUV REV FR HEMATOL 12:835-844

10. BESSIS,M. AND MOHANDAS,N., 1975, DEFORMABILITY OF NORMAL, SHAPE-ALTERED AND PATHOLOGICAL RED CELLS. BLOOD CELLS 1:315-321

11. LA CELLE,P.L. AND KIRKPATRICK,F.H., 1975, DETERMINANTS OF ERYTHROCYTE MEMBRANE ELASTICITY. ERYTHROCYTE STRUCTURE AND FUNCTION BREWER,G.J. ED. 535-557, LISS PUBLISHER, NEW YORK

12. JUNG,C.Y., 1975, CARRIER-MEDIATED GLUCOSE TRANSPORT ACROSS HUMAN RED CELL MEMBRANES. THE RED BLOOD CELL MAC N SURGENOR,D. ED. 705-751, 2ND EDITION,ACADEMIC PRESS, NEW YORK

13. WIDDAS,W.F., 1968, MEMBRANE TRANSPORT OF SUGARS. CARBOHYDRATE METABOLISM AND ITS DISORDERS DICKENS,F., WHELAN,W.J. AND RANDLE,P.J. ED. 1-23, ACADEMIC PRESS, NEW YORK

14. LACKO,L., WITTKE,B. AND GECK,P., 1973, THE TEMPERATURE DEPENDENCE OF THE EXCHANGE TRANSPORT OF GLUCOSE IN HUMAN ERYTHROCYTES. J CELL PHYSIOL 82:213-218

15. EADIE,G.S., MACLEOD,J.J.R. AND NOBLE,E.C., 1923, INSULIN
     AND GLYCOLYSIS. AM J PHYSIOL 65:462-476

16. RIJKSEN,G. AND STAAL,G.E.J., 1976, PURIFICATION AND SOME
     PROPERTIES OF HUMAN ERYTHROCYTE HEXOKINASE. BIOCHIM BIOPHYS
     ACTA 445:330-341

17. BEUTLER,E., 1971, 2,3-DIPHOSPHOGLYCERATE AFFECTS ENZYMES
     OF GLUCOSE METABOLISM IN RED BLOOD CELLS. NATURE (NEW
     BIOL) 232:20-21

18. ROSE,I.A., WARMS,J.V.B. AND KOSOW,D.P., 1974, SPECIFICITY
     FOR THE GLUCOSE-6-P INHIBITION SITE OF HEXOKINASE. ARCH
     BIOCHEM BIOPHYS 164:729-735

19. BEUTLER,E., 1975, RED CELL METABOLISM. A MANUAL OF
     BIOCHEMICAL METHODS 2ND EDITON , GRUNE & STRATTON, NEW YORK

20. BROK,F., RAMOT,B., ZWANG,E. AND DANON,D., 1966, ENZYME
     ACTIVITIES IN HUMAN RED BLOOD CELLS OF DIFFERENT AGE GROUPS.
     ISR J MED SCI 2:291-296

21. ARNOLD,H., HOFFMANN,A., ENGELHARDT,R. AND LOEHR,G.W., 1973,
     PURIFICATION AND KINETIC PROPERTIES OF GLUCOSE-PHOSPHATE
     ISOMERASE FROM HUMAN ERYTHROCYTES. ERYTHROCYTES, THROMBOCYTES,
     LEUKOCYTES GERLACH,E., MOSER,K., DEUTSCH,E. AND WILMANNS,W.
     ED. 177-180, GEORG THIEME, STUTTGART

22. KONRAD,P.N., VALENTINE,W.N. AND PAGLIA,D.E., 1972, ENZYMATIC
     ACTIVITIES AND GLUTATHIONE CONTENT OF ERYTHROCYTES IN THE
     NEWBORN. COMPARISON WITH RED CELLS OF OLDER NORMAL SUBJECTS
     AND THOSE WITH COMPARABLE RETICULOCYTOSIS. ACTA HAEMATOL
     48:193-201

23. STAAL,G.E.J., KOSTER,J.F., BAENZIGER,C.J.M. AND VAN
     MILLIGEN-BOERSMA,L., 1972, HUMAN ERYTHROCYTE
     PHOSPHOFRUCTOKINASE: ITS PURIFICATION AND SOME PROPERTIES.
     BIOCHIM BIOPHYS ACTA 276:113-123

24. BEUTLER,E., SCOTT,S., BISHOP,A., MARGOLIS,N., MATSUMOTO,F.
     AND KUHL,W., 1974, RED CELL ALDOLASE DEFICIENCY AND HEMOLYTIC
     ANEMIA: A NEW SYNDROME. TRANS ASSOC AM PHYSICIANS 86:154-
     166

25. SKALA,H., DREYFUS,J.C., VIVES-CORRONS,J.L., MATSUMOTO,F.
     AND BEUTLER,E., 1977, TRIOSE PHOSPHATE ISOMERASE DEFICIENCY.
     BIOCHEM MED 18:226-234

26. MILLS,G.C. AND HILL,F.L., 1971, METABOLIC CONTROL MECHANISMS
     IN HUMAN ERYTHROCYTES. THE ROLE OF GLYCERALDEHYDE PHOSPHATE
     DEHYDROGENASE. ARCH BIOCHEM BIOPHYS 146:306-311

27. BARTOS,H.R. AND DESFORGES,J.F., 1967, ENZYMES AS ERYTHROCYTE
     AGE REFERENCE STANDARDS. AM J MED SCI 254:862-865

28. YOSHIDA,A. AND WATANABE,S., 1972, HUMAN PHOSPHOGLYCERATE
     KINASE I. CRYSTALLIZATION AND CHARACTERIZATION OF NORMAL
     ENZYME. J BIOL CHEM 247:440-445

29. ROSE,Z.B., 1968, THE PURIFICATION AND PROPERTIES OF
     DIPHOSPHOGLYCERATE MUTASE FROM HUMAN ERYTHROCYTES. J BIOL
     CHEM 243:4810-4820

30. ROSE,Z. AND LIEBOWITZ,J., 1970, 2,3-DIPHOSPHOGLYCERATE
     PHOSPHATASE FROM HUMAN ERYTHROCYTES. GENERAL PROPERTIES
     AND ACTIVATION BY ANIONS. J BIOL CHEM 245:3232-3241

31. HARKNESS,D.R., THOMPSON,W., ROTH,S. AND GRAYSON,V., 1970,
     THE 2,3-DIPHOSPHOGLYCERIC ACID PHOSPHATASE ACTIVITY OF
     PHOSPHOGLYCERIC ACID MUTASE PURIFIED FROM HUMAN ERYTHROCYTES.
     ARCH BIOCHEM BIOPHYS 138:208-219

32. HOORN,R.K.J., FILKWEERT,J.P. AND STAAL,G.E.J., 1974,
     PURIFICATION AND PROPERTIES OF ENOLASE OF HUMAN ERYTHROCYTES.
     INT J BIOCHEM 5:845-852

33. IBSEN,K.H., SCHILLER,K.W. AND VENN-WATSON,E.A., 1968,
     STABILIZATION, PARTIAL PURIFICATION, AND EFFECTS OF ACTIVATING
     CATIONS, ADP, AND PHOSPHOENOLPYRUVATE ON THE REACTION RATES
     OF AN ERYTHROCYTE PYRUVATE KINASE. ARCH BIOCHEM BIOPHYS
     128:583-590

34. BEUTLER,E. AND GUINTO,E., 1974, MECHANISM OF STIMULATION
     OF THE HEXOSE MONOPHOSPHATE SHUNT OF ERYTHROCYTES BY
     PYRUVATE. ENZYME 18:7-18

35. BEUTLER,E. AND TEEPLE,L., 1969, MANNOSE METABOLISM IN THE
     HUMAN ERYTHROCYTE. J CLIN INVEST 48:461-466

36. BLUME,K.G. AND BEUTLER,E., 1971, PURIFICATION AND PROPERTIES
     OF GALACTOKINASE FROM HUMAN RED BLOOD CELLS. J BIOL CHEM
     246:6507-6510

37. BEUTLER,E. AND MITCHELL,M., 1969, UDP GLU CONSUMPTION
     METHODS. GALACTOSEMIA HSIA,D.Y.Y. ED. 72-82, CHAS. C.
     THOMAS, SPRINGFIELD, ILL

38. BEUTLER,E., 1975, UNPUBLISHED

39. BEUTLER,E. AND GUINTO,E., 1973, DIHYDROXYACETONE METABOLISM
     BY HUMAN ERYTHROCYTES: DEMONSTRATION OF TRIOKINASE ACTIVITY
     AND ITS CHARACTERIZATION. BLOOD 41:559-568

40. BEUTLER,E. AND GUINTO,E., 1974, THE REDUCTION OF
     GLYCERALDEHYDE BY HUMAN ERYTHROCYTES. L-HEXONATE DEHYDROGENASE
     ACTIVITY. J CLIN INVEST 53:1258-1264

41. BARRETTO,O.C.O. AND BEUTLER,E., 1975, THE SORBITOL OXIDIZING
     ENZYME OF RED BLOOD CELLS. J LAB CLIN MED 85:645-649

42. KIM,B.K., CHA,S. AND PARKS JR,R.E., 1968, PURINE NUCLEOSIDE
     PHOSPHORYLASE AND HUMAN ERYTHROCYTES. II. KINETIC ANALYSIS
     AND SUBSTRATE-BINDING STUDIES. J BIOL CHEM 243:1771-1776

43. YOSHIDA,A., 1967, HUMAN GLUCOSE-6-PHOSPHATE DEHYDROGENASE:
     PURIFICATION AND CHARACTERIZATION OF NEGRO TYPE VARIANT
     (A+) AND COMPARISON WITH NORMAL ENZYME (B+). BIOCHEM GENET
     1:81-99

44. YOSHIDA,A., 1973, HEMOLYTIC ANEMIA AND G-6-PD DEFICIENCY. SCIENCE 179:532-537

45. TURNER,B.M., FISHER,R.A. AND HARRIS,H., 1974, THE AGE RELATED LOSS OF ACTIVITY OF FOUR ENZYMES IN THE HUMAN ERYTHROCYTE. CLIN CHIM ACTA 50:85-95

46. WALLER,H.D., 1968, GLUTATHIONE REDUCTASE DEFICIENCY. HEREDITARY DISORDERS OF ERYTHROCYTE METABOLISM BEUTLER,E. ED. 185-208, CITY OF HOPE SYMP. SERIES, VOL. I, GRUNE & STRATTON, N.Y.

47. BEUTLER,E. AND MATSUMOTO,F., 1975, ETHNIC VARIATION IN RED CELL GLUTATHIONE PEROXIDASE ACTIVITY. BLOOD 46:103-110

48. BRUNS,F.H., NOLTMANN,E. AND VAHLHAUS,E., 1958, UEBER DEN STOFFWECHSEL VON RIBOSE-6-PHOSPHAT IN HAEMOLYSATEN. I. AKTIVITAETS-MESSUNG UND EIGENSCHAFTEN DER PHOSPHORIBOSE-ISOMERASE. II. DER PENTOSEPHOSPHATE-CYCLUS IN ROTEN BLUTZELLEN. BIOCHEM Z 330:483-496

49. DISCHE,Z. AND SIGEURA,H., 1957, INTERCONVERSION OF RIBOSE-6-PHOSPHATE AND HEXOSE-6-PHOSPHATE IN HUMAN BLOOD. I. ISOMERIZATION OF RIBOSE-5-PHOSPHAE IN HUMAN HEMOLYSATES. BIOCHIM BIOPHYS ACTA 24:87-99

50. BRUNS,F.H., DUNWALD,E. AND NOLTMANN,E., 1958, UEBER DEN STOFFWECHSEL VON RIBOSE-5-PHOSPHAT IN HAEMOLYSATIN III. QUANTITATIVE BESTIMMUNG VON SEDOHEPTULOSE-7-PHOSPHAT UND EINIGE EIGENSCHAFTEN DER TRANSKETOLASE DER ERYTHROCYTEN UND DES BLUTSERUMS. BIOCHEM Z 330:497-508

51. BROWNSTONE,Y.S. AND DENSTEDT,O.F., 1961, THE PENTOSE PHOSPHATE METABOLIC PATHWAY IN THE HUMAN ERYTHROCYTE. II. THE TRANSKETOLASE AND TRANSALDOLASE ACTIVITY OF THE HUMAN ERYTHROCYTE. CAN J BIOCHEM 39:533-545

52. BARTLETT,G.R., 1968, GLUCOSE AND MANNOSE DIPHOSPHATES IN THE RED BLOOD CELL. BIOCHIM BIOPHYS ACTA 156:231-239

53. DALE,G.L. AND POPJAK,G., 1976, PURIFICATION OF NORMAL AND INACTIVE GALACTOSEMIC GALACTOSE-1-PHOSPHATE URIDYLTRANSFERASE FROM HUMAN RED CELLS. J BIOL CHEM 251:1057-1063

54. TEDESCO,T.A., 1972, HUMAN GALACTOSE 1-PHOSPHATE URIDYLTRANSFERASE. PURIFICATION, ANTIBODY PRODUCTION AND COMPARISON OF THE WILD TYPE, DUARTE VARIANT, AND GALACTOSEMIC GENE PRODUCTS. J BIOL CHEM 247:6631-6636

55. NOLTMANN,E. AND BRUNS,F.H., 1959, UEBER DIE PHOSPHOGLUCOMUTASE DER ERYTHROCYTEN UND DES SERUMS. HOPPE SEYLERS Z PHYSIOL CHEM 313:194-200

56. MOSES,S.W., CHAYOTH,R., LEVIN,S., LAZAROVITZ,E. AND RUBINSTEIN,D., 1968, GLUCOSE AND GLYCOGEN METABOLISM IN ERYTHROCYTES FROM NORMAL AND GLYCOGEN STORAGE DISEASE TYPE III SUBJECTS. J CLIN INVEST 47:1343-1348

57. YOSHIKAWA,H., 1968, NON-GLYCOLYTIC METABOLISM OF CARBOHYDRATE IN RED BLOOD CELLS. METABOLISM AND MEMBRANE PERMEABILITY OF ERYTHROCYTES AND THROMBOCYTES DEUTSCH,E., GERLACH,E. AND MOSER,K. ED. 38-42, GEORG THIEME VERLAG, STUTTGART

58. WANG,Y.M., PATTERSON,H.J. AND VAN EYS,J., 1971, THE POTENTIAL
     USE OF XYLITOL IN GLUCOSE-6-PHOSPHATE DEHYDROGENASE DEFICIENCY
     ANEMIA. J CLIN INVEST 50:1421-1428

59. BEUTLER,E. AND MATHAI,C.K., 1968, GENETIC VARIATION IN RED
     CELL GALACTOSE-1-PHOSPHATE URIDYL TRANSFERASE. HEREDITARY
     DISORDERS OF ERYTHROCYTE METABOLISM BEUTLER,E. ED. 66-86,
     CITY OF HOPE SYMP. SERIES, VOL. I, GRUNE & STRATTON, N.Y.

60. GUARINO,A.J. AND SABLE,H.Z., 1955, STUDIES ON PHOSPHOMUTASES
     II. PHOSPHORIBOMUTASE AND PHOSPHOGLUCOMUTASE. J BIOL CHEM
     215:515-526

61. GIBLETT,E.R., ANDERSON,J.E., COHEN,F., POLLARA,B. AND
     MEUWISSEN,H.J., 1972, ADENOSINE DEAMINASE DEFICIENCY IN
     TWO PATIENTS WITH SEVERELY IMPAIRED CELLULAR IMMUNITY.
     LANCET 2:1067-1069

62. AGARWAL,R.P., CRABTREE,G.W., PARKS JR,R.E., NELSON,J.A.,
     KEIGHTLEY,R., PARKMAN,R., ROSEN,F.S., STERN,R.C. AND
     POLMAR,S.H., 1976, PURINE NUCLEOSIDE METABOLISM IN THE
     ERYTHROCYTES OF PATIENTS WITH ADENOSINE DEAMINASE DEFICIENCY
     AND SEVERE COMBINED IMMUNODEFICIENCY. J CLIN INVEST 57:1025-
     1035

63. MEYSKENS,F.L. AND WILLIAMS,H.E., 1971, ADENOSINE METABOLISM
     IN HUMAN ERYTHROCYTES. BIOCHIM BIOPHYS ACTA 240:170-179

64. ROTHMAN,I.K., ZANJANI,E.D., GORDON,A.S. AND SILBER,R.,
     1970, NUCLEOSIDE DEAMINASE: AN ENZYMATIC MARKER FOR STRESS
     ERYTHROPOIESIS IN THE MOUSE. J CLIN INVEST 49:2051-2067

65. HARRISON,D.E., MALATHI,V.G. AND SILBER,R., 1975, ELEVATED
     ERYTHROCYTE NUCLEOSIDE DEAMINASE LEVELS IN GENETICALLY
     ANEMIC W/WV AND SL/SLD MICE. BLOOD CELLS 1:605-614

66. KIM,B.K., CHA,S. AND PARKS JR,R.E., 1968, PURINE NUCLEOSIDE
     PHOSPHORYLASE FROM HUMAN ERYTHROCYTES. I. PURIFICATION AND
     PROPERTIES. J BIOL CHEM 243:1763-1770

67. AGARWAL,R.P. AND PARKS JR.,R.E., 1969, PURINE NUCLEOSIDE
     PHOSPHORYLASE FROM HUMAN ERYTHROCYTES. J BIOL CHEM 244:644-
     647

68. VAN HEUKELOM,L.H.S., STAAL,G.E.J., STOOP,J.W. AND
     ZEGERS,B.J.M., 1976, AN ABNORMAL FORM OF PURINE NUCLEOSIDE
     PHOSPHORYLASE IN A FAMILY WITH A CHILD WITH SEVERE DEFECTIVE
     T-CELL-AND NORMAL B-CELL IMMUNITY. CLIN CHIM ACTA 72:117-
     124

69. GIBLETT,E.R., AMMANN,A.J., WARA,D.W., SANDMAN,R. AND
     DIAMOND,L.K., 1975, NUCLEOSIDE-PHOSPHORYLASE DEFICIENCY IN
     A CHILD WITH SEVERELY DEFECTIVE T-CELL IMMUNITY AND NORMAL
     B-CELL IMMUNITY. LANCET 1:1010-1013

70. NISHIZAWA,T., NISHIDA,Y. AND AKAOKA,I., 1976, ERYTHROCYTE
     ADENOSINE KINASE ACTIVITY IN GOUT. CLIN CHIM ACTA 67:15-20

71. PAGLIA,D.E. AND VALENTINE,W.N., 1975, CHARACTERISTICS OF
     A PYRIMIDINE-SPECIFIC 5'-NUCLEOTIDASE IN HUMAN ERYTHROCYTES.
     J BIOL CHEM 250:7973-7979

72. TORRANCE,J.D., WHITTAKER,D. AND BEUTLER,E., 1977, PURIFICATION AND PROPERTIES OF HUMAN ERYTHROCYTE PYPIMIDINE 5'-NUCLEOTIDASE. PROC NATL ACAD SCI USA 74:3701-3704

73. ORRINGER,E.P. AND PARKER,J.C., 1973, ION AND WATER MOVEMENTS IN RED BLOOD CELLS. PROG HEMATOL 8:1-23

74. NAKAO,T., NAGANO,K., ADACHI,K. AND NAKAO,M., 1963, SEPARATION OF TWO ADENOSINE TRIPHOSPHATASES FROM ERYTHROCYTE MEMBRANE. BIOCHEM BIOPHYS RES COMMUN 13:444-448

75. ZAIL,S.S. AND VAN DEN HOEK,A.K., 1976, STUDIES ON CALCIUM TRANSPORT AND CALCIUM-DEPENDENT ADENOSINE TRIPHOSPHATASE ACTIVITY OF ERYTHROCYTE MEMBRANES IN HEREDITARY SPHEROCYTOSIS. BR J HAEMATOL 34:605-611

76. HSIEH,H.-.S. AND JAFFE,E.R., 1975, THE METABOLISM OF METHEMOGLOBIN IN HUMAN ERYTHROCYTES. THE RED BLOOD CELL SURGENOR,D.M. ED. 2:799-824, 2ND EDITION, ACADEMIC PRESS, NEW YORK

77. SCOTT,E.M., 1968, CONGENITAL METHEMOGLOBINEMIA DUE TO DPNH-DIAPHORASE DEFICIENCY. HEREDITARY DISORDERS OF ERYTHROCYTE METABOLISM BEUTLER,E. ED. 102-113, CITY OF HOPE SYMP. SERIES, VOL. I, GRUNE & STRATTON, N.Y.

78. BEUTLER,E. AND BALUDA,M.C., 1963, METHEMOGLOBIN REDUCTION. STUDIES OF THE INTERACTION BETWEEN CELL POPULATIONS AND OF THE ROLE OF METHYLENE BLUE. BLOOD 22:323-333

79. SASS,M.D., CARUSO,C.J. AND FARHANGI,M., 1967, TPNH-METHEMOGLOBIN REDUCTASE DEFICIENCY: A NEW RED-CELL ENZYME DEFECT. J LAB CLIN MED 70:760-767

2

GLUCOSE-6-PHOSPHATE DEHYDROGENASE DEFICIENCY

2.1. History

It has long been recognized that certain ordinarily salutary drugs may produce an acute hemolytic anemia in some susceptible individuals. The 8-aminoquinoline antimalarial, pamaquine (plasmoquine), was such a medication. It was the investigation of the hemolytic effect of pamaquine and its derivatives which led to the recognition that hereditary red cell enzyme deficiencies could produce hemolytic disease.

When Mühlens[1] first described the use of pamaquine in the treatment of malaria in 1926, he wrote:

> That plasmoquine has no damaging effect on the red blood cells themselves is suggested to me not only by the significant increase in hemoglobin during treatment and the often rapid significant regression of splenomegaly but also by its use in cases of blackwater fever . . .

In the same year, the first cases of acute hemolytic anemia produced by pamaquine were described by Cordes.[2] Initially he observed four cases, one fatal, among 72 black patients receiving pamaquine. These and two additional cases in a series totaling 250 were presented in greater detail in later publications.[3,4] Blood smears from one of the patients were examined by Professor Victor Shilling, who observed marked anisocytosis and poikilocytosis, many normoblasts, and some polychromatophilia. Professor F. D. Mallory performed a necropsy on one of the patients and observed numerous red cells in endothelial leukocytes of the spleen. During the next few years many additional cases of pamaquine-induced hemolytic anemia were reported.[5-34] As early as 1928 Heinz bodies were observed in the red cells of a patient with probable mild hemolytic anemia occurring during pamaquine treatment.[8] Routine hematologic examination of the blood of patients undergoing pamaquine-induced hemolysis failed to shed light on its cause. Osmotic fragility tests, Donath–Landsteiner test, and bleeding and clotting times were reported to be normal, and immersing the patient in cold water did not elicit further hemolysis.[19] The administration of pamaquine 26 days[19] or 3 months[35] after the original exposure caused recurrent hemolytic episodes. In 1943 Mann[21] observed the presence of a nonspecific hemagglutinin in the serum of one patient, and conjectured, incorrectly, that abnormal plasma factors were responsible for hemolysis. In 1946 Dimson and McMartin[27] reported 25 cases of pamaquine-induced hemoglobinuria. *In vitro* studies of red cell hemolysis, and investigation of dermal response to pamaquine failed to disclose the cause of sensitivity to hemolysis. Other studies showed red cell fragility to be normal, and hemolysis could not be reproduced *in vitro* by incubating the patient's cells with homologous plasma, with plasma from a patient who had recently received pamaquine, or with plasma to which varying amounts of pamaquine had been added, or by incubating normal red cells with a patient's plasma.[35] Earle *et al.*[32] measured the mechanical and osmotic fragility of red cells of patients receiving pamaquine, and studied isoagglutinins, hemolysins, cold hemagglutinins, and autoagglutinins without observing any difference between pamaquine-sensitive and -nonsensitive subjects. They also observed no correlation between plasma pamaquine levels and hemolysis. Other similarly fruitless efforts were reported.[33,36-38] The familial nature of pamaquine sensitivity was noted early, and analogies were drawn between this disorder and favism.[30] Racial differences in susceptibility to hemolysis by pamaquine were also recognized by early investigators.[18,22,25,27,32]

As American troops in the Pacific and in Korea were exposed to vivax malaria during World War II and the Korean conflict, an active search for more effective, less toxic antimalarial drugs was carried out. These investigations led to introduction of the 6-methoxy-8-aminoquinoline drug, primaquine.[39] This drug had the capacity to eradicate tissue stages of vivax malaria without causing appreciable toxic side effects in the vast majority of soldiers who ingested it. But as had been the case with primaquine, approximately 11% of black soldiers who were given primaquine developed an acute hemolytic anemia. This potentially serious toxic side effect of an important drug was no longer merely a scientific curiosity, but became an important practical problem. Beginning in 1952 systematic studies were undertaken at the Army Malaria Research Unit at the Stateville Penitentiary in Joliet, Illinois to determine the cause of this type of drug sensitivity.

To determine whether sensitivity to primaquine was due to abnormal metabolism of the drug, on the one hand, or to an intrinsic abnormality of the red cells, on the other, cross-transfusion studies were carried out with ^{51}Cr-labeled erythrocytes.[40] Red cells from primaquine-sensitive donors were tagged with ^{51}Cr and transfused into nonsensitive recipients. When these recipients were given 30 mg of primaquine daily, accelerated destruction of the labeled cells from primaquine-sensitive donors was readily demonstrated (Fig. 3). The converse experiment was also carried out. Red cells from nonsensitive donors were labeled and transfused into sensitive recipients. Administration of primaquine to these recipients produced a hemolytic anemia, but the tagged red cells from nonsensitive donors were not destroyed. These studies clearly established that primaquine sensitivity was due to an intrinsic abnormality of the erythrocyte.

Attention was now directed to investigation of the nature of the red cell abnormality. As had been shown in earlier studies of pamaquine-sensitive subjects, primaquine-sensitive red cells appeared normal when examined by conventional hematologic techniques; osmotic fragility, mechanical fragility, *in vitro* susceptibility to lysis by primaquine, antigenic

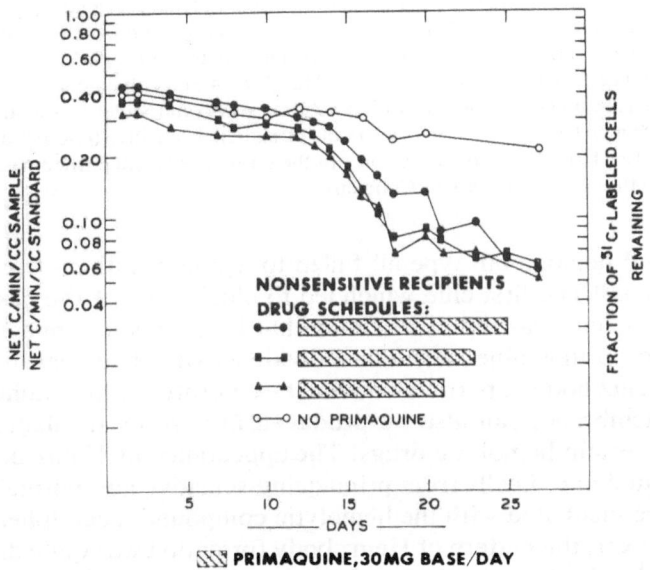

FIGURE 3. The effect of the administration of 30 mg of primaquine daily on ^{51}Cr-labeled red cells from a primaquine-sensitive (G-6-PD-deficient) donor transfused into normal recipients. The administration of primaquine resulted in accelerated destruction of the transfused cells. (Reprinted from Dern *et al.*,[40] through the courtesy of the authors and Mosby Company.)

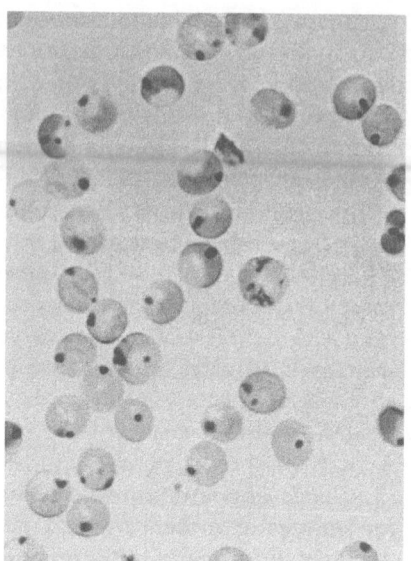 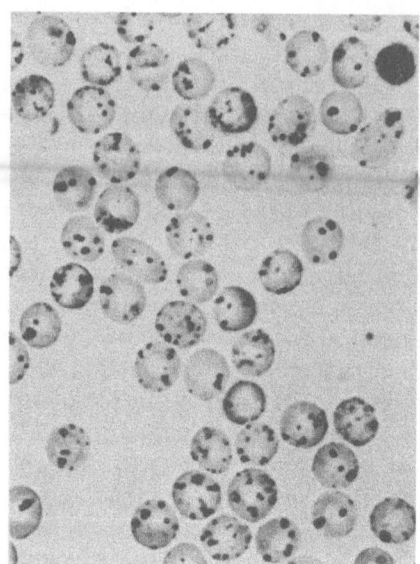

FIGURE 4. *In vitro* Heinz body formation in normal (left) and primaquine-sensitive (G-6-PD-deficient) (right) red cells. Whole blood, 100 μl, was added to 2 ml of a 100 mg/100 ml acetylphenylhydrazine solution in 67 mM sodium phosphate buffer, pH 7.6. The suspension was mixed and aerated immediately and after 2 hr. After 4 hr incubation the suspension was stained for Heinz bodies by mixing with a solution of crystal violet in slightly hypotonic saline. Many small Heinz bodies are seen in the primaquine-sensitive (G-6-PD-deficient) red cells while a few large Heinz bodies stained in the normal cells. (Reprinted from Beutler *et al.*,[42] through the courtesy of Mosby Company.)

pattern, and hemoglobin type all failed to distinguish them from normal erythrocytes.[41] The first clue which led to elucidation of the basic defect of these red cells was the observation that Heinz bodies appeared in the red cells of primaquine-sensitive individuals who had ingested primaquine.[41] Heinz bodies, particles of denatured protein which adhere to the red cell membrane, can also be produced *in vitro* by incubation of red cells with certain hemolytic drugs. The appearance of Heinz bodies was demonstrated in red cells from primaquine-sensitive and normal subjects which were incubated with the hemolytic compound, acetylphenylhydrazine. However, the pattern of Heinz body formation was quite different in the normal cells than in those of primaquine-sensitive subjects. Most normal erythrocytes developed only one or two large Heinz bodies, whereas many small Heinz bodies formed in most of the primaquine-sensitive erythrocytes (Fig. 4).[42] This finding made possible for the first time the identification *in vitro* of primaquine-sensitive individuals. It also opened the door to the broader study *in vitro* of the hemolytic phenomenon.

Red cells were subsequently incubated with a variety of metabolic inhibitors. The pattern of Heinz body formation which was characteristic of primaquine-sensitive cells developed when normal erythrocytes were treated with iodoacetate and arsenite.[42] Because both of these compounds are sulfhydryl inhibitors, attention turned to the sulfhydryl compounds of the red cell. The content of reduced glutathione (GSH) was found to be lower in primaquine-sensitive red cells than in normal cells.[43] More importantly, it was noted that primaquine-sensitive cells incubated with acetylphenylhydrazine were unable to maintain their GSH content. Estimation of the GHS level of red cells incubated with acetylphenylhydrazine, the "GSH stability test," made it possible to identify primaquine-sensitive persons accurately.[44] It also focused further attention on the pathways which maintain GSH in the reduced state. The reduction of oxidized glutathione (GSSG) to GSH is catalyzed by glutathione reductase, and requires NADPH as a hydrogen donor (see Chapter 1). The hexose monophosphate pathway was examined, since it serves as a source of NADPH. Primaquine-sensitive red cells proved to be deficient in the first enzyme of this pathway, glucose-6-phosphate dehydrogenase (G-6-PD).[45] Quite independently of these investigations, Waller and co-workers[46] noted an absence of G-6-PD in the erythrocytes of an Iranian student who had undergone an apparently spontaneous hemolytic episode.

The availability of the glutathione stability test also made family studies possible, and the mode of inheritance of GSH instability was soon defined as a sex-linked characteristic.[47] Males were normal or fully affected, while females usually manifested an intermediate degree of GSH instability; some obligate heterozygous females were fully affected or not affected at all. Results similar to those observed with the GSH stability test were obtained when G-6-PD activity was measured in erythrocytes. Ohno's demonstration that one of the two X chromosomes of females was heterochromatic,[48] a form of chromatin known to be genetically inactive in insects,[49] led to our suggestion that only one of the two X chromosomes of females was active; we proposed that one X chromosome randomly selected was inactivated early in embryogenesis.[50,51] This hypothesis was advanced to explain the occurrence of identical levels of G-6-PD activity in normal males and females and the variability observed in the expression of G-6-PD activity among different heterozygous females. It was confirmed by demonstrating that heterozygotes for G-6-PD deficiency had two red cell populations, one deficient and one normal.[52] It was advanced independently by Lyon to account for variegate coat color patterns in mice bearing X-linked coat color genes.[53]

The availability of the glutathione stability test and the subsequent recognition of G-6-PD deficiency as the primary defect in primaquine-sensitive red cells stimulated surveys of the incidence of the defect in many parts of the world. It soon became apparent that G-6-PD deficiency was not limited to black American males; GSH instability and G-6-PD deficiency were also found to be common in Mediterranean populations,[54,55] and later in Oriental populations. Marks and Gross pointed out that G-6-PD deficiency in Mediterranean populations was much more severe than that observed in black Americans.[56] With the development of electrophoretic techniques for the study of red cell G-6-PD,[57,58] it soon became evident that the enzyme deficiency found in the Mediterranean region was quite different from that found among black Americans. Further heterogeneity in G-6-PD deficiency became apparent when Newton and Bass[59] demonstrated G-6-PD deficiency in the red cells of a patient with hereditary nonspherocytic hemolytic anemia (NSHA). Detailed biochemical study of the red cells of such subjects by Kirkman et al.[60] showed that the residual enzyme was different from that of the more common Negro and Caucasian variants, and that the deficient enzyme differed in individual cases. In 1967 procedures for the study of G-6-PD variants were standardized by a World Health Organization scientific group,[61] and it became possible to compare G-6-PD variants reported by many different laboratories. The result has been the discovery of the existence of an astonishing number of distinct G-6-PD variants. Structural studies have made an excellent start toward the understanding of the amino acid sequence of G-6-PD and of the substitutions which lead to some of the known variants.[62,63]

2.2. Genetics and Population Distribution

The initial studies of primaquine sensitivity were carried out in a men's prison. In this population individuals could be clearly divided into those who were sensitive and those who were nonsensitive, whether classification was based on hemolytic response to drug administration, Heinz body formation, GSH stability test, or enzyme assay. When studies were carried out on relatives of G-6-PD-deficient individuals, however, it was found that women often manifested only partial G-6-PD deficiency.[47,64] In most families transmission was from mother to son, and it was proposed that G-6-PD deficiency was a sex-linked disorder.[47,64] Confirmation was provided by the finding that the locus for G-6-PD deficiency is tightly linked to the loci for color blindness.[65-68] Further investigations have shown that the locus for G-6-PD is one of a cluster of genes on the X chromosome which includes those for deutan and protan color blindness, and for hemophilia A (factor VIII deficiency).[69] It also seems to be tightly linked to X-linked optic atrophy.[330] It is located about 10, 14, and 24 map units, respectively, from the loci for Xm serum groups,[69] hereditary sideroblastic anemia,[70] and Becker's muscular dystrophy.[69] It is separated by a considerably greater distance from the loci for Xg,[71-74] ichthyosis, Fabry's disease, retinoschisis,[75] and hypoxanthine guanine phosphoribosyltransferase (HGPRT).[76]

It might have been anticipated that all women who were heterozygous for G-6-PD deficiency would have intermediate levels of G-6-PD activity. It quickly became apparent, however, that this was not the case. For example, a woman who has sons with normal G-6-PD activity must have at least one normal allele for G-6-PD. Yet, some such women had no detectable enzyme activity in their red cells; they were as severely affected as males.[77] Conversely, a woman who has a son with G-6-PD deficiency must have at least one gene for G-6-PD deficiency. Yet some women with deficient sons have completely normal enzyme activity.[78,79] The explanation for this seeming anomaly lies in the principle of X inactivation.[51,53] Both X chromosomes in the female conceptus are active after fertilization.[80] Early in embryonic development, however, one of the two X chromosomes becomes heterochromatic and genetically inactive. The result is a mosaic of X chromosome activity in the human female: some cells transcribe genes on the maternally derived and others on the paternally derived X chromosome. In the erythroid series the final proportion may vary between the extremes of only maternally derived or only paternally derived X chromosomes being active.

A high degree of concordance exists in the expression of the heterozygous state for G-6-PD deficiency in identical twins.[81] While it was suggested[81] that this finding indicated that the inactivating process itself was nonrandom, it is likely that X-linked genes other than those for G-6-PD influence the proliferation of cells after the inactivation process takes place.[82-84] It is easy to calculate that a small proliferative advantage would produce a very large difference in the final proportion of cells with a maternally derived or a paternally derived active X chromosome. If cells with a maternally derived X chromosome had only a 5% advantage per generation over those with a paternally derived X chromosome, the ratio of these cells to one another would be 2.65:1 after 20 cell divisions, and 11.5:1 after 50 cell divisions. An interesting example of selection among red cell populations is provided by heterozygotes for hypoxanthine guanine phosphoribosyltransferase deficiency. In these persons red cell precursors deficient in HGPRT are apparently at a selective disadvantage, and when heterozygosity for G-6-PD is also present, only one or the other allele is expressed in the peripheral blood.[85] The pattern of proliferation may well be tissue specific, since the relative expression of two G-6-PD alleles in different tissues may vary. For example, we have examined a heterozygote for G-6-PD A and B in which both enzyme types were expressed equally in red cells, but only G-6-PD B was found in liver.[86] The fact that X inactivation does occur, and that it involves the locus for G-6-PD, was confirmed by cloning fibroblast cultures from women heterozygous for both G-6-PD A and B. Whereas mixed cultures showed both electrophoretic phenotypes, clones manifested only one or the other type of enzyme.[87] The fact that clones can be identified on the basis of their G-6-PD type has made the G-6-PD polymorphism extremely valuable as a means for tracing the origin of both benign and malignant tumors. Acquired neoplasms generally have a clonal origin.[88-90] However, there are exceptions. In a patient with metastatic colon carcinoma who was heterozygous for G-6-PD A and G-6-PD B, some of the metastases were predominantly G-6-PD A and others predominantly G-6-PD B.[86] Hereditary tumors such as trichoepitheliomas often have multiple origins.[91] The principle of X inactivation involving the locus for G-6-PD has also been used to confirm that the erythrocytes are involved in the neoplastic change in chronic granulocytic leukemia,[92] and to establish that paroxysmal nocturnal hemoglobinuria[93] is a clonal disorder. It has also been demonstrated using this principle that atherosclerotic plaques arise from a single cell.[94,95] The high frequency of the Gd^A gene has assured the availability of cultured cells with the Gd^A/Gd^B genotype. Such cells have been useful in investigations of basic aspects of the inactivation phenomenon. For example, treatments designed to reactivate the inactive X have been applied to clones of such cells[96] without success, and cell hybridization studies using G-6-PD-deficient cells were used to show that two X chromosomes may be active in hybrid cells.[97] Since our original suggestion[51] that the distribution of G-6-PD phenotypes in heterozygotes might provide information regarding the number of primordial cells present at the time of inactivation, a number of estimates of this cell number have been made.[98,99] However, these estimates generally do not take into account the effect of selection between cell populations upon determination of the final phenotype.[82,84]

Unfortunately, no satisfactory animal models for G-6-PD deficiency are available. An electrophoretic polymorphism exists in swine.[100] Partial (50%) deficiency of G-6-PD was documented in one dog,[101] with no apparent clinical effects. There were no offspring or known littermates, and further studies were not possible. A G-6-PD-deficient strain of rats has been lost.[102] Certain mammals, such as sheep and goats,[103] have G-6-PD levels in the range found in the A− type of deficiency. However, the enzyme is apparently sufficiently active *in vivo* to provide protection against the hemolytic stress imposed by primaquine injection.[104] G-6-PD deficiency was reported to occur in cattle,[105] but the apparent deficiency, based on results obtained using a screening procedure, proved to be a deficiency of NADPH diaphorase; considerable G-6-PD activity was demonstrated in red cells of cattle.[106]

Very extensive polymorphisms involving G-6-PD are known to occur in many populations. Most surveys have been limited to the detection of G-6-PD deficiency. Since expression of G-6-PD deficiency in females is so variable, and detection unreliable, gene frequency figures are meaningful only when derived from males. Table III summarizes available data concerning the incidence of G-6-PD deficiency in many populations. Although the precise incidence of different G-6-PD variants has rarely been defined in population surveys, available data suggest that among African populations deficiency is usually due to G-6-PD A−. In Mediterranean countries such as Greece, Turkey, Israel, Egypt, and Italy, G-6-PD Mediterranean appears to be most prevalent, although careful analysis has shown that a number of different severely deficient variants are present,

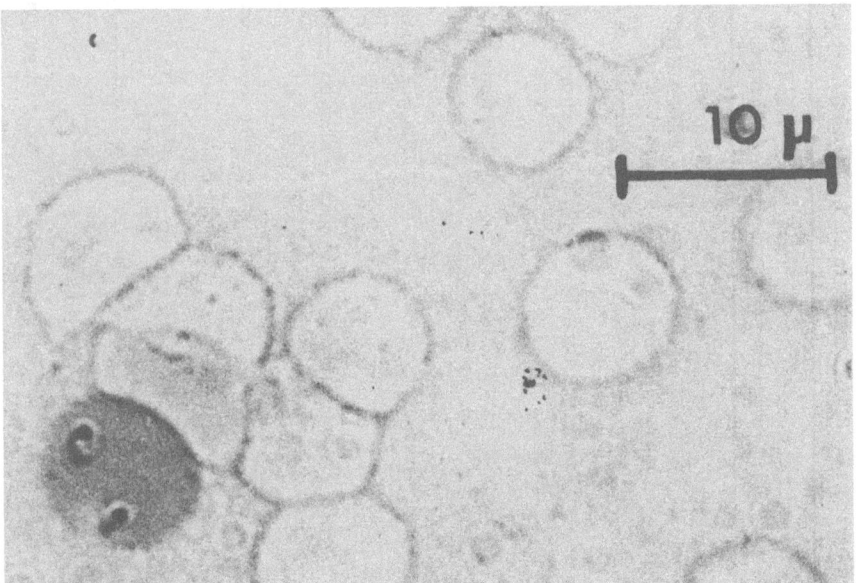

FIGURE 5. The distribution of malaria parasites in the peripheral blood of a woman heterozygous for G-6-PD deficiency. G-6-PD-deficient cells were identified by a methemoglobin elution technique, so that normal cells appear to be filled with hemoglobin, while G-6-PD-deficient cells appear as empty ghosts. Normal cells are more actively parasitized than are G-6-PD-deficient cells.[250] (Reproduced through the courtesy of Dr. Lucio Luzzatto.)

TABLE III

The Incidence of G-6-PD Deficiency or of G-6-PD Electrophoretic Phenotypes in Males of Various Populations

Geographical location	Population	Method	Incidence[a]	Sample size
w World				
Bolivia	Caucasian: Mestizo	BCB[b]/MRT[b]	0	44 [107]
	Caucasian: White	BCB/MRT	0	26 [108]
	Indian: Aymara		0.75	268 [108]
	Indian: Quechua		1.5	67
Brazil	Fathers of 380 families	Electrophoresis	10.53 A 5.26 A− 84.21 B	380 [109]
	Light mulatto or darker	Electrophoresis	8.73 A 8.53 A− 82.73 B	996 [109]
	Light or dark yellow	Electrophoresis	3.15 A 7.87 A− 88.98 B	127 [109]
	Unspecified sons of 380 families	Electrophoresis	6.06 A 7.73 A− 86.21 B	1501 [109]
	White	Electrophoresis	3.64 A 4.70 A− 91.67 B	660 [109]
	Caucasian	MTT[c]	3.9	102 [110]
	Negro	MTT	12.3	316 [110]
	Sao Paulo Caucasian	Assay/electrophoresis	1.39 def. 0 A 100 B	72 [111] 60 60
	Japanese	Assay/electrophoresis	0 def. 0 A	43 [111] 42

Country	Population	Method	%	Reference
	Negro	Assay/electrophoresis	100 B	42
			8.16 def.	49[111]
			10.42 A	48
			89.58 B	48
Canada	Chinese Canadians	BCB	4.71	361[112]
	Southeastern Ojibwa	Electrophoresis	0	59 (all B+)[113]
Colombia	Caucasian	BCB	2.52	119[114]
	Indian		0	45
	Mestizo		1.41	213
	Negro		15.45	123
Cuba	Caucasian	Electrophoresis	3.23 A	155[115]
			0.65 A−	
			95.48 B	
	Mulatto	Electrophoresis	11.03 A	145[115]
			8.97 A−	
			79.31 B	
	Negro	Electrophoresis	19.05 A	168[115]
			16.07 A−	
			63.69 B	
	Habana Province	Electrophoresis	4.44 A	405[116]
			2.47 A−	
			92.84 B	
Curacao	Negro	BCB	12.8	573[117]
Dutch Guiana	Brokopondo	Assay	19.4	336[118]
	Negro (Upper Surinam)		20.2	311[118]
	Northern areas		7.0	115[118]
	Tapanahony		15.9	88[118]
	Negro (Surinam)	Electrophoresis	1.95 def.	256[119]
			11.33 A	
			1.95 B	

(continued)

Percent of deficiency or of electrophoretic phenotype.
BCB = Brilliant cresyl blue decolorization test; MTT = MTT tetrazolium spot test; DCIP = dichlorophenolindophenol decolorization test; MRT = methemoglobin reduction test.

TABLE III (continued)

Geographical location	Population	Method	Incidence[a]	Sample size
Jamaica	Kingston	Methylene blue	14.75 def.	217 [120]
		Assay	20.79 A	202 [120]
		Electrophoresis	13.86 A −	202 [120]
			65.35 B	202 [120]
Mexico	Jewish	Electrophoresis	4.21 (Medit.)	95 [120]
	Indian:			
	Costa Sierra	BCB	0	48 [122]
	Maya		0	20 [122]
	Mixteco		3.57	56 [122]
	Nahua		0	124 [122]
	Tarahumara		0	79 [122]
	Tarasco		0	55 [122]
	Tzotzil-Tzeltales		0	14 [122]
	Yaqui		0	66 [122]
	Mestizo:			
	Diverse locations	BCB	0	82 [122]
	Indian:			
	Mazateco	?	0	138 [123]
	Mixteco		1.39	144 [123]
	Nahua		1.32	303 [123]
	Tarahumara		0	79 [123]
	Tarasco		0	55 [123]
	Yaqui		0	66 [123]
	Zapoteco		0	111 [123]

Country	Group		Method	% / type	n [ref]
	Indian:				
		Chinanteco	?	0	21 [123]
		Chol		0	152 [123]
		Chontal		2.02	99 [123]
		Huasteco		0	72 [123]
		Maya		0	20 [123]
		Mixe		0	32 [123]
		Popoloco		0	17 [123]
		Totonaco		0	86 [123]
		Tzeltal-Txotzil		0	14 [123]
	Non-Indian				
		Cuajinicuilapa	BCB	6.22	418 [124]
		Ometepec		2.22	405 [124]
		Pochutla		0.29	346 [124]
		San Pedro Mixtepec		1.79	335 [124]
	Indian		BCB	0.92	218 [125]
Nicaragua	Creole		?	18.2	313 [126]
	Indian			19	174 [126]
Peru	Indian (no Spanish blood)		BCB	0	154 [127]
	Indian:				
		Cerro de Pasco workers	Electrophoresis	0 def. / 100 B	41 [128]
		Lima	Electrophoresis	0 def. / 100 B	33 [128]
		Province of Danier Carrion	Electrophoresis	0 def. / 100 B	109 [128]
Trinidad	East Indian		BCB	13.73	153 [129]
	Negro (West Africa origin)		BCB	13.14	175 [129]
United States	Indian (Seneca)		Assay	0	105 [130]
	Negro		Assay/electrophoresis	9.89 A−	182 [131]
	Negro (Memphis)		BCB	16.49	97 [132]
	Negro		DCIP	10.56	521 [133]
	White		DCIP	0	328 [133]
	Negro		Assay/fluorescent	12.6	20,810 [134]

(continued)

TABLE III (continued)

Geographical location	Population	Method	Incidence[a]	Sample size
United States (continued)	Negro (Cook County)	BCB	11.38	624 [135]
	Negro	Electrophoresis	16.08 A+ 17.68 A- 66.24 B+ 0 def. 100 B	311 [136]
Venezuela	Makiritare Indians	Electrophoresis		70 [137]
	Mestizo (Barquisimeto)	MRT	7.0	300 [138]
	Mestizo (Caracas)	BCB	2.0	300 [138]
	Indian (Paraujanos)	BCB	0	57 [139]
	Negro (Tapipa)	BCB	11.5	26 [139]
Congo	Nontribal Bantu	GSH-Stab.	21.46	522 [140]
	Leopoldville	BCB	20.33	300 [141]
	Hamitic and Sudanese tribes	BCB	5.52	326 [142]
	Nontribal Bantu	BCB	18.03	477
	Tribal Bantu	BCB	20.05	843 [142]
East Africa (Kenya, Uganda, Rwanda, Tanzania)	Acholi	BCB	8.70	23 [143]
	Ankole		3.17	63 [143]
	Ganda		12.50	424 [143]
	Kiga		1.85	54 [143]
	Luo		6.67	45 [143]
	Nyoro		11.11	18 [143]
	Soga		7.14	14 [143]
	Teso		9.52	21 [143]
	Toro		8.57	35 [143]
	Bondei	BCB	27.27	121 [144]
	Digo		23.08	26 [144]

Region	Population	Method	Value	n [ref]
	Ganda		15.00	40 [144]
	Giriama		16.83	101 [144]
	Kikuyu		2.86	70 [144]
	Luo		28.00	50 [144]
	Masai		1.69	59 [144]
	Sambaa		20.69	29 [144]
	Zigua		23.08	26 [144]
E. Senegal	Niokolonko	Electrophoresis	7.81 A-	192 [145]
Egypt	Lower Egypt	MRT	31.22	205 [146]
	Met. Cities		15.96	94 [146]
	Unclassified		25.30	83 [146]
	Upper Egypt		27.12	118 [146]
Ethiopia	Fallasha	?	0	208 [147]
	Fallasha	GSH-Stab/BCB	0	824 [148]
	Nonselect	DCIP	0.49	1019 [133]
Gambia	Gambian	BCB	15.53	103 [149]
	Keneba villagers	DCIP	8.30	289 [150]
Ghana	Ghanian	Electrophoresis	21.0 A 13.0 A- 56.0 B 5.0 B-like 5.0 O enzyme	39 [151]
	Accra:			
	Typhoid patients	MTT	38.89	36 [152]
	Viral hepatitis patients		43	200 [152]
	Southern Ghana	BCB	23.96	96 [149]
	Southern Ghana	MRT/electrophoresis	25.6 A+ 15.9 A- 57.3 B+ 1.2 other	851 [153]
Kenya	(see E. Africa)			
Madeira	Portuguese	BCB	0.87	458 [154]
Malagasy Republic	Nonselect	MTT spot test	1.59	279 [155]

(continued)

TABLE III (continued)

Geographical location	Population	Method	Incidence[a]	Sample size
Nigeria	W. Nigeria (90% Yoruba)	Electrophoresis	22.95 A 21.64 A− 55.41 B	1451 [156]
	Abua	BCB	22.22	81 [157]
	Kalabani		10.71	56 [157]
	Ogoni		27.37	179 [157]
	Southern Ibo		20.92	153 [157]
	85% Yoruba	BCB	20.43	93 [158]
	N. Nigeria	BCB	20.59	136 [149]
	Yoruba	Electrophoresis	21.99 A+ 21.99 A− 56.03 B+	141 [136]
Rwanda	Rwandan (see E. Africa)	BCB	3.01	133 [143]
S. Africa	Bantu	GSH-Stab	3.23	310 [129]
	Bushmen		3.45	29 [129]
	Cape Malay		3.77	53 [129]
	Indian		0	100 [129]
	Bantu	GSH-Stab	4.89	757 [159]
	European		0	250 [159]
	Indian (Tamil, Hindu, Urdu, Moslem)		0.67	149 [159]
	Malay	GSH-Stab	2.00	50 [159]
	Indian	BCB	2.00	50 [159]
Tanzania	Ifakara	MRT	18.35	109 [160]
	Mountain areas		8.47	59 [160]
	Various regions		14.46	408 [160]

Region	Location	Method	Value	
Uganda	Aura	BCB	8.96	67 [161]
	Bundebugyo		18.46	65 [161]
	Fort Portal		11.00	100 [161]
	Gulu		12.00	100 [161]
	Kabale		2.78	180 [161]
	Mbale		14.00	100 [161]
	Mbarara		9.00	100 [161]
	Moroto		13.33	60 [161]
	Soroti		13.00	100 [161]
urasia				
Bangladesh	Bengali Moslem	Electrophoresis	4.00 def. 96.00 B+	150 [162]
Borneo	Mostly from Djkarta (see Malaysia)	BCB/MRT	1.07	466 [163]
Brunei				
Ceylon	(see Sri Lanka)			
China	Nonselect	GSH-Stab	0	41 [164]
	Kwangtung Province	MRT	4.50	200 [165]
	Nonselect (examined in Singapore)	BCB	2.33	301 [166]
Cyprus	Syrianochori	BCB	6.99	229 [168]
	Troodos		0	476 [168]
	Yialousa		10.62	339 [168]
Czechoslovakia	Nonselect	MRT/GSH-Stab	0	112 [99]
Fiji Islands	Fijian	Assay	0.11	913 [169]
	Indian		1.23	974 [169]
Great Britain	British and Irish	Glut-Stab	0	116 [170]
	West Scotland (Glasgow)	MRT	0	404 [171]
Greece	Crete	GSH-Stab	2.91	206 [172]
	Cyprus		3.23	310 [172]
	Nonselect	GSH-Stab and BCB	0.69	580 [172]
	Aegean Islands	BCB	2.91	378 [173]
	Asia Minor		1.78	225 [173]

(continued)

TABLE III (continued)

Geographical location	Population	Method	Incidence[a]	Sample size
Greece (continued)	Athens		2.50	120 [173]
	Black Sea coast		0	72 [173]
	Central Greece		5.56	827 [173]
	Crete		3.85	390 [173]
	Epirus		3.61	305 [173]
	Immigrants (Egypt, Russia, Rumania)		0	54 [173]
	Ionian Islands		2.92	171 [173]
	Macedonia		6.35	1418 [173]
	Peloponnese		5.93	911 [173]
	Salonica		5.41	74 [173]
	Thessaly		9.04	553 [173]
	Thrace		2.46	203 [173]
	Alexandra	BCB	2.93	786 [174]
	Lesbos		4.94	1317 [174]
	Rhodes		12.50	496 [174]
	Chalkidhiki	BCB	32.35	102 [175]
	Crete		8.23	158 [175]
	Greece (total)		18.35	665 [175]
	Rhodes		31.82	198 [175]
	Arta District	BCB	8.39	441 [176]
	Corfu (Ionian Islands)		5.52	888 [176]
	Elasson (N.E. Thessaly)		6.70	194 [176]
	Karditsa (S.W. Thessaly)		11.22	392 [176]
	Petromagoula (Central Greece)		14.50	200 [176]

Country	Population	Method	%	n
	Nonselect	BCB	1.79	56 [177]
	Nonselect	MTT	3.35	986 [178]
	Petromagoula and surrounding villages	BCB	14.50	200 [179]
	Pyrgos, Amalias, and surrounding villages	BCB	6.21	290 [179]
	Arta District	BCB	9.96	532 [180]
	Lemnos	BCB	13.50	200 [181]
	Thrace (Greek)		2.00	100 [181]
	Thrace (Turkish)		2.00	100 [181]
	Aegean Islands and Crete	BCB	3.70	135 [182]
	Athens		2.05	146 [182]
	Peloponnese		3.65	192 [182]
	Sterea, Hellas, Euboea		2.60	192 [182]
	Others		2.48	121 [182]
Guam	Chamorros (from all Guam)	BCB	0.41	246 [183]
Hawaii	Chinese	BCB	3.61	83 [184]
	Filipino		5.97	67 [184]
	Hybrid		0	62 [184]
Hong Kong	From Kwantung and Fu-Kien Province	BCB	3.74	1177 [185]
Hungary	Bodrogkoz	MRT	3.90	233 [186]
India	Parsees of Bombay	BCB	19.00	100 [187]
	Bombay	BCB	7.41	81 [188]
	Maharashtra	MRT	10.00	100 [189]
	Nonselect (examined in Singapore)	BCB	0	13 [166]
	Unspecified	BCB	3.26	92 [166]
	South India (Nilgiri Hills)	GSH-Stab	5.00	60 [70]
	Irula	Electrophoresis	8.99	89 [190]
	Kurumba		12.50	16 [190]
	Toda		0	48 [190]

(continued)

TABLE III (continued)

Geographical location	Population	Method	Incidence[a]	Sample size
India (continued)	North:			
	Punjab	BCB/MRT	7.50	1748 [191]
	Sind	BCB	3.13	90 [191]
	Uttar Pradesh	GSH-Stab/MRT	6.50	1457 [191]
	South:			
	Andhra Pradesh	BCB	4.70	443 [191]
	Kerala		0.27	256 [191]
	Tamil Nadu (Madras States)		9.00	100 [191]
	East:			
	Bengali (Calcutta)	Assay	4.73	485 [191]
	West:			
	Bombay	BCB	5.50	501 [191]
	Gujarati-speaking	BCB	6.30	1247 [191]
	Konkani-speaking	BCB	0.66	290 [191]
	Nagpur	MRT	11.70	554 [191]
	Marathi-speaking	BCB/MRT	2.00	2796 [191]
Iran	Armenian	GSH-Stab/BCB	0.60	158 [192]
	Basseri		13.30	83 [192]
	Ghashghai		11.30	133 [192]
	Mamassani		20.00	91 [192]
	Moslem		7.90	984 [192]
	Zoroastrian		0	146 [192]
	Armenian (New Julfa)	GSH-Stab	0.66	152 [193]
	Moslem	GSH-Stab	9.78	358 [194]
	Unspecified	DCIP	9.78	409 [133]

	Population	Method	%	n
Iraq and Persia	Jewish	GSH-Stab	40.00	15 [186]
Israel	Afghanistan	GSH-Stab ?	10.3	29 [147]
	Algiers and Tunisia		0.9	112 [147]
	Arab		4.4	264 [147]
	Ashkenazim		0.4	819 [147]
	Atlas Mountains		4.35	23 [147]
	Bukhara		0	46 [147]
	Caucasus		28.0	25 [147]
	Central Iran		10.80	370 [147]
	Circassian		0	57 [147]
	Druze		4.4	92 [147]
	Egypt		3.8	112 [147]
	Gerba		0	52 [147]
	Greece and Bulgaria		0.7	152 [147]
	India (Bnei Israel)		2.0	102 [147]
	India (Cochin)		10.3	58 [147]
	Iran		15.1	557 [147]
	Iraq		24.8	902 [147]
	Iraq (Baghdad)		24.48	286 [147]
	Iraq (Mosul, Erbil, Kirkuk)		52.00	34 [147]
	Karaite		0	18 [147]
	Kurdistan		58.2	196 [147]
	Kurdistan (Iraq–W. Iran)		35.09	59 [147]
	Kurdistan (N. Iraqi Border)		70.64	126 [147]
	Libya		0.9	219 [147]
	Morocco		0.5	219 [147]
	Other European Sephardim		2.2	93 [147]
	Samaritan		0	69 [147]
	Syria and Lebanon		6.3	80 [147]
	Turkey		1.9	256 [147]
	Western Iran		44.40	45 [147]
	Yemen and Aden		5.3	415 [147]
	Afghanistan	Fluorescent	17.9	39 [195]

(continued)

TABLE III (continued)

Geographical location	Population	Method	Incidence[a]	Sample size
Israel (continued)	Arab		0	49 [195]
	Ashkenazim		0.8	1208 [195]
	Balkan		5.7	226 [195]
	Egypt		11.3	80 [195]
	India		6.3	16 [195]
	Iraq		27.9	484 [195]
	N. Africa		0.7	571 [195]
	Persia		12.0	291 [195]
	Syria and Lebanon		6.4	233 [195]
	Turkey		4.8	291 [195]
	Unknown		0	62 [195]
	Yemen and Aden		7.4	297 [195]
	Ashkenazi parents	Fluorescent	1.80	944 [196]
	Israeli parents		2.68	635 [196]
	Non-Ashkenazi:			
	Arab	Fluorescent	1.45	758 [196]
	Bulgaria–Greece		2.04	98 [196]
	Circassian		0	2 [196]
	Druze		0	2 [196]
	Georgia (USSR)		7.50	80 [196]
	India–Pakistan		4.48	201 [196]
	Iran		13.48	89 [196]
	Iraq		25.30	332 [196]
	Kurdistan		50.0	4 [196]
	North Africa		1.62	1786 [196]
	Syria–Lebanon		0	23 [196]
	Turkey		4.27	234 [196]

Country	Location	Method	Value	n	Ref
Italy	Yemen	MRT	5.43	313	[196]
	Central Italy	?	0	1557	[197]
	Sardinia				
	0–300 m alt. (31 villages)		19.94	3224	[198]
	300–600 m alt. (15 villages)		18.43	2263	[198]
	600–1000 m alt. (6 villages)		5.38	836	[198]
	Nonselect	GSH-Stab	13.11	61	[199]
	Lecce Province	BCB	2.18	275	[200]
	Sardinia:				
	Benetutti	BCB	9.00	100	[201]
	Cabras		35.0	200	[201]
	Desulo		3.10	313	[201]
	Fonni		3.00	100	[201]
	Galtelli		12.00	175	[201]
	Gergei		18.5	92	[201]
	Isili		9.0	100	[201]
	Lanusei		4.00	100	[201]
	Lode		29.40	163	[201]
	Luras		7.00	100	[201]
	Orosei		14.00	180	[201]
	Siniscola		11.30	198	[201]
	S. Giusta		30.9	42	[201]
	Suni		14.30	98	[201]
	Terralba		30.0	100	[201]
	Teulada		16.9	101	[201]
	Tonara		4.00	148	[201]
	Tortoli		16.00	50	[201]
	Usini		6.10	99	[201]
Japan	Tokyo	DCIP/MTT	0	2107	[202]
Korea	South Korea	BCB	0.13	742	[203]
Lebanon	Beirut	?	2.58	155	[204]
	Bekaa		1.49	67	[204]

(continued)

TABLE III (continued)

Geographical location	Population	Method	Incidence[a]	Sample size
Lebanon *(continued)*	Mount Lebanon		2.86	210 [204]
	North Lebanon		0	29 [204]
	South Lebanon		6.82	88 [204]
	Armenian	BCB	0	36 [205]
	Chiites		4.95	101 [205]
	Druzes		0	105 [205]
	Greek Orthodox and Catholic		1.15	87 [205]
	Maronites		4.27	117 [205]
	Sunnites		6.19	97 [205]
Malaya	(see Malaysia)			
Malaysia	Aboriginal	BCB	17.00	607 [206]
	Brunei: Malay	BCB	6.31	317 [207]
	Malaya:			
	Chinese	BCB	2.42	207 [208]
	Indian		0.98	204 [208]
	Malay		2.02	346 [208]
	Subah:			
	Bajau	BCB	3.45	58 [207]
	Bisaya		16.67	6 [207]
	Kadazan		12.12	165 [207]
	Malay		4.11	73 [207]
	Murut		24.24	33 [207]
	Miscellaneous		0	63 [207]
	Sarawak:			
	Land Dayak	BCB	5.26	133 [209]
	Sea Dayak	BCB	5.00	100 [209]

Location	Method	%	N
Sarawak:			
Iban	BCB	5.36	56 [207]
Land Dayak		0	24 [207]
Malay		11.58	95 [207]
Sea Dayak		1.25	80 [207]
Miscellaneous		0	38 [207]
Singapore (W. Java):			
Chinese	BCB	2.50	240 [210]
Eurasian		3.70	27 [210]
European		0	80 [210]
Indian		3.03	132 [210]
Jewish		37.50	16 [210]
Malay		0.65	155 [210]
Singapore:			
Chinese	BCB	3.35	3312 [211]
Malay		2.02	1384 [211]
Malta	BCB	4.03	2062 [212]
Gozo		6.52	230 [212]
Urban, rural, and mixed populations	BCB	2.70	1145 [213]
Phillipines			
Unspecified (examined in Baltimore, U.S.A.)	?	13.33	15 [214]
Nonselect	BCB	6.63	407 [215]
Rumania			
Husi			
(Patients and normal subjects)	MRT	0.67	890 [216]
Sabah			
(see Malaysia)			
Sarawak			
(see Malaysia)			
Saudi Arabia			
Eastern Province			
Al-Hasa Oasis			
Mansura	BCB	53.26	92 [217]
Qarah		24.04	104 [217]
Unspecified		4.69	64 [217]

(continued)

TABLE III (continued)

Geographical location	Population	Method	Incidence[a]	Sample size
Saudi Arabia (continued)	Eastern Province			
	Quatif Oasis			
	Al Ajam	BCB	65.38	104 [217]
	Safwah		64.71	51 [217]
	Unspecified		34.23	111 [217]
	Other	BCB	2.94	34 [217]
	Western provinces	BCB	4.12	97 [217]
Singapore	(see Malaysia)			
Spain	North (Biscay)	MRT	1.11	180 [218]
	North (Corunna)		0.33	304 [218]
	South (Huelva)		0.74	269 [21]
	South (Murcia)		0.49	205 [218]
	Central (Madrid)		0.75	266 [218]
	West (Badajos)		0.51	195 [218]
	West (Caceres)		1.54	130 [218]
	Balearic Islands (Mallorca)	BCB	1.24	242 [219]
	Balearic Islands (Menorca)		0.47	212 [219]
	Central and North		0	170[219]
	East coast (Ebro Delta)		0	96 [219]
	East coast (Murcia)		0	221 [218]
	East coast (Valencia)		0.20	504 [218]
	South (Cadiz)		0	309 [218]
	South (Malaga)		0	424 [218]
	West (Caceras)		0	342 [218]

Country	Location/Group	Method	%	n
Sri Lanka (Ceylon)	Colonies:			
	Kandalama	BCB/MRT	3.74	107 [220]
	Tijeapura		3.48	115 [220]
	Schools:			
	Sinhalese	BCB/MRT	5.23	153 [220]
	Moor (Moslem)		5.00	120 [220]
	Tamil		0	160 [220]
	Sinhalese:			
	Hirigollegama	BCB/MRT	7.08	113 [220]
	Nonselect		5.30	132 [220]
	Tihara Bulankulama		20.86	139 [220]
Taiwan	Taipeh, Chi-Chi, and Chung-Li	BCB	3.00	300 [221]
	Hakka Chinese	BCB	5.47	1535 [222]
	Mainland Chinese		1.77	282 [222]
	Taiwanese Chinese		0.29	343 [222]
Thailand	Nonselect	BCB/MRT	11.45	131 [223]
	Nakorn	BCB	14.80	266 [224]
	Rayong	BCB	13.20	253 [224]
	N. Thailand	Electrophoresis	12.86 def. 87.14 B+	482 [225]
	N.E. Thailand	Electrophoresis	14.33 def. 85.67 B+	649 [225]
	Central Thailand	Electrophoresis	13.57 def. 86.43 B+	199 [225]
	S. Thailand	Electrophoresis	2.83 def. 97.17 B+	247 [225]
Turkey	N.E. Thailand	BCB/spot test	12.62	832 [226]
	Adana and Tarsus (Eti-Turkish)	Spot test	11.43	105 [227]
	Armenian		0	44 [227]
	Black Sea Coast (Rize)		0	109 [227]
	Diyurbakir: Kurdish-speaking		1.92	208 [227]
	Greek (Istanbul)		0	37 [227]
	Izmir (Western seacoast)		0.94	212 [227]

(continued)

TABLE III (continued)

Geographical location	Population	Method	Incidence [a]	Sample size
Turkey (continued)	Jewish		0	29 [227]
	Random		0.50	1000 [227]
	Turkish Cyprus		3.50	200 [227]
USSR	Arkhangelsk Region	?	2.14	279 [228]
Vietnam	S. Vietnam			
	Montagnards (Ra tribe)	BCB	1.64	122 [229]
	Vietnamese (Da Nang)	BCB	1.62	495 [229]
	South Vietnam	DCIP	4.14	362 [133]
	North	BCB	5.80	138 [230]
	Central	BCB	1.89	53 [230]
	South	BCB	1.37	510 [230]
Yugoslavia	Dalmatian Coast	BCB	0.78	387 [231]
	Gypsies of Skopje (Macedonia)	BCB	5.88	34 [231]
	Macedonia	BCB	0	72 [231]
Oceania				
Australia	Gazelle Peninsula: New Britain:	BCB		
	Baining		12.00	108 [232]
	Sulka		15.00	102 [232]
	Tolai		0.80	122 [232]
	Linguistic groups: Eastern Highlands:	BCB		
	Auyana		5.00	40 [232]
	Fore		0	39 [232]
	Gadsup		0	39 [232]
	Kukukuku		0	116 [232]
	Tiarora		1.10	88 [232]

		Method	%	n
Sepik River District:				
	New Guinea:			
	Abelam	BCB	8.00	49 [232]
	Sause		0.90	324 [232]
Australian	Aborigines (all Australia)	BCB	0	435 [233]
Micronesia	Angaur	BCB	8.62	58 [234]
	Ifalik		5.88	34 [234]
	Koror		8.33	24 [234]
	Ulithi		0	117 [234]
New Guinea	Costal Papua:	Assay		
	Kerema District		10.30	97 [235]
	Rigo District		9.47	95 [235]
	Netherlands			
	Mulia (Dani speaking)	BCB	0	25 [236]
	Papuan	Assay	7.63	799 [237]
	Eastern Highlands	BCB	0.78	383 [238]
	Gazelle Peninsula	BCB	17.62	94 [238]
	(see Australia)			
New Zealand	Maori	DCIP	0.19	540 [239]
Polynesia	Cook Island	DCIP	0	110 [239]
	Nive Island		0	34 [239]
	Samoa		0	86 [239]
	Tokelau Island		0	10 [239]
	Tonga		0	7 [239]

possibly at polymorphic levels.[240-243] In the Orient G-6-PD Canton and Hong Kong-Pokfulam appear to be particularly common, although many other variants have also been detected.

Because of its tropical distribution and because it affects primarily red blood cells, the suggestion has been made that G-6-PD deficiency may have reached high gene frequencies among some populations by conferring some degree of immunity to falciparum malaria.[144,244-246] Results of population studies, however, were inconclusive and sometimes contradictory.[247-249] The first convincing evidence of the effect of G-6-PD deficiency on malarial infection was provided by Luzzatto et al.[250] in an ingenious study of falciparum malaria-infected women heterozygous for G-6-PD A−. After treating their subjects' blood with sodium nitrite and reducing methemoglobin in the presence of Nile blue sulfate, these investigators identified G-6-PD-deficient cells histochemically using the methemoglobin elution technique. They observed many more parasites in G-6-PD-normal than in G-6-PD-deficient erythrocytes (Fig. 5). This suggested that either the G-6-PD-deficient environment was an inhospitable one for the malaria parasite or, alternatively, that deficient cells that had been parasitized by malaria were rapidly sequestered by the spleen, depriving the malaria parasite of the opportunity to multiply and to infect other erythrocytes.

Fewer surveys of the frequency of electrophoretic phenotypes of G-6-PD have been carried out than those in which enzyme deficiency has been detected. The major electrophoretic mutant is G-6-PD A. It occurs among black Americans with a frequency of approximately 16%.[57]

2.3.   Glucose-6-phosphate Dehydrogenase

2.3.1.   Purification

With recognition of the clinical importance of G-6-PD, effects were soon undertaken to purify the enzyme to homogeneity. Early attempts resulted in 80-fold,[60] 500-fold,[251] and 8300-fold[252] purification. Kirkman achieved 10,000-fold purification from large volumes of outdated bank blood. The resulting preparation had an activity of 64 U/mg protein, indicating that it was approximately one-third pure.[253] Soon afterward, Chung and Langdon[254] were able to purify the enzyme to a specific activity of 113 U/mg protein, and believing that the enzyme was nearly homogeneous, carried out terminal amino acid analyses. They found two different amino terminals, tyrosine and alanine, and concluded that the enzyme was made of dissimilar subunits. However, Chung and Langdon's preparation was apparently not homogeneous. Actual purification of the enzyme to homogeneity was accomplished by Yoshida.[255] Specific activity of the crystalline enzyme preparation was approximately 180 U/mg, and even higher levels were measured when the enzyme was activated by extreme concentration.

Yoshida's original method required 12 purification steps and provided a yield of nearly 50%. Subsequently, a variety of simplified methods for obtaining essentially pure G-6-PD were reported. Rattazzi achieved purification with an overall yield of about 60% using only three steps: DEAE-Sephadex chromatography, recycling gel filtration on Sephadex G-100, and CM-Sephadex chromatography with specific elution with substrate glucose-6-phosphate.[256] Specific elution with the substrate[257] NADP⁺ or the substrate analog[258] 6-phosphogluconate has also been used to good advantage. Affinity chromatography has been carried out on NADP-Sepharose[259,260] and with an N-(aminohexyl)adenosine-2′,5′-biphosphate column.[261]

2.3.2. Subunit Structure

Even before it was possible to purify G-6-PD to homogeneity, the importance of NADP⁺ in its stability and structure had become apparent. Marks et al.[251] had shown that NADP⁺ stabilized the enzyme against inactivation by heating or by dilution. Fluorescence spectra of highly purified enzyme indicated that tightly bound NADP⁺ was present,[251,253,262] and that its removal resulted in loss of activity and dissociation of the enzyme into monomeric subunits.[263] Although enzyme dissociated with urea–guanidine hydrochloride was first reported to have a subunit with a molecular weight of 43,000 daltons,[255] most subsequent estimates of subunit size were somewhat larger. Measurements carried out using a variety of methods showed subunit molecular weight values of 52,500,[263] 53,000,[264] and 55,000–60,000.[265] It is quite generally agreed that the molecular weight of the active dimer, containing one molecule of bound NADP⁺, is about 110,000 daltons; reported values based on various methods are 105,000,[263] 104,000,[266] 123,000,[255] and 110,000.[265] Measurements carried out on crude hemolysates[266] indicate that in vivo the enzyme probably exists primarily as a dimer with a molecular weight of about 105,000. However, formation of a tetramer or even larger aggregates appears to occur at low salt concentration at pH 6 to 7.[264,267,268] It has been suggested that the dissociation of the active dimer with bound NADP⁺ is promoted by the presence of NADPH.[267] The appearance of monomers and their association into dimers and tetramers has also been studied with the use of the electron microscope. These investigations indicated that the monomer has an axial ratio of about 2.0 with dimensions of 68 × 34 Å.[269]

The question of whether the subunits of G-6-PD were identical or were the products of two separate gene loci was approached originally through hybridization of rat and human,[270,271] rat and bovine,[272] or different human variants[273] of G-6-PD. Several alternative interpretations of the results were possible, and they were believed to be compatible with a heteropolymeric structure of G-6-PD.[272] However, the question was resolved by study of the electrophoretic mobility of subunits from G-6-PD A and G-6-PD B. In both cases the isolated subunits moved as a single band, indicating that only one type of polypeptide chain was involved.[265] This conclusion was supported by the existence of a single amino terminal and a single carboxy terminal for the enzyme.[265] Further evidence for the subunit structure of G-6-PD was obtained by the study of human oocytes which had the Gd^A/Gd^B phenotype. Since at this stage inactivation has not yet occurred, both alleles were active in each cell. Consequently, a single hybrid band was found midway between the bands for G-6-PD A and G-6-PD B.[80]

2.3.3. Kinetic Properties

The K_m of G-6-PD for $NADP^+$ is very low and therefore difficult to determine. Using sensitive spectrofluorometric techniques K_m values of approximately 2×10^{-6} M[253] and $1.3-2.6 \times 10^{-6}$ M[252] were obtained. Less sensitive spectrophotometric methods yielded somewhat higher K_m values, e.g., 4.2×10^{-6} M,[251] and it was suggested that the enzyme has sigmoid kinetics with respect to NADP.[274,275] These results, however, are not clearly established, since they are not found using spectrofluorometric techniques,[253,276] at least when $NADP^+$-stabilized enzyme is examined.

The K_m of the enzyme for glucose-6-phosphate is higher, and is therefore easier to determine. Values of 39×10^{-6} M,[277] 63×10^{-6} M,[252] 21×10^{-6} M,[60] and 35×10^{-6} M,[251] have been reported under various conditions. The enzyme is specific for the β-anomer of glucose-6-phosphate, and does not appear to utilize the α-anomer.[278] G-6-PD is also able to use certain substrate analogs, albeit at a rate considerably lower than that expressed toward the natural substrates, $NADP^+$ and glucose-6-phosphate. NAD^+,[253] galactose-6-phosphate,[253] 2-deoxyglucose-6-phosphate,[279] deamino NADP $^+$,[279] and glucose[278,280] are all utilized by the enzyme. Utilization of glucose is markedly stimulated by the presence of bicarbonate.[280] The enzyme is strongly inhibited by NADPH[253,267,274,275 281,282] and by ATP.[283–286]

When examined in a tris–phosphate–glycine buffer system using fixed substrate concentrations the pH–activity curve may be described as truncate. The activity rises rapidly until a pH of 7.5 is reached. It then increases very slowly until the pH of the mixture is 9.0 to 9.5, when the activity again steeply declines.[60] When the V_{max} of the enzyme is estimated at different pH levels in tris or borate buffers, a continual increase in activity is observed.[287] Under somewhat different conditions, the V_{max} in tris–borate buffer shows a rise in the range between pH 6 and 7–8 with no further change after this level.[268]

The K_i of the normal enzyme for NADPH is 9 μM in 0.05 M tris pH 7.3 at a concentration of 60 μM glucose-6-phosphate at 25° C.[286] Inhibition by ATP is competitive with glucose-6-phosphate and has been reported to have a K_i of 1 mM at pH 7.3 in the presence of 80 μM NADP.[286] Dehydro-isoandrosterone, pregnenolone, and certain related steroids at concentrations of 1 μM or less inhibit G-6-PD.[288,289] The effect of a series of synthetic steroids and steroid conjugates has been investigated, and it was concluded that the inhibitory activity depends on a negative charge of the oxygen and C-3 of the steroid moiety as well as on the presence of an oxo group at C-17 or C-20.[290]

2.3.4. Biochemical Properties of Variants

Within a few years of the discovery of G-6-PD deficiency, it became evident that the severity of the defect was much greater in Mediterranean populations than in Afro-Americans.[56] The development of electrophoretic systems made possible determination that the electrophoretic mobility of the residual enzyme of Mediterranean men with G-6-PD deficiency was normal, but that in Negro men it was faster than normal. The kinetic properties of the enzyme appeared to be normal in Negro subjects, whereas those in Mediterranean subjects proved to be grossly abnormal.[291] Initially, the Negro type of enzyme deficiency was designated as the A− type, while that observed in Mediterranean subjects was designated as the B− type. The letters denoted the relative mobility of the enzyme, and the minus signs indicated that the variant was a deficient one. However, when it became apparent that many G-6-PD variants with properties quite distinct from those of Mediterranean subjects also had normal electrophoretic mobility, the designation B− was abandoned by international agreement,[61] and the enzyme was renamed G-6-PD Mediterranean. In addition to mutant enzymes producing G-6-PD deficiency, electrophoretic variation of the enzyme also occurs. The most common of such variants is G-6-PD A, occurring with a gene frequency of approximately 0.16 in the American black population.[57] Although the average enzyme activity of males with G-6-PD A is only approximately 84% of those with G-6-PD B,[292] this difference is of no clinical significance, and no stigmata of G-6-PD deficiency are encountered. The apparent properties of G-6-PD obviously depend on the method of purification employed and the conditions under which the properties of the enzyme are tested. Until standardization of methodology was achieved, it was impossible to determine whether an enzyme purified in one laboratory was the same as that which had been examined elsewhere. Side-by-side comparison is rendered very difficult because of the instability of many G-6-PD variants. In 1967 international agreement was reached regarding methods of standardization, and since that time, over 150 variants have been described. The characteristics of those variants which are presumed to be distinct are summarized in Table IV. Since laboratory reagents differ from batch to batch, even when obtained from the same supplier,[396] and because minor differences may exist in methodology, it is not a certainty that each of these variants is actually structurally unique. Furthermore, because of the limited number of enzyme characterisitcs which have been standardized, variants which seem to be identical using standard techniques may be different when examined in another manner. For example, although G-6-PD B, A, and A− have the same pH–activity curves measured in triple buffer, certain pH-dependent differences between these enzymes have been observed using advanced kinetic techniques.[268] Many variants have been described which are not included in Table IV either because they seem to be identical to one previously described, or because characterization was carried out using nonstandard methodology. Unfortunately, some laboratories rely on Cellogel electrophoresis.[399] Although simple and in many ways satisfactory, this is not a standard technique for G-6-PD characterization, and the results cannot be compared with those obtained with starch gel electrophoresis in tris–EDTA–borate and tris–HCl systems. In addition to the standard methods used for G-6-PD characterization, many other procedures for the study of G-6-PD variants have been described. Electrophoretic techniques abound, and include the use of Cellogel,[399] cellulose acetate strips,[400–402] agar gel,[401,403,404] and polyacrylamide gel.[405] Column techniques[406,407] and thin-layer chromatographic methods[408] have also been described.

Variants of G-6-PD are divided into five classes. *Class 1* includes those which are regularly associated with nonspherocytic hemolytic anemia. In *class 2* variants the residual enzyme activity is less than 10% of normal, but this severe enzyme deficiency is not associated with chronic hemolytic disease, except in unusual instances. *Class 3* G-6-PD variants are those which produce moderate to mild enzyme deficiency, with residual G-6-PD activity between 10 and 60% of normal. As in class 2 variants, hemolysis is not ordinarily present. *Class 4* variants are mutations in which the enzyme activity is within the normal range. *Class 5* variants are those in which enzyme activity is increased.

It is of special interest that the residual G-6-PD activity of class 1 variants is often higher than that of class 2 variants. Yet class 1 variants are characterized by chronic hemolysis, whereas class 2 variants are not. The functional impairment of G-6-PD activity in class 1 variants is in

TABLE IV

Glucose-6-phosphate Dehydrogenase Variants

Variant	Population origin	Electrophoretic mobility (% of normal)	Activity (% of normal)	K_m G-6-P (μM)	K_m NADP (μM)	2-Deoxy-G-6-P (% of G-6-P)	Deamino-NADP (% of NADP)	Heat stability	pH optimum	K_i NADPH (μM)
Deficiency associated with nonspherocytic hemolytic anemia:										
Electrophoretically fast:										
St. Louis (Paris) [293]	France	125 (tris) 130 (PO4)	0	130	—	8-20	50	Very labile	Normal	—
Baudelacque [294]	France	113 (TEB)	15	38	—	5	43	Very labile	Normal	—
Ohio [295]	Italy	110 (tris-glycine)	2-16	Slightly increased	Slightly increased	<4	—	Very labile	—	—
Charleston [296]	African	103 (tris) 104-107 (TEB) 107 (PO4)	14	30-40	5.5-13	5.2-7.0	81-86	Very labile	—	—
Lincoln Park [297]	Puerto Rican	112 (tris) 106 (TEB) 104 (PO4)	6.5	33	8.1	7.3	13.4	Labile	Monophasic with peak at 8.5	21.75
Grand Prairie [298]	U.S.—white	100 (tris) 105 (TEB) 88 (PO4)	17	48	3.9	3.4	72.1	Very labile	Normal	—
Lawndale [299]	African	104 (tris)	0	188	17.5	—	—	Very labile	Normal	—
East Harlem [300]	African	102 (tris) 104 (TEB) 102 (PO4)	10	107	8.2	2.1	34.5	Labile	—	—
Torrance [301,282]	U.S.	103 (PO4)	2.4	48-60	2.4	—	—	Very labile	8.0-8.5	3.0
Seian [302]	Japanese	103 (TEB) 116 (PO4)	8-9	130 ± 20	5.5 ± 1.5	18	76	—	Slightly biphasic 7.0 and 8.8	—
San Diego [303]	African	103 (tris)	20-40	45	—	2.2	—	Normal	Normal	—
Jackson [304]	U.S.—white	100 (tris) 102 (TEB) 104 (PO4)	20	33	6.1	2.8	66.7	Normal	Normal	—
Chinese [305]	Chinese	101 (TEB) 100 (PO4)	0-14	29-88	—	2.7-5.0	50-70	Normal	Normal	—

(continued)

TABLE IV (continued)

Variant	Population origin	Electrophoretic mobility (% of normal)	Activity (% of normal)	K_m G-6-P (μM)	K_m NADP+ (μM)	2-Deoxy-G-6-P (% of G-6-P)	Deamino-NADP (% of NADP)	Heat stability	pH optimum	K_i NADPH (μM)
Electrophoretically normal:										
Bat-Yam [308]	Iraq—Jewish	100 (TEB)	0	27	—	40-45	—	Very labile	Biphasic 6.5 and 10.5	—
Albuquerque [307]	U.S.—white	100 (tris, TEB, PO4)	1	115	11	0	—	Very labile	Sharp peak at 8.5	—
Bangkok [308]	Thailand	100 (tris, TEB, PO4)	5	60	5.3	8.4	—	Very labile	8-8.5	—
Oklahoma [309,310]	W. Europe	100 (tris)	4-10	127-200	20	<4	—	Labile	Narrow peak at 8.2	—
Duarte [307]	U.S.—white	100 (tris, TEB, PO4)	8.5	58	5	5.4	—	Very labile	7.0	—
Hong Kong [311]	Chinese	100 (TEB, PO4)	0-15	Half of normal	Normal	Slightly increased	—	Normal	Normal	—
Chicago [312]	W. Europe	100 (tris)	9-26	58-76	3.1-3.7	<4	—	Very labile	Normal	—
Boston [313]	Polish-Jewish	100 (TEB)	5	18-21	1.7-2.2	12	200	Labile	Sharp	—
Englewood [314]	N. Italy	100 (tris)	0.5	56	0.5	29.6	—	Labile	Biphasic 6.5 and 10.0	—
New York [314]	Black-Italian	100 (tris)	0.6	51	3	15.7	—	Labile	Abnormal 7.5	—
Hawaii [278]	U.S.—white	100 (tris, TEB)	23	39	9.7	2.9	37.9	Very labile	Biphasic 7.0 and 8.5	28.6
Cornell [315]	U.S.—white (Dutch, Irish, German, Indian)	100 (TEB, PO4)	5	55	11.8	3.2	51	Very labile	7.0	—
Tokushima [316]	Japanese	100 (TEB, PO4)	3	50	27	2.0	52	Very labile	Normal	6.0
Hayem [305]	France	100 (tris)	0	32	—	51-65	100-120	Unstable	Normal	26.0
Missoula [317,318]	U.S.—white	100 (PO4)	5	37	4.3	0	36.5	Very labile	Abnormal peak at 6.0	55.0

Variant	Origin									
au [310]	Swiss	100 (TEB, PO₄)	7	37.9	6.5	7.1	80.1	Very labile	Biphasic 7.0 and 8.5	—
iinki [320,321]	Finland	Normal	10–20	38.7±8	(N = 8) 3.73 1.7	Normal	Normal	Normal	Normal	—
jga [322]	Russian	100 (TEB)	20	40	1.7	—	—	Normal	Biphasic 7.5 and 9.5	—

lectrophoretically slow:

Variant	Origin									
g Prairie [323]	U.S.—white	98–99.5 (tris), 98–99 (TEB), 99 (PO₄)	2.3–7.7	24–29	3.1–4.7	8.3–9.2	107–111	Very labile	Monophasic, optimum at 9.0–9.5	—
ima [324]	Sephardic Jewish	99 (tris), 98 (TEB), 95 (PO₄)	6	9–59	2.5	30	266	Labile	Biphasic 6.5 and 10.0	23.5
igton Heights [297]	U.S.—white	99 (tris), 100 (TEB), 88 (PO₄)	8	179	5.1	1.3	15.2	Very labile	Peaked at 8.5	—
ler [764,382]	U.S.—white	97 (tris), 97 (TEB), 90 (PO₄)	35	30	—	3.7	62.4	Very labile	Slightly biphasic	2.6
mbra [325,282]	Finland–Sweden	95 (tris), 96 (TEB), 85 (PO₄)	9–20	55	2.6	2	—	Labile	Abnormal	3.3
nta [326]	U.S.—black	87 (tris), 93 (TEB), 83 (PO₄)	25	63	4.5	3.2	44.5	Very labile	Normal	(N = 7.6–30.9) 5.5
g Kong–akfulam [305,327]	Chinese	92 (TEB)	0–3	59–69	—	2.2–3.6	72	Normal	Normal	—
Jod [306]	N. Africa—Jewish	90–92 (TEB)	10	100	—	40	—	Labile	Biphasic 6.5 and 10.0	—
aukee [328]	Puerto Rico—white	92 (tris)	0.5	224	—	3.7	—	—	8.0	—
iat Gan [306]	Iraq—Jewish	90–92 (TEB)	0	35	—	40	—	Very	Biphasic 6.5 and 10.0	—
chester [329,282]	England	90 (TEB)	20–25	64	6	3.5	79	Labile	Slightly biphasic	—
yo [316]	Japanese	90 (tris), 90 (TEB), 70 (PO₄)	4.4	65	5.5	2.5	55.2	Very labile	Normal	(N = 1.3–12.1) 6.2
cester [330]	U.S.—white	86 (TEB)	0	11.2	61	<2	21	Very labile	Sharp peak at 8.0	—

(continued)

TABLE IV (continued)

riant	Population origin	Electrophoretic mobility (% of normal)	Activity (% of normal)	K_m G-6-P (μM)	K_m NADP+ (μM)	2-Deoxy-G-6-P (% of G-6-P)	Deamino-NADP (% of NADP)	Heat stability	pH optimum	K_i NADPH (μM)
iburg [331,332]	Germany	85 (TEB) 90 (PO4)	10-20	87-118	4	—	—	—	Biphasic 7.0 and 9.0	—
tterdam [314]	Dutch	95	1.9	23	3.3	6	—	Normal	Biphasic 7.0 and 9.5	—
iannesburg [333]	S. Africa— W. Europe	Slow	17	80	1.7	<4	51	Labile	Normal	—

Severe enzyme deficiency usually without nonspherocytic hemolytic anemia
Electrophoretically fast:

alien-Chi [334]	Taiwan	110 (tris) 120 (PO4)	1	10.1	—	42	—	Normal	Biphasic 6.3 and 10.0	—
1 Jose [335]	Costa Rica	112 (TEB) (pH 8.7)	0	Normal	Normal	10	52-55	Normal	Normal	Increased
1 Juan [336]	Puerto Rico	110 (tris) 105 (PO4)	10	16.2 ± 0.7	—	21.6	—	Very labile	Biphasic 7.0 and 9.5	—
kara [337,338]	Turkey	109 (tris)	8.0	52	15	<4	(. N 40-60) 69	Labile	Slightly biphasic 7.5 and 9.0	(N = 23 ± 3) 42.0
blin [339]	Polish	105-110 (tris pH 8.4)	0.4	26	16-22	2.3	—	Normal	—	—
ion [340,282]	Philippines	107 (tris, PO4)	<3	8-12	3.6-5.2	180	400	Labile	Biphasic 5.5-9.0	37
rkham [341,282]	New Guinea	105-108 (tris)	1.5-10.0	4.4-6.3	—	162-222	—	Labile	Biphasic 6.0 and 9.5-10.0	16.0
wan-Hakka [342]	Hakka Chinese	105 (tris) 110 (PO4)	2-9	10.7-12.2	—	9.8-21.1	—	Normal	Biphasic 7.0 and 9.5-10.0	—
alien [334]	Taiwan	105 (tris)	0	8.7	—	72.2	—	Very labile	Biphasic 6.5 and 9.75	—
rara [343]	N. Italy	106 (tris) 105 (TEB) 117 (PO4)	5	28-29	2.8-3.9	12-23	65-85	Very labile	Normal	—
leran [334]	Iran	100 (tris) 110 (PO4)	<1	46.8	—	<4	—	Normal	Biphasic 5.5 and 10.0	—

Electrophoretically normal:

donesia [344]	Indonesia	100 (tris)	<5	25–52	4–9	—	—	Slightly labile to normal	Slightly biphasic	—
mpbellpore [345]	Pakistan	100 (tris) 100 (PO₄)	2–7	11.4–13.9	—	5.6–16.4	—	Very labile	Biphasic 7.5 and 9.5	—
editerranean [346,347,382]	Greece Sardinia Sephardic Jews	100 (tris. TEB, PO₄)	0–7	19–26	1.2–1.6	23–27	350	Labile	Biphasic 6.5 and 9.5	16.0
rinth [348]	Greece Mediterranean S.E. Asia	100 (TEB, tris. PO₄)	0–7	19–26	1.2–1.6	23–27	55–60	Labile	Biphasic 6.5 and 9.5	—
Fayoum [340]	Egypt	100 (TEB, PO₄)	6	41.4 ± 1.3	—	26.3	229	Labile	Biphasic 7.0 and 9.0	—
thidol [349]	Thailand	100 (tris, PO₄)	3.5–31.0	27–53	—	0.8–4.6	43–76	Normal	Truncate	—
gdad [350,351]	Iraq—Jewish	100 (tris, PO₄)	0–5	70–77	20–25	45	—	—	Biphasic 6.5 and 9.0–9.5	—
Morro [336]	African	100 (tris, TEB)	10	35.6	—	11.0	90	Labile	Biphasic 7.0 and 9.5	—
atam [352]	African	100 (TEB)	<1	16–18	2.6	23	170	Labile	Biphasic with sharp peak at 9.5	80–100
rami [353]	France	100 (tris)	4	20	6	4.6	230	Labile	Biphasic 6.0 and 9.0	—
rovograd [354]	Russian	100 (tris, TEB) 98 (PO₄)	0	6.5	3.1	—	—	Labile	Sharp peak at 8.5	—
mm [355]	Germany	100 (TEB, PO₄)	1.4	38.2	4.8	46.4	230	Very labile	Abnormal flat below 7.5, peak at 8.5	—
rsus [355]	Turkey	100 (TEB, PO₄)	5.2	27.9	11	33.2	261	Labile	Abnormal flat below 7.5, peak at 9.5	—
iraj [356]	Thailand	100 (tris, PO₄)	6–15	18–28	—	13–16	124–177	Labile	Biphasic 6.5–7.5 and 9.0–10.0	—
ori [357]	Japanese	100 (tris, TEB. PO₄)	3.5	40	5.0	3.4	67.7	Normal	Normal	—

(continued)

TABLE IV (continued)

ariant	Population origin	Electrophoretic mobility (% of normal)	Activity (% of normal)	K_m G-6-P (μM)	K_m NADP$^+$ (μM)	2-Deoxy-G-6-P (% of G-6-P)	Deamino-NADP (% of NADP)	Heat stability	pH optimum	K_iNADPH (μM)
Electrophoretically slow:										
rchomenos [358]	Greece	100 (tris, TEB) 92–94 (PO₄)	0–7	11	2.1	105	350	—	Biphasic 6.0 and 9.5	—
ammu [359]	Kashmir Indian	99 (tris, TEB) 101 (PO₄)	5	53	9	3.8	57	Normal	Normal	—
titanon [360]	Thailand	98 (TEB)	10.4	70	2.1	0	40.7	Normal	Slightly biphasic	—
oulouse [361]	France–Italy	100 (tris) 97 (TEB) 96 (PO₄)	3	55	1.2–3	13	220	Very labile	Slightly biphasic	—
anay [362]	Philippines	96 (tris, PO₄)	5	30	4.7	Normal	—	Slightly labile	Biphasic	—
hitomir [364]	Russian	90–98 (TEB) 78–84 (PO₄)	0	5.4–8.3	1.4–3.1	53	350	Labile	Biphasic 6.5 and 9.0	—
noda [363]	Japanese	93 (tris) 95 (TEB) 94 (PO₄)	3.5	20	3.0	12.6	180	Labile	Biphasic 7.0–7.5 and 9.0–9.5	12.7
oznan [364]	Polish	94 (tris)	0	13–30	0.5–1.1	17–44	—	Labile	Biphasic 6.5 and 10.0	—
achen [365]	Germany	92–94 (tris)	3	60–70	20–25	<4	40–60	Very labile	Normal	7.0
ifta [306]	Iraq-Jewish	87–90 (TEB)	0	25	—	60	—	Very labile	No clear pH optimum	—
arswell [366]	Ireland	92 (tris) 48 (TEB) 78 (PO₄)	10	44	6.4	3.5	—	Normal	Normal	—
Moderate to mild enzyme deficiency										
Electrophoretically fast:										
arbieri [367]	Italy	135 (tris, pH 7.6)	24–40	Increased	Increased	—	—	Normal	Normal	—
uerto Rico [336]	Puerto Rico	112 (tris)	38	18.6	—	2.7	—	Labile	Normal	—
— [368,369,370,58,382]	Black	110 (tris, TEB) 115 (PO₄)	8–20	50–70	2.9–4.4	<4	50–60	Normal	Normal	13.0

rousse [371,372]	Arab	110 (tris)	20	19–29	1.9–3.3	4–11	—	Normal	Normal	—
tere [373]	French	107 (tris) 108 (TEB) 112 (PO₄)	50–60	48	5.3	4	45	Labile	Slightly biphasic 7–9	—
onto [374]	N. European	105 (TEB) 107–109 (tris)	10–20	40	5.5	8	63	Labile	Normal	(N = 17–31) 37–57
e [375]	Japanese	107–108 (TEB) 112–115 (PO₄)	33–45	50–55	5–6	2.5–3.0	53–57	Normal	Normal	
buto [376]	Negro Bantu	108 (TEB) 109 (PO₄)	20	30	8.2	<4	—	Labile	Normal	—
tilla [357]	Spanish	108 (TEB) 110 (PO₄)	20	50	4.5	4–5	68–74	Labile	Normal	Strongly inhibited by NADPH
lissa [377]	Greece	105 (tris) 107 (TEB) 105 (PO₄)	25	18.1–22.0	3.1–3.7	3.7	59–65	—	Truncate	—
pei-Hakka [342]	China	105 (tris) 110 (PO₄)	6–9	28–43	3.3–5.4	—	—	Labile	Normal	—
ton [378]	S. China	105 (tris, PO₄)	4–24	18–38	—	4–15	—	Labile	Biphasic 6.5–7.0 and 9.0–9.5	—
byle [379]	Algeria	104 (TEB) 110 (PO₄)	14–36	68	—	Normal	—	Normal	Normal	—
tta [240]	Egypt	103 (tris, PO₄)	27	39.1	—	5.9	77.6	Labile	Biphasic 7.0, 8.5–9.0	—
letri [380]	Italian	100–105 (tris, PO₄)	21	140	4.4	33	330	Very labile	Biphasic 6.0 and 9.0	(N = 40–60) 30
n [381]	Thai	102 (TEB)	10.4	—	—	35.8	137–160	Very labile	—	—
lura [372]	Italy	100 (TEB) 103 (PO₄)	15	40	4.5	<2	90	Moderately labile	Normal	72
Electrophoretically normal:										
lumbus [295]	Negro	100 (tris)	36	Normal	Normal	Normal	—	Normal	—	—
fu [382]	Japanese	100 (tris, TEB)	12	25	5.0	5.2	105	Normal	Normal	(N = 1.3–12.1) 13.0
Kharga [240]	Egypt	100 (TEB, PO₄)	11	60.5 ± 3.8	—	6.1	50.7	Labile	8.5–9.0	—
ant [381]	Thai	100 (TEB)	18	41.7	—	18.6–19.2	80.8–107.8	Normal	Normal	—

(continued)

TABLE IV (continued)

riant	Population origin	Electrophoretic mobility (% of normal)	Activity (% of normal)	K_m G-6-P (μM)	K_m NADP+ (μM)	2-Deoxy-G-6-P (% of G-6-P)	Deamino-NADP (% of NADP)	Heat stability	pH optimum	K_i NADPH (μM)
Electrophoretically slow:										
hens [241]	Greece	98 (TEB)	20–25	16–19	2.5–6.5	10–15	125	Labile	Slightly biphasic	—
va [240]	Egyptian	98 (TEB, PO₄)	12	15–18	—	26	200	Labile	5.5 and 9.0–9.5	—
s Angeles [383]	U.S.—white	94.6 (tris) 97.5 (TEB) 85.7 (PO₄)	34	16.66	11.05	6.05	11	Normal	Biphasic (5.5 and 10.0)	(N = 19.2 ± 5.8) 9.3
ashington [334]	Negro	95 (tris)	16–33	49–57.4	—	1.6	—	Normal	Normal	—
nevento [336]	Italy	93 (tris)	13	4.6	—	245	—	Labile	Biphasic 5.5 and 9.75	—
inacria [384]	Sicilian	93 (TEB) 90 (PO₄)	20–25	20–26	2.5	6–7	125–145	Labile	Biphasic 7.0 and 9.0	—
exandra [348]	Italian	90–93 (TEB) 88–90 (PO₄)	75	26	3	3.5	50	Normal	Normal	—
mperdown [348]	Maltese	90–93 (TEB) 88–90 (PO₄)	15	17.5	2.6	18	150	Normal	Slightly biphasic	—
st Bengal [387]	Asiatic Indian	82 (tris) 90 (TEB)	9	31	6.6	4.0	—	Normal	Normal	—
ianyama [333]	Africa	95 (tris)	73	(N = 29+0.9) 19.9	2.8	8	62	—	Normal	—
xico [833]	Mexico	91 (tris) 85–88 (TEB) 90 (PO₄)	10–22	32–40	2–3	130–160	—	—	Normal	—
rt Royal [385]	Sicily	85 (TEB)	50–75	20	—	7.5	10	Labile	—	—
attle [386]	Welsh–Scotch	90 (tris) 80 (TEB)	8–21	15–25	2.4–2.8	7–11	—	Normal	Slightly biphasic	—
rala [387]	Asiatic S.E. India	75 (TEB) 90 (tris)	50	23	1.5	7.4	—	Normal	Biphasic 6.5 and 9.5	—
rbandar [388]	Indian	74 (tris) 68 (TEB) 89 (PO₄)	78	4.9	1.0	12–19	110	Normal	Normal	—
Very mild or no enzyme deficiency *Electrophoretically fast:*										
ambane [376]	Bantu African	112 (TEB) 115 (PO₄)	100	38	4.7	<4	—	Normal	Slightly biphasic	—

acom [389]	Negro	110 (TEB) / 107 (PO₄)	100	62	3.	<4	—	Normal	Normal	—
Saint ...uveur [390]	France	118 (tris) / 109 (TEB) / 114 (PO₄)	60–70	40	2.2–4.0	4	90–100	Normal	Normal	—
70.369.277.282	Negro	110 (tris, TEB) / 115 (PO₄)	80–100	50–70	2.9–4.4	<4	50–60	Normal	Normal	6.7
...dia [391]	Greece	104 (tris) / 107 (TEB) / 108 (PO₄)	100	40.6	3.5	2.6	60	—	Normal	—
enzo ...rquez [376]	Bantu African	106 (TEB, PO₄)	100	66	4.3	<4	—	Normal	Normal	—
County [348]	Negro	105 (TEB)	100	61	4	6	—	—	Normal	—
...ctrophoretically normal: normal) [255.263.57.282]	Various	100	100	50–70	2.9–4.4	<4	55–60	Normal	Normal	9.0
...ctrophoretically slow: aly [392]	Greece	105 (tris) / 98 (TEB) / 98 (PO₄)	100–110	28.5	12.3	9.7	70		Normal	—
...ista [377]	Greece	95 (tris, TEB) / 91–92 (PO₄)	85	24.7	6.5	6.5	52.4	—	Normal	—
...ern [393]	Greece	95 (TEB, PO₄)	60	38	2.2	3.6	42	—	Normal	—
...na [393]	Negro	94 (TEB) / 80–82 (PO₄)	100	66	4	2.6	69	—	Normal	—
nore- ...itin [394.136]	Negro	90 (tris)	75	65	3.1	<4	—	Normal	Normal	—
acase [376]	Bantu African	90 (TEB, PO₄)	100	141	3.8	<4	—	Normal	Normal	—
...Ode [287]	Negro	85 (TEB)	100	60	24	—	—	Labile	Slightly biphasic	—
...i Gerais [397]	Brazil	82 (PO₄)	<70	41	4	9	—	—	Normal	—
...na [395]	Negro	80 (PO₄)	70–80	32	3.5	Normal	—	—	Normal	—
n-Austin [394.136]	Negro	80 (tris)	72	62–72	3.3	<4	—	Normal	Normal	—
...le [394]	Negro	65 (TEB)	100	91	3.3	—	—	Labile	Normal	—
reased enzyme activity ...en [398]	U.S.—white	100 (tris, TEB) / 120 (PO₄ pH 6.5)	400	51	3.0	3.0	44	Normal	Normal	—

many cases much greater than is suggested by the results of assay of mixed red blood cells under standard conditions. The reason for this discrepancy is not always apparent. In a number of variants associated with nonspherocytic hemolytic anemia the residual enzyme shows marked sensitivity to the inhibitory effect of NADPH.[282] In some of these the enzyme is quite active when assayed *in vitro* at low NADPH concentrations, but may be nearly devoid of activity under *in vivo* conditions. Other factors which might play a role are susceptibility to inhibition by ATP[283,285] and very high Michaelis constants for NADP$^+$ and/or glucose-6-phosphate.[309,310] Instability is a characteristic that is particularly common in class 1 variants.[314] In some cases sufficient enzyme is present in very young erythrocytes to account for a moderate amount of residual activity in hemolysates, but disappears totally after the red cells reach 5 or 10 days of age. The absence of enzyme might account for the vulnerability of red cells to destruction in the circulation.

Human G-6-PD is quite antigenic when injected into rabbits. Marks and Tsutsui[409] first demonstrated the properties of anti-human erythrocyte G-6-PD by injecting rabbits with partially purified enzyme. Both soluble and insoluble combinations of enzyme were formed, and NADP$^+$ was found to affect the enzyme–antiserum combination. The antiserum inhibited human red cell G-6-PD, and G-6-PD from mouse, rat, and sheep, but not from rabbit or yeast. With the development of homogeneous prepara-

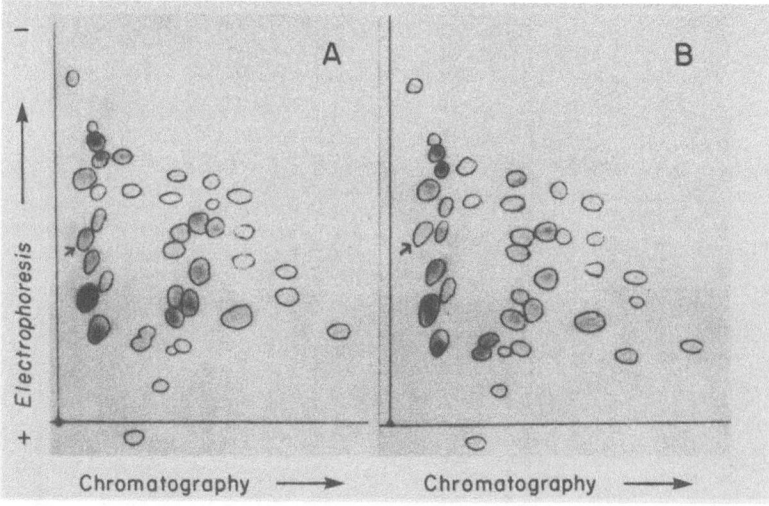

FIGURE 6. "Fingerprints" of G-6-PD A and B. A single peptide difference can be seen. The cause of this difference has been identified as a substitution of aspartic acid for asparagine. (Reproduced through the courtesy of Dr. A. Yoshida.)

tions of human G-6-PD, it has been possible to investigate, by a variety of techniques, the amount of G-6-PD antigen in the erythrocytes of patients with various types of G-6-PD deficiency. Using enzyme neutralization curves[368] and electroimmune diffusion,[410] G-6-PD A− exhibited approximately normal specific activity.[368] In contrast, the specific activity of G-6-PD Mediterranean[279,410,411] was diminished. Less common G-6-PD mutants have also been examined. West Bengal,[410] Seattle,[410] and Worcester-like[410] variants had normal specific activity, whereas Mali,[410] Fort de France,[410] Kerala,[410] Matam,[410] Benevento-like,[410] Union,[340] Port Royal,[411] Canton,[411] Toronto,[374] and Manchester[329] all had diminished specific activity. However, caution must be used in interpreting the results of immunologic studies. Different antisera may give different results.[412]

Fingerprinting of normal G-6-PD (G-6-PD B), G-6-PD A, and G-6-PD Hektoen has been carried out using crystallized homogeneous enzyme purified from erythrocytes. A single peptide difference has been observed in each case. The amino acid substitution in the case of G-6-PD A has been identified as that of aspartic acid for asparagine[63] (Fig. 6). Because of the large subunit size of G-6-PD, identifying the amino acid sequence of the protein is a very difficult task which has not yet been completed. Sequencing of many of the peptide fragments has, however, been carried out.

2.4. Physiology and Pathophysiology

The many variants of G-6-PD reflect a full spectrum of disease states ranging from deficiency so severe that no enzyme is detectable in circulating red cells, to a state in which G-6-PD activity in red cells is actually increased (Table V). It has been estimated that approximately 100 million people are G-6-PD deficient.[413] The vast majority of G-6-PD-deficient individuals go from cradle to grave without ever being aware of any difference from their nondeficient kin and neighbors. Under normal circumstances they are not anemic, although a few exceptions have been noted in the case of G-6-PD Mediterranean.[307,414,415] Increased red cell destruction ordinarily occurs only under special conditions. Hemolysis may be induced by the administration of certain drugs such as primaquine, by various infections, by diabetic acidosis, by unknown precipitating factors in the neonatal period, and by ingestion of fava beans.

2.4.1. The Steady State

2.4.1.1. Red Cells. Although the activity of G-6-PD in red cells is diminished, it is usually possible to detect some residual activity.

Deficiency of the enzyme is most marked in the older members of the

TABLE V

Clinical Manifestations of the Different Classes of G-6-PD Variants

	Class 4 (nondeficient)	Class 3 (mild deficiency)	Class 2 (severe deficiency)	Class 1 (NSHA)
G-6-PD activity (%)	Over 60	10–60	0–10	0–35
Example	A Barbieri	A⁻	Mediterranean Canton	Duarte Oklahoma Alhambra
Drug-induced hemolysis	0	+	+	+
Infection-induced hemolysis	0	+	+	+
Diabetic acidosis-induced hemolysis	0	+	+	+
Favism	0	0	+	+
Icterus neonatorum	0	±	+	+
Red cell life span in absence of stress	N	N or sl →	N or sl →	→
Anemia in the absence of stress	0	0	0	+

red cell population. This finding is particularly prominent in the case of G-6-PD A−, in which the enzyme activity of newly formed erythrocytes is probably almost normal. As the red cells age, G-6-PD activity declines until it is virtually absent from senescent erythrocytes.[416-418] The reduced glutathione content of G-6-PD-deficient erythrocytes is diminished,[43,419] and the concentration of oxidized glutathione is increased.[419] However, the total glutathione content is decreased,[419] probably because erythrocytes have the capacity to extrude GSSG actively,[420-422] a process that appears to depend markedly on the level of GSSG within the erythrocyte.[423] Unstressed red cells with G-6-PD A− metabolize glucose through the HMP at a normal or near-normal rate.[424,425] Unlike normal erythrocytes in which the NADPH/NADP$^+$ ratio is maintained at such a high level that G-6-PD is severely inhibited,[274,275,426] the lower steady state NADPH/NADP$^+$ ratio of G-6-PD-deficient cells[426] allows the enzyme to function at a rate much closer to its V_{max} in these erythrocytes. When methylene blue is added to erythrocytes, it oxidizes the enzyme NADPH diaphorase, which in turn oxidizes red cell NADPH.[427] In normal cells the resulting decrease in NADPH level and increase in NADP$^+$ level releases G-6-PD from inhibition and provides substrate for its activity. Consequently, a marked increase in the rate of HMP metabolism occurs. Methylene blue treatment of G-6-PD A− cells only slightly increases the rate of HMP metabolism, as measured by CO_2 evolution.[281,424,425] This is probably due in large part to the fact that NADPH levels are already low in G-6-PD-deficient cells.[426,428] It has also been suggested that the G-6-PD in these cells operates under some as yet undefined metabolic restraint.[429] The rate of metabolism through the HMP can also be estimated by linking the reduced methylene blue (leukomethylene blue) to the reduction of methemoglobin. Leukomethylene blue reacts nonenzymatically with methemoglobin, reducing it to hemoglobin.[427] Normal cells therefore have the capacity to accelerate methemoglobin reduction greatly in the presence of methylene blue, but G-6-PD-deficient red cells cannot do so. Because the main route of reduction of methemoglobin in red cells, the NADH-linked pathway, is unimpaired in G-6-PD-deficient cells, steady state methemoglobin levels are normal. In a patient with combined NADH diaphorase deficiency and G-6-PD deficiency the level of methemoglobin was slightly higher than that in a sib who had only NADH diaphorase deficiency,[430] but the reported difference is of doubtful significance.

Minor differences have been observed between G-6-PD-deficient and normal cells stored in blood bank preservative solutions. 2,3-DPG levels appear to be better maintained[431] and pyruvate accumulates more rapidly in G-6-PD-deficient than in normal cells.[432] It has been suggested that the viability of G-6-PD-deficient red cells stored in adenine-containing preservative media may be inferior to that of nondeficient cells.[433] The proposal has occasionally been made that G-6-PD-deficient blood not be used for transfusion purposes,[117,434,435] or used only when fresh.[436] This position appears to be based largely on one anecdotal report of an acute febrile hemolytic reaction occurring in a patient who had received 100 ml of G-6-PD-deficient blood.[117] In point of fact, follow-up examination of the donor blood in a laboratory experienced in studying G-6-PD variants revealed that it was not even enzyme deficient.[437] In another report[435] the recommendation is based merely on the fact that chromated G-6-PD-deficient red cells were destroyed, as might have been expected, when nitrofurantoin was administered intravenously. It is difficult to agree with the conclusion drawn from this study:

> The above reported data stress the necessity in blood banks of screening for deficient G-6-PD erythrocytes among the populations with a high frequency of the defect. The use of sensitive donor blood must be avoided in emergencies and in surgical practice for in these cases the recipients have more chances to receive potentially hemolytic drugs. The wide range of such drugs in the many fields of their therapeutic indications makes the use of sensitive donor blood inadvisable in all cases.

Clinical evaluation of 23 patients who received 24 units of G-6-PD-deficient blood failed to reveal any deleterious effects.[437] There are no firm data to support a view that the G-6-PD blood should be segregated or not used for transfusion purposes. Indeed, proscribing donation of blood by G-6-PD-deficient donors would seriously and unnecessarily impair the supply of human blood. Even in populations in which the gene frequency for G-6-PD deficiency is very high only a fraction of the blood received by multiply transfused recipients would be G-6-PD deficient. Only in exchange transfusion of infants does the possibility of accelerated destruction of G-6-PD-deficient cells adding to an already high bilirubin load warrant serious concern.

Certain well-defined changes in enzymes other than G-6-PD are also found in these cells. The activity of NADPH diaphorase is decreased,[438,539] and that of glutathione reductase (GR) is increased[440–443] in spite of one report to the contrary.[439] Less than normal augmentation of GR activity occurs when G-6-PD-deficient hemolysates are incubated with flavine adenine dinucleotide (FAD). The increased GR activity may be due to higher saturation with FAD,[443,444] and average FAD levels in G-6-PD-deficient erythrocytes are about 1.5 times those of nondeficient cells.[441] It is also possible that because of the higher levels of GSSG in G-6-PD-deficient red cells[419] a larger proportion of GR is present in the oxidized form, which may be less susceptible to destruction than is the reduced form. It spite of a report to the contrary,[442] red cell glutathione peroxidase activity is usually increased in G-6-PD deficiency, and it has been suggested that this enzyme might be induced by increased peroxide levels.[445]

The increases which have been reported to occur in red cell GAPD,[446] aldolase,[447-449] hexokinase,[450] catalase,[451] and lactic dehydrogenase[446] have not been confirmed in other studies.[43,447,452-456] It has been suggested that transketolase and transaldolase levels are increased in G-6-PD-deficient cells.[448] A report of diminished red cell acid phosphatase activity in black males with G-6-PD deficiency[457] could not be confirmed in an Oriental population,[458] in Mediterranean,[456] or black[456] G-6-PD-deficient subjects. The different frequencies of acid phosphatase electrophoretic phenotypes found in patients with G-6-PD deficiency[459] are difficult to explain, and could not be confirmed.[456] The activity of inorganic pyrophosphatase is decreased in Mediterranean G-6-PD-deficient red cells,[460] and it nearly disappears when the red cells are incubated with acetylphenylhydrazine. Believed to be a sulfhydryl enzyme, pryrophosphatase is apparently stabilized by glutathione,[461] and the decreased activity in G-6-PD-deficient cells may be a reflection of the lower glutathione level, but conflicting data have been published.[456]

A small decrease in protein sulfhydryl groups seems to be present in G-6-PD-deficient red cells.[462] The pattern of metabolic intermediates in G-6-PD-deficient cells is normal.[463] In G-6-PD-deficient patients with nonspherocytic hemolytic anemia ATP levels declined on autoincubation,[463,464] but were stable in persons with G-6-PD A−. Incubation of G-6-PD-deficient cells with phenylhydrazine resulted in loss of GSH as well as in rapid destruction of ATP.[465]

Although Tarlov et al.[466] reported decreased total lipid content of enzyme-deficient cells, most observations suggest that the lipid content of G-6-PD-deficient erythrocytes is normal,[447,467,468] except for minor differences in phosphatide levels.[469] Membrane sulfhydryl groups do not appear to be compromised in G-6-PD deficiency.[462] Morphologic abnormalities have been described in the membranes of G-6-PD-deficient cells, but whether such abnormalities actually exist in vivo is unknown.[470] Deformability of G-6-PD-deficient cells has been found to be unimpaired.[471]

Individuals with the common types of G-6-PD deficiency are not anemic in the absence of stress, with a few unexplained exceptions.[307,414,415] Some shortening of red cell life span may occur in the steady state, although the published data are quite ambiguous. Calculations of the ^{51}Cr $t_{1/2}$ from early published studies[40] give values of 34.6, 28.0, 25.0, and 22.1 days for four G-6-PD A− subjects, giving a mean of 27.4 days and a standard deviation of 5.4 days. These values tend to be in the lower portion of the normal range of 25 to 32 days.[472] A surprisingly large deviation from these originally reported values was reported subsequently, with ^{51}Cr $t_{1/2}$ values of 18, 24.5, and 18 days.[473] If such a short ^{51}Cr red cell life span were actually to exist in G-6-PD A− subjects, clinical evidence of a hemolytic state, including an elevated reticulocyte count, would surely be present. Since such stigmata of hemolysis are not evident in G-6-PD-deficient persons, it seems likely that the very short ^{51}Cr red cell life spans were due to technical factors. Indeed, in the same study, [^{32}P]diisopropylfluorophosphate (DFP) red cell life-span values of 38 to 58 days, a more modest shortening, were observed.[473] Furthermore, in persons with the much more severe Mediterranean deficiency the ^{51}Cr $t_{1/2}$ red cell life span in 18 subjects averaged 29 days.[474] In other studies, two subjects had $t_{1/2}$ values of 30 and 33 days,[475] and six subjects values of 21 to 24.5 days.[476] A moderately shortened mean ^{51}Cr $t_{1/2}$ of 22.8 ± 3.9 days (mean ± standard deviation) was reported for red cells of five subjects with G-6-PD Canton, 21.3 ± 2.1 days for three subjects with G-6-PD Chinese, and a normal life span for those with G-6-PD Hong Kong–Pokfulam.[477] Cases of G-6-PD deficiency combined with hereditary spherocytosis,[478,479] glucose phosphate isomerase deficiency,[480,481] heterozygous pyruvate kinase deficiency,[482] autoimmune hemolytic anemia,[483] Gilbert's disease,[484] and elliptocytosis[485,486] have been observed; in none of these cases was there any obvious interaction between G-6-PD deficiency and the independently inherited disorder. One of the patients with G-6-PD deficiency and elliptocytosis had mild shortening of red cell life span,[485] which could have been attributed either to elliptocytosis or to the enzyme deficiency. A patient with hereditary spherocytosis and G-6-PD deficiency had a satisfactory response to splenectomy.[479]

2.4.1.2. *White Cells.* The synthesis of leukocyte G-6-PD is regulated by the same gene as that of red cell G-6-PD. It is therefore not surprising that the kinetic properties of enzyme partially purified from leukocytes are very similar to those of enzyme obtained from erythrocytes.[487–489] Recent studies suggest that the enzyme from leukocytes has slightly different properties on isoelectric focusing probably because of posttranslation modification.[490] Because leukocytes have a shorter life span, moreoever, the expression of unstable variants of G-6-PD is much less severe in leukocytes than in long-lived erythrocytes. Modest decreases in leukocyte enzyme activity occur in patients with G-6-PD A−,[56,491,492] G-6-PD Mediterranean,[56,487–489,493] G-6-PD-deficient Chinese males,[494] and a number of less common variants.[338,487,491,495–499] The decrease in activity is much greater in G-6-PD Mediterranean than in G-6-PD A−. The relatively modest decrease in leukocyte G-6-PD levels which are observed in such instances do not appear to result in any functional abnormality of the white cells.[489] However, marked decreases in G-6-PD in certain severely deficient variants have been associated with an abnormality in the killing function of the leukocytes.[495-497] A reported[500,501] decrease in thermal stability of G-6-PD in chronic granulomatous disease (CGD) has been shown to be due not to an abnormal G-6-PD,[502] but rather to the absence of stabilizing factors in CGD leukocytes. In two families very low leukocyte G-6-PD activity was recorded in the presence of normal[492] or only modestly lowered[496] red cell enzyme levels. Leukopenia has occasionally been noted in G-6-PD deficiency with nonspherocytic hemolytic anemia.[304,307,503]

2.4.1.3. Platelets. Reduced platelet G-6-PD activity has been reported in individuals with G-6-PD A−,[491,504] G-6-PD Mediterranean,[320,491,505-507] in Chinese males with G-6-PD deficiency,[494] and in patients with other types of severe G-6-PD deficiency.[293,338,352,491,498] Although there appears to be general agreement that G-6-PD-deficient patients do not have a bleeding tendency, somewhat conflicting data have been reported concerning platelet function measurements. According to Schwartz et al.[507] G-6-PD-deficient patients manifested a reduction in availability of platelet factor 3, in prothrombin consumption time, and in platelet retention in a glass bead column. However, Gray et al.[498] found platelet factor 3 recalcification time to be normal in platelets which had no detectable G-6-PD activity. Both groups of investigators found that platelet aggregation and platelet counts were normal.

2.4.1.4. Other Tissues. Diminished G-6-PD activity has been recorded in many tissues and in the body fluids of G-6-PD-deficient persons. Included are cultured fibroblasts,[508] liver,[509,510] kidney,[494,511] lens,[512,513] adrenal,[494] saliva,[514] milk,[515] and hair roots.[516] The latter represent individual clones of cells and may therefore be useful in heterozygote detection.

2.4.2. Association of Various Disease States with G-6-PD Deficiency

2.4.2.1. Nonhematologic Changes. Population studies have shown that certain disorders occur more frequently in G-6-PD-deficient individuals than in nondeficient control groups. For example, it has been reported that the systolic and diastolic blood pressures and serum creatinine levels are higher in deficient males than in controls.[517] It has also been suggested that overall fitness is less in G-6-PD-deficient individuals than in controls because the incidence of G-6-PD deficiency appeared to decrease with increasing age.[518] A statistically significant lower incidence of G-6-PD deficiency among champion athletes than in the general population was interpreted to indicate that G-6-PD deficiency may prevent the performance of outstanding athletic feats.[519] Coronary artery disease was found to be more frequent among black males with G-6-PD A or G-6-PD A− than in those with G-6-PD B.[520] In one study[521] abnormal standard glucose tolerance tests were found in G-6-PD deficiency, but no difference was reported in the incidence of diabetes mellitus.[520] On the other hand, it is claimed in another report that cortisone-modified glucose tolerance tests, but not standard glucose tolerance tests, gave higher 1- and 2-hr blood sugar levels in G-6-PD-deficient than in control males.[522] Such correlations are suspect because they do not take into account the wide variation in the proportion of African genes present in individual U.S. blacks. Some have well under 20%, whereas others may have in excess of 90% of genes of African origin. The average proportion of non-African genes in blacks living in the California area was estimated to be 22%.[523] Any disorder which is more prevalent in persons with large numbers of African genes is likely to be correlated with the incidence of G-6-PD deficiency in a racially mixed population. The high incidence of G-6-PD deficiency in persons with sickle cell disease elicited the suggestion that the presence of G-6-PD deficiency might improve survival of sicklers.[524] However, the association was probably spuriously derived at least partially from the association of Gd^A with other genes of African origin in a racially mixed population. Indeed, a study which took this factor into account[130] showed that the incidence of G-6-PD deficiency was no higher in individuals with sickle cell disease than in their brothers with sickle trait or with hemoglobin A. No correlation between sickling and G-6-PD deficiency was found in another study carried out in the United States,[525] nor in one carried out in Africa.[526] The results of earlier African studies which suggested that G-6-PD deficiency improved survival in sickling were probably due to faulty methodology.[527] Indeed, it has been suggested that hemolytic crises which are sometimes encountered in patients with sickle disease may be due to G-6-PD deficiency.[528]

The suggestion that seizure disorders may be more common in G-6-PD deficiency[328,529] has not been statistically validated. In a study of a large number of black subjects with schizophrenia, the overall incidence of G-6-PD deficiency was no different from that observed in a control group. However, patients with catatonic schizophrenia exhibited an unusually high incidence of G-6-PD deficiency, whereas a low incidence was observed in patients with paranoid schizophrenia.[530] The possibility was considered that the expression of a schizophrenic disorder is influenced by the presence or absence of G-6-PD deficiency, but subsequent studies failed to confirm the original observations.[531]

A moderate decrease in G-6-PD activity of the lens occurs in individuals with G-6-PD A−.[532] Cataractous lenses extracted from Mediterranean patients with G-6-PD deficiency showed an absence of enzyme, while activity was detected in cataractous lenses from nondeficient controls.[513] However, there is no evidence that the incidence of cataracts is increased in the common types of G-6-PD deficiency. On the other hand, cataracts have been reported to occur in some patients with functionally severe G-6-PD deficiency and nonspherocytic hemolytic anemia.[328,533,534] Optic atrophy has been observed in at least two patients with G-6-PD deficiency[330,535] but it is likely that, in each case, the association was a coincidental one.

A number of investigators have claimed that the incidence of G-6-PD deficiency is lower in cancer patients than in controls,[536,541] and have concluded that G-6-PD deficiency may provide some degree of protection against cancer. Unfortunately, in all of these investigations G-6-PD deficiency was detected either by undefined or by grossly inadequate methodology. Since cancer is often associated with shortened red cell life span, ascertainment of G-6-PD deficiency which does not take into account red cell age is likely to provide spurious results. An adequate investigation of the incidence of G-6-PD deficiency in cancer would be of value.

Renin release is reportedly exhausted in G-6-PD-deficient subjects but not in normal subjects after six consecutive 30-min periods of upright posture stimulation.[542] Attention has also been directed to steroid metabolism in G-6-PD-deficient individuals because of the role which NADPH plays in this process. Increased excretion of cortisol and of cortisol derivatives not reduced in the A ring was observed in one study.[543] However, in another investigation[510] no differences were observed in plasma cortisol levels or in total 17-oxogenic urinary steroid excretion during a 24-hr period, either before or after maximal stimulation with corticotrophin. A preliminary report of a modest fall in serum cholesterol levels during primaquine-induced hemolysis in two G-6-PD A− subjects[544] is difficult to evaluate.

One patient with G-6-PD A− twice suffered necrosis of skin flaps being used in a grafting procedure, and a possible association between the enzyme deficiency and this complication was postulated.[545] Minor differences between red cell lead concentrations in G-6-PD A− children and normal control children have been reported. There were no significant differences in blood lead concentrations, and only when the data were "corrected" for hematocrit was any difference observed.[546]

2.4.2.2. Drug-Induced Hemolytic Anemia.   The clinical course of primaquine-induced hemolysis has been studied under carefully controlled conditions in men with the A− type of G-6-PD deficiency.[547] The daily administration of 30 mg of primaquine results in little or no evidence of hemolysis for 2 or 3 days. However, Heinz bodies appear in the erythrocytes and then the hemoglobin concentration of the blood falls and the urine begins to darken. Sometimes no other abnormalities are noted by the patient; in more severe cases, weakness and abdominal and back pain occur, the patient becomes icteric, and the urine turns nearly black. A mild decrease in plasma cholesterol levels during hemolysis has been reported to occur[544] and red cell lipid levels have been reported to show a mild decline.[466] Sequestration of red cells occurs both in liver and spleen,[548] and Heinz bodies disappear as the hemoglobin concentration of the blood approaches its nadir.[547] Reticulocytosis develops, and polychromatophilia is observed in the blood film. Regardless of the severity of the anemia precipitated by drug administration, the acute hemolytic phase ends spontaneously in about 1 week, even if drug administration is continued. Now, the "recovery phase" begins. The patient feels better and the color of the urine becomes normal. The hemoglobin concentration of the blood rises to normal and the reticulocyte count declines. The self-limited nature of the hemolytic anemia is readily explained by the fact that only the older members of the red cell population are destroyed during drug challenge.[549] It is these cells which are most enzyme deficient[64,418]; the newly produced erythrocytes contain nearly normal levels of G-6-PD, which enables them to resist drug-induced destruction.

The hemolytic effect of primaquine in subjects with G-6-PD Mediterranean has also been carefully studied. Severe anemia occurs after the administration of 30 mg of primaquine daily, and even those cells not destroyed in the initial hemolytic episode are still susceptible to destruction when challenged with drug in a normal recipient.[551,610] Cohort labeling of red blood cells with ^{59}Fe showed that even young red cells were susceptible to destruction.[550] Approximately equal sequestration of red cells in liver and in spleen was observed.[551,552] The erythropoietic response in persons with the Mediterranean type of G-6-PD deficiency was shown to be unimpaired.[553] When hemolysis is very severe, renal failure may result.[511,554]

Primaquine is only one of a large number of drugs which can precipitate hemolytic anemia in primaquine-sensitive individuals (Table VI). Closely related 8-aminoquinoline antimalarials also have the capacity to do so. Older 8-aminoquinoline antimalarials such as pamaquine (plasmoquin) produce particularly severe hemolytic anemia, and fatalities were sometimes observed when this drug was in common use.[3,4] Since infectious diseases can themselves precipitate hemolytic anemia in G-6-PD-deficient individuals (see Section 2.4.2.3), evaluation of the hemolytic potency of drugs based on the effects of their clinical use may be quite misleading. When a patient who is given a drug during management of an infection develops a hemolytic episode, a cause-and-effect relationship has often been assumed to exist between administration of the drug, on

TABLE VI
Drugs and Chemicals Which Have Clearly Been Shown to Cause Clinically
Significant Hemolytic Anemia in G-6-PD Deficiency

Acetanilid	Pentaquine
Methylene blue	Sulfanilamide
Nalidixic acid (Negram)	Sulfacetamide
Naphthalene	Sulfapyridine
Niridazole (Ambilhar)	Sulfphamethoxazole (Gantanol)
Nitrofurantoin (Furadantin)	Thiazolesulfone
Phenylhydrazine	Toluidine blue
Primaquine	Trinitrotoluene (TNT)
Pamaquine	

the one hand, and the hemolytic response, on the other. In point of fact, the hemolytic anemia may have resulted from the infection. Unfortunately, in many instances investigators have attempted to verify their conclusions that a drug had hemolytic potency in G-6-PD deficiency by substituting the drug in question for acetylphenylhydrazine in a modified GSH stability test. Thus, GSH stability tests have been carried out using nitrofurantoin,[555] naphthol,[556] sulfamethoxypyridazine,[557] aspirin,[558] vitamin K,[559] niridazole,[560] sulfadiazine, sulfanilamide, sulfapyridine, and trisulfa.[561] The response of red cell GSH levels in such studies did not always correspond to the known hemolytic effect of the drugs involved. For example, sulfanilamide and sulfapyridine, both known to produce hemolysis in G-6-PD-deficient cells, did not decrease GSH levels.[561] Yet, even ascorbic acid, not hemolytic in ordinary doses (see Section 2.4.2.2), caused a fall in the GSH level of primaquine-sensitive cells in initial studies of the glutathione stability test.[44] Obviously, the metabolism of a drug and its levels in the blood play such an important role in its potential production of an oxidative challenge that the substitution of the drug for acetylphenylhydrazine in an in vitro test tells us little about its hemolytic potency. A more complex and possibly more promising approach to the evaluation of the hemolytic potency of drugs in G-6-PD deficiency is measurement of the effect of plasma drug metabolites on oxidative metabolism of normal erythrocytes. This method is based on the reasonable assumption that a hemolytic drug is one that stresses the hexose monophosphate pathway of erythrocytes. Preliminary investigations of this technique seem promising,[562,563] but it has not been extensively used.

The most reliable data concerning the hemolytic potency of drugs have been obtained by administration of putative hemolytic agents to normal volunteers transfused with ^{51}Cr-labeled G-6-PD-deficient erythrocytes. Most of the drugs discussed in the following paragraphs have been blamed at one time or another for the occurrence of hemolytic anemia in G-6-PD-deficient individuals. Uncritical compilations based on isolated or inconclusive observations are often given to G-6-PD-deficient patients with a warning that all drugs on the list must be avoided. Careful scrutiny of the evidence, however, suggests that many can be given with impunity to deficient subjects (Table VII).

Acetanilid is a moderately potent hemolytic agent when given to volunteers with G-6-PD A−. One-quarter to one-half of the red cells of such recipients were destroyed during a 7-day course of 3.6 g acetanilid daily, and a volunteer receiving this dose manifested a fall in hemoglobin level from 14.8 to approximately 10 g/100 ml in 2 weeks.[564] Presumably, hemolysis would be more severe in individuals with class 2 variants such as G-6-PD Mediterranean or Canton.

The administration of *acetaminophen (Paracetamol; Tylenol; Tralgon; hydroxyacetanilid)* in combination with a muscle relaxant was associated with a hemolytic episode in a G-6-PD-deficient subject.[511] However, 2 g daily of this drug has been given experimentally to persons with G-6-PD Canton[477] and 3.6 g daily to those with G-6-PD A−[565] without producing hemolysis. Therefore, it does not appear that a cause-and-effect relationship exists between acetaminophen administration and hemolytic anemia.

Acetophenetidine (phenacetin) appears to be a relatively mild hemolytic agent. Only 10 to 20% of labeled red cells from G-6-PD A− donors were destroyed after administration of 3.6 g of phenacetin daily for 8 days.[564] The effect of this drug is apparently quite mild even in the more severe types of G-6-PD deficiency[566]; severe hemolysis following administration of this drug to G-6-PD-deficient subjects[567] may well represent the result of infection, rather than phenacetin-induced hemolysis, except in one instance when 25 g of the drug was ingested.[568] Furthermore, phenacetin-induced hemolytic anemia has also frequently been documented in individuals shown not to be G-6-PD deficient.[569]

Acetylsalicylic acid (aspirin) is often included in lists of drugs that produce hemolysis in G-6-PD-deficient individuals. If it were indeed a hemolytic agent, it would be clinically extremely important. Neither aspirin nor its breakdown product, gentisic acid, stimulated the HMP of normal red cells.[570] Although high concentrations of o-salicylate inhibit the HMP, no inhibition can be demonstrated at levels which are attained *in vivo*.[571] Indeed, the administration of 3.6 g of aspirin daily failed to produce hemolysis of G-6-PD A− ^{51}Cr-labeled cells[565]; even doses ranging from 4 to 12 g/day appear to produce only very mild hemolysis without anemia in subjects with G-6-PD A−.[572] Only when 25 g of aspirin was ingested with 25 g of phenacetin by a G-6-PD-deficient black male, pre-

TABLE VII

*Drugs Which Can Probably Safely Be Given in Normal Therapeutic Doses to
G-6-PD-Deficient Subjects (without Nonspherocytic Hemolytic Anemia)*

Acetaminophen (Paracetamol, Tylenol, Tralgon, Hydroxyacetanilid)
Acetophenetidine (phenacetin)
Acetylsalicylic acid (aspirin)
Aminopyrine (Pyramidone, Amidopyrine)
Antazoline (Antistine)
Antipyrine
Ascorbic acid (vitamin C)
Benzhexol (Artane)
Chloramphenicol
Chlorguanidine (Proguanil, Paludrine)
Chloroquine
Colchicine
Diphenylhydramine (Benedryl)
Isoniazide
L-Dopa
Menadione sodium bisulfite (Hykinone)
Menapthone
p-Aminobenzoic acid
Phenylbutazone
Phenytoin
Probenecid (Benemid)
Procaine amide hydrochloride (Pronestyl)
Pyrimethamine (Daraprim)
Quinidine
Quinine
Streptomycin
Sulfacytine
Sulfadiazine
Sulfaguanidine
Sulfamerazine
Sulfamethoxypyriazine (Kynex)
Sulfisoxazole (Gantrisin)
Trimethoprim
Tripelennamine (Pyribenzamine)
Vitamin K

sumably in a suicide attempt, was severe hemolysis observed.[568] With the
more severe enzyme deficiencies encountered among Oriental subjects
the ^{51}Cr red cell survival was shortened only to a $t_{1/2}$ of 16 days after
administration of 6 g of calcium aspirin daily.[477] In a total of 203 challenges with aspirin, there were only two instances in which it appeared
that the aspirin might have been implicated in a hemolytic reaction.[573]
Since these patients were febrile, it seems most likely that the infection

rather than the aspirin was the precipitating factor. Similarly, a case report of hemolysis following aspirin administration[558] is difficult to interpret; it is likely that the hemolysis which was observed was due to a viral infection for which the patient was being treated, rather than to the aspirin itself. Frank hemolysis due to aspirin administration seems only to have been described in individuals with nonspherocytic hemolytic anemia due to unusual G-6-PD variants,[293,314,315,328,574] and even there one cannot always be certain that other factors might not have played a role. The ^{51}Cr survival of red cells with G-6-PD Milwaukee was shortened from a $t_{1/2}$ of 6.5 days to one of 1.7 days when 1.8 g of aspirin and to only 23 hr when 225 mg of gentisic acid were given daily.

Aminopyrine (pyramidone; amidopyrine) is included in most lists of agents which produce hemolysis in G-6-PD deficiency. The putative hemolytic effect of aminopyrine was erroneously attributed to Sartori and Panizon[575] in an early review[576] which was subsequently[467] cited as a source. We are not aware of any valid observations implicating aminopyrine in hemolytic anemia in G-6-PD-deficient individuals, and indeed hemolysis has been observed in nondeficient patients.[577] *Antipyrine,* closely related to aminopyrine, was mentioned by Kimbro *et al.*[555] as one of several components of a proprietary drug ingested by a patient who developed hemolytic anemia. As a result it, too, has generally been included in lists of hemolytic drugs. Again, we know of no evidence that there are any cases in which a cause-and-effect relationship between the ingestion of antipyrine and hemolytic anemia has been established. In a recent study[573] two hemolytic episodes occurred in 171 challenges of 129 G-6-PD-deficient patients with aminopyrine, and one hemolytic episode occurred in 85 challenges with antipyrine. In each case these drugs were given to febrile patients in combination with other drugs. Accordingly, it seems that both aminopyrine and antipyrine must be considered to be harmless in G-6-PD-deficient individuals. There is a single report of a patient developing a hemolytic anemia after surgery for renal colic. This patient had received, prior to surgery, injections of 5 g daily of *methapyrone (Novalgine),* an analgesic closely related to aminopyrine.[578] The temporal relationship between the administration of this drug and hemolysis is quite suggestive of drug-induced hemolysis, but the stress of surgical manipulation and of possible infection could also have been responsible for hemolysis.

p-Aminosalicylic acid (PAS) is often mentioned as a possible hemolytic agent because of early, anecdotal accounts[555,579–582] of hemolysis occurring in patients receiving this drug. In one report,[581] for example, two G-6-PD-deficient patients with tuberculosis were reported to undergo hemolysis when 15 g of PAS was given intravenously. The data presented indicated that only one of these patients actually experienced a well-documented hemolytic episode. This patient, however, failed to develop hemolysis when PAS was given in the same dose 5 months later. In another report[582] PAS was readministered to one of two patients who had developed explosive hemolytic episodes with an onset shortly after the administration of PAS. During this course of treatment, there was little fall in hematocrit, although the bone marrow seemed to show increased erythroblastic activity. Moreover, acute hemolysis has also been reported in non-G-6-PD-deficient persons who developed hemolytic anemia when receiving PAS,[583,584] and challenge of ^{51}Cr-labeled red cells *in vivo* with PAS failed to result in their destruction.[477,585] It would therefore seem unlikely that PAS should be regarded as a cause of hemolytic anemia in G-6-PD deficiency.

Amodiaquin (Camoquin), an antimalarial, failed to produce hemolysis in a G-6-PD-deficient Papuan subject.[586] However, the same subject failed to develop hemolysis when challenged with primaquine, a finding difficult to reconcile with the low red cell G-6-PD levels which were repeatedly recorded.

The initial studies of the GSH stability test[44] demonstrated that incubation of G-6-PD-deficient red cells with *ascorbic acid (vitamin C)* results in a decline of GSH levels. Ascorbate has also been shown to produce oxidative denaturation of hemoglobin.[587-589] The administration of ascorbic acid in unspecified doses did not destroy ^{51}Cr-labeled G-6-PD-deficient cells,[565] but some destruction of G-6-PD-deficient cells resulting from daily 1.5-g doses of ascorbic acid has been claimed.[61] *In vitro* incubation of human G-6-PD-deficient red cells with ascorbic acid decreased their life span when they were transfused into rats.[590] A dramatic effect of ascorbic acid administration was noted in a 68-year-old black male with G-6-PD deficiency of the A− type. He had been hospitalized for treatment of second-degree burns, and for unspecified reasons was given 80 g of ascorbic acid intravenously on each of two consecutive days. The patient developed an episode of possible disseminated intravascular coagulation. The hemoglobin level of the blood, which had been normal prior to treatment, fell to 5.8 g/100 ml, he became comatose, and developed a right-sided hemiparesis. Anuria developed, but hemodialysis produced little change in his status, and the patient died.[591]

When G-6-PD A− erythrocytes were labeled with ^{51}Cr and challenged with *chloramphenicol*, no shortening of their survival was observed.[565] However, Larizza et al.[592] reported that hemolytic anemia occurred in G-6-PD-deficient subjects, ostensibly with G-6-PD Mediterranean, who were given therapeutic courses of chloramphenicol. Subsequently, other case reports appeared. A G-6-PD-deficient Hindu

subject developed a possible, although hardly clear-cut, hemolytic episode when given chloramphenicol in treatment of a febrile disease.[593]
Severe hemolysis was observed in two Asian Indian children receiving
chloramphenicol in treatment of typhoid fever.[594] Since typhoid itself
produces hemolytic anemia in G-6-PD deficiency, it is difficult to ascribe
the hemolysis to the treatment. Careful studies by Chan et al.[477,595] and
McCaffrey et al.[475] appear to have clarified the status of chloramphenicol.
In patients with severely deficient Oriental variants of G-6-PD, including
three subjects with G-6-PD Canton and two subjects with G-6-PD
Chinese, transfused G-6-PD-deficient red cells had a shortened red cell
survival in patients with untreated typhoid fever,[595] and the red cell life
span appeared to be normalized by chloramphenicol therapy. A similar
situation was observed in two Egyptian children with G-6-PD Mediterranean who developed hemolytic anemia during treatment of typhoid fever
with chloramphenicol. After the patients had recovered, ^{51}Cr survival
studies were carried out, establishing a baseline survival, after which 35
mg chloramphenicol/kg body weight was given daily. The pretreatment
^{51}Cr $t_{1/2}$ was normal at 33 and 30 days, respectively, for the two patients.
The administration of chloramphenicol shortened the ^{51}Cr $t_{1/2}$ to 17 and 16
days (Fig. 7). Calculation of the percentage of cells destroyed by chloramphenicol administration was estimated at 13 and 14.5% of the red cell

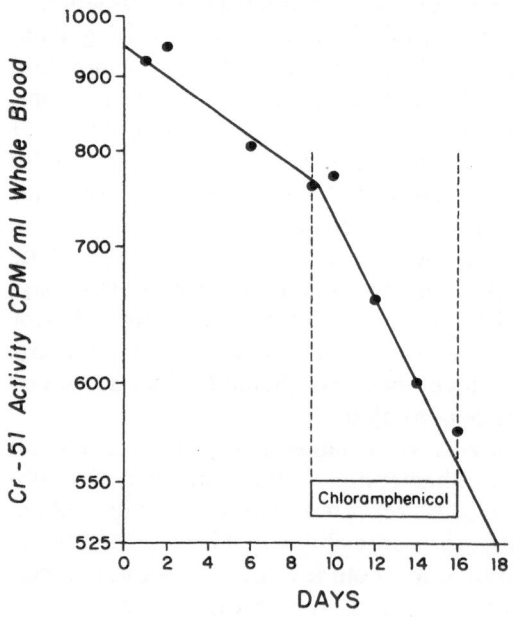

FIGURE 7. A ^{51}Cr red cell survival curve of an Egyptian patient,
presumably with G-6-PD Mediterranean, given 35 mg chlorampheni-
col/kg body weight. (Redrawn from
McCaffrey et al.,[475] through the
courtesy of the author and the
American College of Physicians.)

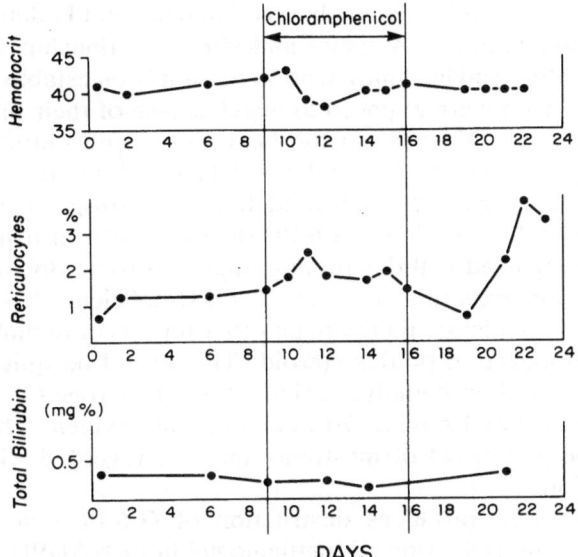

FIGURE 8.   The effect of administration of chloramphenicol, 35 mg/kg body weight, to the same subject whose ⁵¹Cr survival curve is depicted in Figure 7. Only minimal hematologic changes were observed. (Redrawn from McCaffrey *et al.*,[475] through the courtesy of the author and the American College of Physicians.)

population.[475] The level of destruction observed in these patients is of the same magnitude as that observed with the administration of 3.6 g of phenacetin daily[564]; it would not produce anemia in a person with normal marrow function. Indeed, administration of chloramphenicol to these subjects after their recovery from typhoid fever resulted neither in an appreciable change in hematocrit nor in a rise in serum bilirubin level.[475] (Fig. 8).

Chloroquine, a 4-aminoquinoline antimalarial, has also been implicated in an anecdotal report[582] in the origin of hemolysis. However, it is nonhemolytic with respect to G-6-PD A−,[565] G-6-PD Mediterranean,[562] and G-6-PD Canton[477] red cells.

L-*Dopa* is a major constitutent of the fava bean. It is oxidized to dopaquinone, a potent oxidant substance, and it was therefore suggested that it might be the active hemolytic principle in this bean.[596,597] However, challenge of G-6-PD-deficient cells by L-dopa has shown that this material is not hemolytic.[477,598] Indeed, it has been proposed that L-dopa may protect hemoglobin against oxidation by acting as a free radical trap,[599] and it was shown that catalase served as an L-dopa peroxidase.[600]

A hemolytic crisis has been observed in one G-6-PD-deficient patient with *lead* intoxication.[601] A cause-and-effect relationship between the hemolytic reaction and lead intoxication has not been established. Among black children who were exposed to lead because of their proximity to a battery factory no difference in the hemoglobin concentration was observed among G-6-PD-deficient and -nondeficient children.[546]

A preliminary report[602] indicated that the estrogenic steroid *mestranol* produced hemolysis of G-6-PD-deficient cells in a heterozygous woman. Although red cell destruction appeared to be documented with cross-transfusion experiments using G-6-PD-deficient ^{51}Cr-labeled red cells in normal recipients, there are no other reports of hemolytic responses related to ingestion of this steroid. This would be quite unlikely if mestranol were in fact hemolytic, since it is the estrogen in such widely used preparations as Enovid, Orthonovum, and Ovulen. Therefore, the putative hemolytic effect of mestranol must be regarded with considerable reservation.

Methylene blue produces destruction of G-6-PD-deficient cells.[603] This dye links the reduction of methemoglobin to NADPH produced in the HMP. It is therefore used very successfully in the treatment of toxic methemoglobinemia. However, when methylene blue was given to a G-6-PD-deficient individual with toxic methemoglobinemia, it not only failed to lower the methemoglobin concentration of the blood but also precipitated an acute hemolytic episode.[604]

Nalidixic acid (Negram) seems to be capable of inducing hemolytic anemia in at least some G-6-PD-deficient individuals. An unpublished case occurring in a G-6-PD-deficient Negro subject was mentioned by Belton and Jones in 1965.[605] Subsequently, a dramatic hemolytic episode was observed in a G-6-PD-deficient West Indian boy receiving this drug,[606] and a milder episode in an Italian worker exposed to nalidixic acid dust in the pharmaceutical industry.[607] Another report of a possible hemolytic episode contained no satisfactory evidence that the patient was actually G-6-PD deficient[608]; furthermore, hemolysis did not occur until the 20th day of treatment, an unlikely sequence of events for drug-induced hemolysis in G-6-PD deficiency.[608]

The hemolytic effect of *naphthalene* in G-6-PD deficiency has been documented through numerous clinical observations in infants and children exposed to this compound.[56,78,79,117,556,609–613] Hemolysis has resulted not only from ingestion of naphthalene, but has also been observed in G-6-PD-deficient infants dressed in clothing impregnated with naphthalene or exposed to an atmosphere heavily laden with naphthalene.[556,609] Marked red cell fragmentation is often evident in the peripheral blood film. Hemolytic anemia due to naphthalene exposure has also been documented in children with normal red cell G-6-PD activity.[609]

A single case of hemolysis following *neoarsphenamine* treatment of an African patient with lues probably does not represent drug-induced hemolysis.[614] Some 2 weeks intervened between the beginning of treatment and the mild hemolytic episode which was observed; at the same time, severe hepatocellular damage was present, possibly due to infectious hepatitis. The case is best interpreted as hepatitis-induced hemolysis.

Niridazole (Ambilhar) is a schistosomacide. It has produced hemolytic anemia in individuals with G-6-PD A−,[485,615] G-6-PD Mediterranean,[616] and in undetermined types of G-6-PD deficiency.[560,617] Only moderate shortening of the ^{51}Cr red cell survival has been observed,[616] but severe anemia with a decline in the hemoglobin level to as low as 5.2 g/100 ml was documented.[617]

The administration of *nitrofurantoin (Furadantin)* has been associated with significant hemolysis in patients with G-6-PD A−,[555,618] G-6-PD Mediterranean,[578,619] and in subjects with G-6-PD Canton and G-6-PD Chinese.[477] The shortening of red cell survival by this drug has been demonstrated in experimental subjects transfused with ^{51}Cr-labeled G-6-PD-deficient cells[435,477,620] (Fig. 9), and there is no question that this drug is a potently hemolytic agent. The frequency with which nitrofurantoin-induced hemolytic anemia may occur in clinical practice is emphasized by the finding that acute hemolytic episodes were observed more frequently after the administration of nitrofurantoin than with any other drug when the records of 129 G-6-PD-deficient patients were reviewed in Israel.[573] In contrast to primaquine-induced hemolysis, Heinz bodies do not appear in erythrocytes of G-6-PD-deficient individuals after the administration of nitrofurantoin, nor are they formed after *in vitro* incubation with this compound.[555,621] A closely related drug, *nitrofurazone (Furacin; Nitrofural)*, generally used as a topical agent but occasionally administered systemically in treatment of *Trypanosoma rhodesiense* sleeping sickness, produced anemia in a G-6-PD-deficient subject.[622]

Inhalation of 0.50 ppm of *ozone* by young adults resulted in minimal but statistically significant decreases in red cell GSH levels.[623] A persistent increase in red cell G-6-PD activity was also described,[623] and is very difficult to explain. Because of such data, the speculation has been put forward that exposure to ozone might precipitate hemolytic anemia in G-6-PD-deficient individuals.[624] There is, however, no evidence that this does in fact occur.

Thirty milligrams of *phenylhydrazine* daily, a dose that produces little or no destruction of normal erythrocytes, produced accelerated destruction of G-6-PD-deficient erythrocytes.[564]

Primaquine is the prototype of drugs which produce hemolytic anemia in G-6-PD-deficient persons. The hemolytic effect of this drug occurs

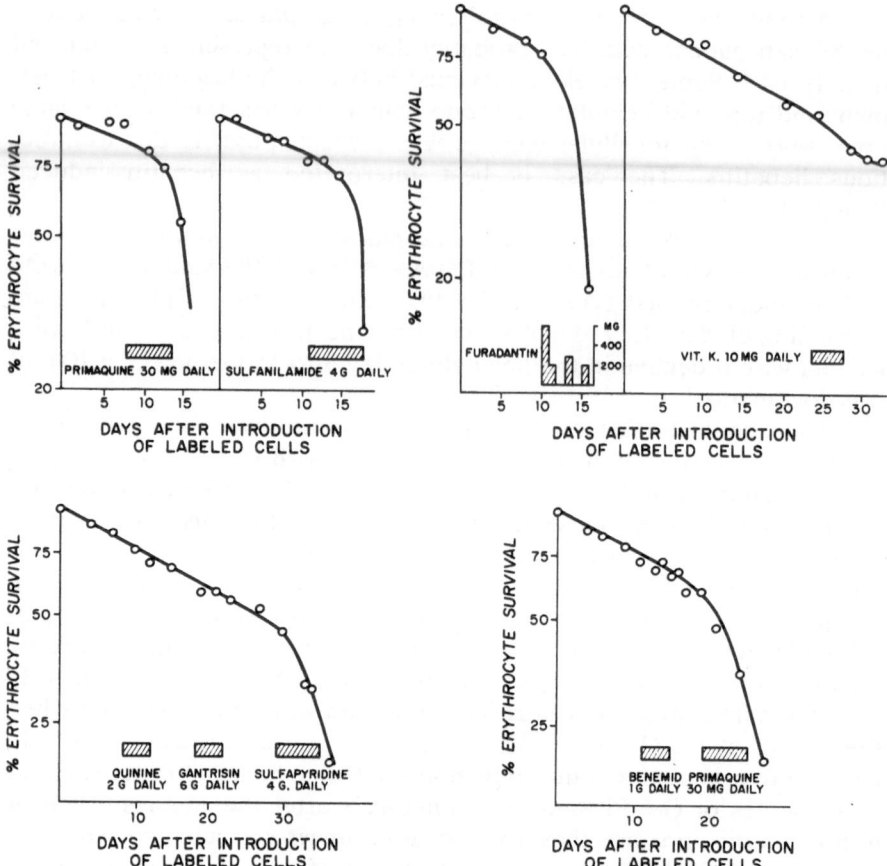

FIGURE 9. ^{51}Cr survival curves of G-6-PD-deficient red cells from Bantu subjects (presumably G-6-PD A) challenged with primaquine, sulfanilamide, Furadantin, menadione sodium bisulfite, quinine, Gantrisin, sulfapyridine, and Benemid, given in the doses indicated. Only primaquine, sulfanilamide, Furadantin, and sulfapyridine produced appreciably accelerated disappearance of labeled erythrocytes. (Redrawn from Zail et al.,[620] with permission of the authors.)

regularly when 30 mg is given daily, and the destruction of G-6-PD-deficient cells has been documented in detail in individuals with G-6-PD A−[564,620,625] (Figs. 3 and 9), with G-6-PD Mediterranean,[550,551,626] and in a Chinese G-6-PD-deficient subject.[477,627] The administration of 45 mg of primaquine once or twice weekly has been used to circumvent serious hemolytic effects of this drug in G-6-PD-deficient individuals. Although this is apparently quite satisfactory in those with the A− type of deficiency,[628] it produces a moderate degree of anemia in persons with more severe, presumably Mediterranean, G-6-PD deficiency.[629] Studies have also been carried out to determine which modifications of the 8-aminoquinoline molecule affect the hemolytic properties of the drug.[565] 4-Amino-1-methylbutylamino, 4-diethylamino-1-methylbutylamino, and 5-isopropylaminoamylamino side chains, forming *primaquine, pamaquine,* and *pentaquine,* respectively, represent compounds highly hemolytic in doses of 30 mg daily. A 4-aminobutylamino or 2-amino-1-methylethylamino side chain, forming *S.N. 3883* and *C.N. 1110,* respectively, formed compounds requiring three to six times the dose of primaquine to cause comparable hemolysis. Alteration of the 6 position substituent in the quinoline nucleus markedly influences hemolytic potency. Pentaquine caused considerable hemolysis when 60 mg/day was administered. *S.N. 15,324,* identical to pentaquine except for substitution of the hydroxy group for a methoxy group in the 6 position of the quinoline nucleus, was less hemolytic. If instead of the 6-methoxy group, a 7-methyl group was present on the quinoline nucleus, the resulting compound (*S.N. 15,305*) had almost no hemolytic potency, even when 500 mg/day was given. *S.N. 3294,* the 4-amino isomer of pamaquine, was nonhemolytic.

Quinacrine (Atabrine) has been reported to produce very mild red cell destruction in G-6-PD deficiency.[572] Although *quinidine*[592] and *quinine*[592,630] have been reported, anecdotally, to cause hemolytic anemia in G-6-PD deficiency, challenge of ^{51}Cr-labeled G-6-PD-deficient cells showed that quinine does not destroy deficient erythrocytes[620] (Fig. 9).

There is probably more confusion about the hemolytic effect of *sulfonamides* in G-6-PD deficiency than about that of any other class of drugs. Sulfonamides are often employed to treat febrile illnesses, and since such illnesses can themselves produce hemolytic reactions in G-6-PD-deficient individuals (see Section 2.4.2.3), it is hazardous to rely upon case reports to determine whether or not a sulfonamide has hemolytic properties in G-6-PD-deficient individuals. Investigations in volunteers have demonstrated that 3.6 to 4 g/day of *sulfanilamide*[564,620] (Fig. 9) or 3.6 g/day *sulfacetamide*[564] had the capacity to destroy ^{51}Cr-labeled G-6-PD A− red cells. A number of other sulfonamides did not produce destruction of G-6-PD A− cells even when administered in large doses. These include *sulfadiazine,* 2 g daily[561] and 5 g daily,[565] *sulfamerazine,* 5 g daily[565] or in *trisulfa*[561] 5 g daily,[565] and *sulfaguanidine* 2 g daily.[561] Although *sulfisoxazole (Gantrisin)* is often listed as a hemolytic drug, this seems to be based on a 1962 review[572] that states that this drug, at a dose of 8 g/day (approximately four times the usual dosage), produces moderate hemolysis. A considerable body of negative evidence is usually ignored. Zail *et* al.[620] challenged ^{51}Cr-labeled G-6-PD A— red cells with 6 g Gantrisin daily and found the drug to be nonhemolytic (Fig. 9). Administration of 4 g Gantrisin daily failed to produce hemolysis or to lower the red cell GSH level of five men with G-6-PD A—.[631] *Sulfamethoxypyridazine (Kynex)* was found to be hemolytic to G-6-PD A— cells, when given a dose of 2 g/day,[572] or 4 g/day.[632] Since this is four to eight times the usual therapeutic dose, it seems doubtful that this observation has any clinical relevance. Furthermore, 2 g/day did not produce hemolysis in Thai patients with G-6-PD deficiency.[557] However, hemolytic anemia has been observed in two G-6-PD-deficient infants whose mothers received Kynex immediately prior to delivery.[633] It was suggested that the slow clearance of this drug by newborns may play a role in their susceptibility to hemolytic anemia. *Sulfamethazine (sulfadimidine)* is mentioned as a cause of hemolysis in a G-6-PD A— subject.[620] *Sulfaphenazol (Depocid)* administration was associated with a severe hemolytic reaction in a patient with G-6-PD deficiency of undetermined type while the patient was being treated for tonsillitis. The relative roles of the drug and infection are not known.[634] *Sulfphormethoxine (Fanasil)* is a long-acting sulfonamide which has been implicated clinically in hemolytic anemia. However, when 1.5 g was administered daily to normal recipients given ^{51}Cr-labeled G-6-PD-deficient red cells of the Mediterranean type, mildly shortened survival of labeled cells was documented.[562] *Sulfamethoxpyrazine (sulfalene)* is another long-acting sulfonamide which has not been implicated in drug-induced hemolytic anemia. However, when G-6-PD Mediterranean red cells were challenged *in vivo* with this drug,[562] a modest shortening of red cell lifespan was observed. Based on these data, one would not expect significant hemolysis to occur clinically with the use of these two drugs. *Sulfasymazine,* in a dosage of 500 mg/day, produced a significant reticulocytosis in patients with G-6-PD A— who had urinary tract infections, but not in those receiving placebo or in nondeficient individuals.[635] *Sulfapyridine*[561] seems to have been responsible for a hemolytic reaction of all of three G-6-PD-deficient Mediterranean subjects who were carefully monitored during therapy. In one case blood transfusion was required. The hemolytic effect of this drug was confirmed in ^{51}Cr survival studies of G-6-PD A— red cells transfused into normal subjects[620] (Fig. 9). A 24-year-old Caucasian male with burns on only 10% of his body developed a fatal hemolytic reaction while being treated topically with 10% *mafenide acetate (Sulfamylon)*. Although there were no other obvious causes for hemolysis, the absence of other reports of hemolytic anemia following the use of this drug makes a cause-and-effect relationship uncertain.[554] *Sulfacytine* did not produce any signs of hemolysis when 2 g/day was given to five men with G-6-PD A—.[631] The administration of 4.0 g daily for 2 days of *sulfi-*

somidine (Domian; Elkosin) to a patient with nonspherocytic hemolytic anemia produced increased signs of hemolysis with fall of the hemoglobin from 9.7 to 7.5 g/100 ml.[566] In another patient[464] with nonspherocytic hemolytic anemia an acute hemolytic crisis appeared to result from the administration of an unspecified dose of this drug. Salicylazosulfapyridine (Azulfidine) has been reported to be hemolytic in the A— type of deficiency.[572] Of the currently used sulfonamides, sulfamethoxazole (Gantanol),[477,627,633-638] a component of the widely used antibacterial combination Septra or Bactrim, is probably the most hemolytic. One gram daily of the latter drug produced severe hemolytic reactions in both G-6-PD A— and G-6-PD Mediterranean subjects.[636] Studies with ^{51}Cr-labeled red cells have confirmed its hemolytic potency.[477]

The sulfone, sulfoxone (Diasone), was shown to produce some destruction of primaquine-sensitive cells when given at a dose of 0.3 g daily. However, the extent of destruction of labeled cells was so slight that it is unlikely that clinically significant anemia would result from this dosage of drug in the A— type of deficiency.[564] A daily dose of 2.4 g produced hemolytic anemia in a patient with normal red cell G-6-PD levels; preferential destruction of older red cells was observed.[639] Thiazolesulfone produced a variable response, rapidly destroying G-6-PD A— cells in some recipients and failing to destroy them in others.[564] The degree of destruction of labeled cells was correlated with other side effects experienced by the recipient, and appears to have been due to individual variation in metabolism of this sulfone. One subject given only 3 g of thiazolesulfone daily developed severe methemoglobinemia, abdominal pain, nausea, and headache and rapidly destroyed ^{51}Cr-labeled G-6-PD A— cells. Cells from the same donor were not hemolyzed in another recipient who was given 18 g of thiazolsulfone daily without experiencing any toxic signs. The hemolytic effect of diaphenylsulfone (DDS; Dapsone) has been carefully documented.[640] Accelerated red cell destruction was observed in normal volunteers given 300 mg of diaphenylsulfone daily. Similar degrees of destruction occurred in black G-6-PD-deficient volunteers receiving only 100 mg of the drug daily. Red cell sequestration appeared to take place primarily in the spleen. Even at dose levels as high as 200 mg daily the amount of destruction of G-6-PD-deficient cells was modest and anemia was mild. Case reports of hemolysis occurring in black soldiers receiving 25 mg of DDS daily along with single weekly doses of 45 mg of primaquine showed the additive effect of DDS and primaquine.[641] It has been speculated that the active hemolytic principle in patients receiving DDS might be 4-amino-4'-hydroxyaminodiphenylsulfone.[642]

A single G-6-PD-deficient volunteer developed a greater degree of anemia when given the diformyl derivative of DDS than did nondeficient volunteers.[643] This drug was shown to accelerate destruction of G-6-PD Mediterranean cells when 400- to 1200-mg single doses were given, but 800-mg doses were required to destroy G-6-PD A— cells.[644]

Toluidine blue, a dye that closely resembles methylene blue in structure, produced a severe hemolytic reaction in a black woman with G-6-PD deficiency who was given 7 mg dye/kg body weight to visualize the parathyroid glands.[645]

Exposure to *trinitrotoluene (TNT)* has been associated with hemolytic episodes in at least six workers.[592,646] In some cases hemolysis recurred on reexposure to TNT. The temporal relationship between TNT exposure and the development of severe hemolysis is strongly suggestive of a cause-and-effect relationship. Szeinberg *et al.*[589] observed mild reticulocytosis in an Iraqui G-6-PD-deficient subject exposed to TNT.

It was first suggested in 1955[647,648] that water-soluble *vitamin K derivatives* might cause hemolytic anemia and kernicterus in premature infants. The findings that vitamin K could lower the GSH level of erythrocytes *in vitro* and that a 5-day-old Negro G-6-PD-deficient child developed severe hemolysis after receiving 10 mg of *menadione sodium bisulfate*, led to the suggestion that these substances could produce hemolysis in G-6-PD deficiency.[559] A case report[649] tended to verify this assumption. However, evidence that vitamin K derivatives actually have this effect is scant. In a study of 30 full-term G-6-PD A— infants given either no vitamin K prophylaxis or doses varying from 1 to 18.75 mg during their first 24 hr of life there was little difference in bilirubin levels. Indeed, G-6-PD-deficient infants receiving *vitamin K (Konakion)* had somewhat lower bilirubin levels than those of control infants.[650] The administration of 1 mg of *menaphthone* to G-6-PD-deficient infants in Nigeria failed to produce any increase in the incidence of neonatal jaundice.[651] The administration of vitamin K derivatives to adult volunteers has also failed to produce hemolysis. Forty milligrams of *menadione sodium bisulfite (Hykinone)* failed to hemolyze G-6-PD Canton erythrocytes.[477] The administration of 10 mg of this compound daily did not appreciably shorten the life span of ^{51}Cr-labeled G-6-PD A— red cells[620] (Fig. 9).

Hemolytic anemia has been described in a G-6-PD-deficient subject who was exposed to the fungicide, *zinc ethylene bisdithiocarbamate*. However, since the patient also has severe hypocatalasemia and had been given the known hemolytic agent, methylene blue, the cause-and-effect relationship between fungicide and hemolytic anemia is by no means clear.[652]

Chromium-51 labeled G-6-PD-deficient red cells have been challenged with a large number of other drugs to determine their sensitivity to destruction. In some cases anecdotal clinical accounts have implicated some of these drugs in hemolytic episodes. The following drugs given daily in the indicated doses were found not to be hemolytic: 30 mg *aniline*,[565] 100 mg *p-aminophenol*,[565] 8 g *p-aminobenzoic acid*,[565] 300 mg *diphenylhydramine (Benedryl)*,[565] 400 mg *antazoline (Antistine)*,[565] 3 g *procaine amide hydrochloride (Pronestyl)*,[565] 300 mg *tripelenamine (Pyribenazmine)*,[565] 300 mg *chlorguanidine (Proguanil; Paludrine)*,[477] 600 mg *phenylbutazone*,[477] 1.5 mg *colchicine*,[477] 6 mg *benzhexol (Artane)*,[477] 1 g *streptomycin*,[477] 300 mg *isoniazid*,[477,585] 18 mg/kg *trimethoprim*,[477] 300 mg *phenytoin*,[477] 1 g *probenecid (Benemid)*[477,620] (Fig. 9), and 25 mg weekly *pyrimethamine (Daraprim)*.[477,565]

The mechanism or mechanisms through which certain drugs shorten the life span of G-6-PD-deficient erythrocytes have not been clearly defined. It is likely that denaturation of hemoglobin into insoluble precipitates—Heinz bodies—and damage to the erythrocyte membrane are the final events preceding the removal of the erythrocyte from the circulation by a perceptive filtering system; the exact sequence of events which lead to such damage is not clear. Although some potentially hemolytic drugs have the capacity to inhibit G-6-PD *in vitro*,[653,654] the concentrations required are so high that it is quite improbable that this phenomenon is of any physiological significance. Many of the drugs which cause the destruction of G-6-PD-deficient cells have the capacity to generate hydrogen peroxide,[655,656] possibly through superoxide[657] when interacting with oxyhemoglobin. Glutathione detoxifies hydrogen peroxide through the glutathione peroxidase reaction, but G-6-PD-deficient cells are unable to maintain their GSH level because of their limited capacity to reduce NADP$^+$ to NADPH. The hydrogen peroxide which accumulates in G-6-PD-deficient cells may then produce oxidative denaturation of hemoglobin and of membrane, leading to the formation of Heinz bodies and ultimately to destruction of the red cells. The GSSG formed may itself be damaging, producing mixed disulfides with hemoglobin and inhibiting enzymes such as hexokinase.[658] It has been suggested that lipid peroxidation may play a role in the sequence of events leading to the destruction of G-6-PD-deficient cells.[578] Non-G-6-PD-deficient patients treated with diphenylsulfone, a compound that produces hemolysis in G-6-PD deficiency (page 89), manifested evidence of lipid peroxidation.[659] However, malonaldehyde production in G-6-PD-deficient cells treated with hydrogen peroxide was no greater than that in other patients with elevated reticulocyte counts.[651]

The role of methemoglobin in the sequence of events leading to hemolysis has been subject to controversy. Many drugs that produce hemolytic anemia in G-6-PD-deficient patients also have the capacity to induce some degree of methemoglobinemia. Heme is much less firmly bound in methemoglobin than in oxyhemoglobin,[660] and heme-free globin is particularly vulnerable to denaturation. However, induction of methemoglobinemia with nitrite does not make rats more susceptible to phenylhydrazine-induced hemolysis.[661] Furthermore, an inverse relationship appears to exist between the hemolytic potency of drugs, on the one hand, and their capacity to form methemoglobin, on the other.[662,663] Whether or not methemoglobin plays a role in the process, treatment of hemoglobin with phenylhydrazine results in production of denatured globin hemochromogens. First pointed out by Warburg in 1931,[664] this phenomenon has been studied using more sophisticated techniques in recent years.[665,666] It has also been suggested that phenylhydrazine and its derivatives produce hemochromogens with the heme of hemoglobin.[667-671] Such a reaction would also result in denaturation of hemoglobin and possibly in the generation of superoxide radicals which are decomposed to hydrogen peroxide.

2.4.2.3. *Hemolytic Anemia Induced by Infection.* Although the prototype of hemolytic anemia in G-6-PD deficiency is the destruction of red cells induced by the administration of drugs, hemolysis precipitated by infectious diseases is probably the more common source of morbidity in G-6-PD-deficient individuals. Typically, the anemia is discovered as the patient is being treated for an infection. Relatively few febrile patients have not been given aspirin- or phenacetin-containing medications, and these are often blamed for the hemolytic episode. Yet G-6-PD-deficient volunteers who were given such drugs did not develop clinically significant hemolysis. It therefore seems likely that in such instances the hemolysis is actually the result of the febrile disorder rather than the drug administration.

Hemolysis resulting from infection is usually mild but occasionally may be very severe. In a number of cases acute renal failure has resulted from infection-induced hemolytic episodes[356,672-679]; in some of these instances the administration of potentially hemolytic drugs may also have played a role. Recovery of the hemoglobin level to normal is often delayed by the marrow suppression which ordinarily accompanies infection. Many different organisms have been implicated; in some instances the illness is an influenza-like infection in which no offending organism is isolated. One of the most common causes of hemolysis in G-6-PD-deficient persons is bacterial pneumonia. At least 19 of 102 G-6-PD-deficient patients admitted to a New York hospital developed hemolytic episodes complicating such an infection.[680] In another survey, one-half of G-6-PD-deficient patients who became anemic in the course of infection suffered from pneumonia.[68] A number of additional reports emphasize the role of pneumonia in precipitating hemolysis in G-6-PD-deficient individuals.[673,682–684] Typhoid fever also commonly precipitates hemolysis in G-6-PD deficiency.[475,593–595,673,678,685–687] Other infections associated with hemolysis include those caused by *Salmonella*,[314,688,689] *Proteus*,[690] *Escherichia coli*,[680] β-streptococci,[681] staphylococci,[681] tuberculosis,[681] and rickettsiae.[674] When red cells from volunteer donors with G-6-PD Canton were infused into chloramphenicol-treated patients with typhoid fever, cholangitis, fever of unknown origin, or perirectal abscess, no shortening of red cell survival was noted.[595] Presumably antibiotic treatment was sufficient to prevent any red cell destruction which might otherwise have occurred.

Increased red cell destruction may be particularly noticeable in G-6-PD-deficient patients with viral hepatitis. Modest shortening of red cell survival and mild anemia has been observed in many patients with acute infectious hepatitis,[691] but frank anemia usually does not develop.[447,692] In patients with G-6-PD deficiency, in contrast, anemia seems to be common in infectious hepatitis. In one study of 125 children with viral hepatitis 23% of those with normal G-6-PD activity experienced hemolysis while 87% of the group with G-6-PD Mediterranean developed hemolytic anemia.[692] In some instances the anemia is quite severe; hemoglobin values of three black patients studied by Salen *et al.*[693] ranged from 5.4 to 7.7 g/100 ml. The accelerated destruction of red cells imposes a bilirubin load on the damaged liver which results in a marked increase in the plasma bilirubin level. The high bilirubin levels which are encountered may suggest to the physician that the patient is suffering from extensive hepatic necrosis and may soon die of fulminating hepatitis. However, in point of fact the outlook in such patients seems to be quite good,[694] and high bilirubin levels in G-6-PD-deficient patients with hepatitis do not necessarily portend a grave prognosis. Leukocytosis and thrombocytosis appear regularly to accompany the hemolytic reaction of G-6-PD-deficient patients with hepatitis.[677,693,695] Azotemia has also been observed,[673,677,693,695] although it is not clear whether this complication is more common in patients with G-6-PD deficiency than in those without. It has been suggested that hepatitis may stimulate hemolysis by permitting the circulation of "oxidant" compounds which might otherwise be detoxified by the liver.[693] Indeed, old data of questionable reliability suggest that GSH levels may be decreased in patients with hepatitis.[696] Further study will be required to identify the mechanism of hepatitis-induced hemolysis in G-6-PD deficiency.

2.4.2.4. Hemolytic Anemia in Diabetic Acidosis. Diabetic acidosis appears to have the capacity to elicit hemolytic reactions in G-6-PD-deficient persons. The relatively small number of cases which have been reported[689,697,698] probably underestimates the frequency with which this reaction occurs. Hemolysis varies greatly in severity and it disappears when normal metabolic balance is restored. The mechanism through which hemolysis occurs in these patients is not clear. The supply of red cell NADPH may be limited by (1) the effect of pH on the hexokinase reaction[699]; (2) the effect of elevated glucose concentrations acting through L-hexonate dehydrogenase[700,701]; (3) the effect of high concentrations of pyruvate acting as an effective substrate for LDH at low pH levels.[702] None of these mechanisms, alone, appears to be sufficient to account for the observed hemolysis. Perhaps a combination of factors precipitates hemolysis.

2.4.2.5. Neonatal Icterus. Determination of red cell G-6-PD activity of Mediterranean and Oriental newborns with jaundice of unknown origin has shown that a high proportion of them are enzyme deficient.[117,174,177,223,286,649,703–709] The infants are usually moderately anemic; however, severe jaundice with kernicterus has been described frequently.[174,177,350,703–707,710–712] Anisocytosis, poikilocytosis, and normoblastosis have been described.[713] Haptoglobin and hemopexin levels appear to be normal.[709]

Hyperbilirubinemia appears to be quite common in infants with severely deficient G-6-PD variants. Among 23 Chinese G-6-PD-deficient male infants,[704] peak bilirubin levels of over 20 mg/100 ml occurred in 9, and one of these died of kernicterus. Similarly, in another study of 62 Oriental G-6-PD-deficient infants,[711] 13 developed plasma bilirubin levels of over 19 mg/100 ml. Six of these infants were exchange transfused and one developed severe kernicterus before exchange transfusion could be carried out. In a study of Thai infants,[223] 2 of 51 (4%) G-6-PD-deficient infants had bilirubin levels of over 17 mg/100 ml, a degree of bilirubinemia encountered in only 0.3% of 629 male infants with normal G-6-PD activity, when other causes of jaundice were excluded. The incidence of severe jaundice in newborns with G-6-PD Mediterranean is more difficult to determine, and may vary from area to area. Szeinberg *et al.*[714] found that the incidence was no different in Israeli communities with a very high frequency of G-6-PD deficiency than in those with a low frequency. However, in a prospective study of over 7000 infants born in Israel, hyperbilirubinemia was found in 14.3% of 265 G-6-PD-deficient infants, but only in 7.2% of 3582 normal infants.[195] One investigation[715] suggested that the use of a dye mixture of brilliant green, gentian violet, and proflavine might possibly play a causal role, since an increase in the incidence of hemolysis was observed when this dye mixture was employed. Marked regional differences have also been detected in the incidence of neonatal jaundice in Greece; in Alexandra only 1 of 23 G-6-PD-deficient newborn infants had a bilirubin value of more than 16 mg/100 ml, while in Lesbos 28 of 65 and in Rhodes 7 of 62 G-6-PD-deficient newborns were severely jaundiced.[174] Greek infants born in Australia had a much lower incidence of hyperbilirubinemia than appears to be the case in Greece. Although 51 out of 2617 Greek babies in Melbourne required exchange transfusions only one of these was G-6-PD-deficient; this is actually less than the gene frequency for G-6-PD deficiency (0.045) found in this population. However, mild jaundice was more common among G-6-PD-deficient infants in Australia.[716]

The occurrence of neonatal jaundice in infants with the mild A− type of deficiency is much more difficult to evaluate. In an early investigation of black newborns, Zinkham[650] found only a minimally increased bilirubin level in 2 or 3 of 10 G-6-PD-deficient infants when compared with 20 normal full-term infants. The addition of vitamin K_3 or K_1 did not increase the bilirubinemia of G-6-PD-deficient infants. Similarly, O'Flynn and Hsia[135] and Perkins[717] failed to find increased serum bilirubin levels in infants with G-6-PD A−. In anecdotal reports it was found that 19[718] and 4[719] full-term black infants developed a neonatal hyperbilirubinemia associated with G-6-PD deficiency. The nature of the control group was not clear, however, and therefore it was difficult to evaluate whether G-6-PD deficiency played an etiologic role in hemolysis observed in these infants. In the United States, hyperbilirubinemia was noticeable in premature G-6-PD-deficient Negro infants;[720] the average maximum bilirubin value in these infants was 17.3 mg/100 ml, compared with 12.2 mg/100 ml in controls.

In full-term black African newborns, unlike those in the United States, G-6-PD deficiency seems to play a significant role in the occurrence of neonatal jaundice.[158,721,722] Among Bantu newborns 14% of babies with increased jaundice were found to be G-6-PD-deficient, whereas only 1.3% of control infants were enzyme-deficient.[721] In Nigeria the incidence of G-6-PD deficiency in all newborn males was found to be 22.5%, but was over 60% in those with serum bilirubin levels of over 20 mg/100 ml. A Nigerian G-6-PD-deficient infant appears to have approximately a 10% probability of developing a serum bilirubin level of about 20 mg/100 ml, whereas a nondeficient infant has only a 1% probability of developing this degree of jaundice.[722]

The cause of the hyperbilirubinemia of newborn G-6-PD-deficient infants is not clear. In individual instances drugs have been held responsible. Quinine, for example, was blamed for hemolysis in one G-6-PD-deficient infant,[630] although it is unlikely that quinine produces this effect in the A− type of deficiency. In other cases, the prenatal administration of Kynex to the mother has been implicated.[633] The possible role of vitamin K derivatives has been emphasized since Zinkham and Childs'[723] demonstration that these compounds could affect glutathione stability.

However, as indicated earlier, the putative effect of this vitamin on neonatal jaundice seems to be purely anecdotal in nature. Controlled studies seem to provide no evidence of hemolytic effect. That shortened red cell life span may play a role is suggested by the lower hemoglobin values and higher reticulocyte counts observed in G-6-PD-deficient infants.[174,286] The suggestion has also been made that impaired detoxification in the liver in combination with somewhat accelerated hemolysis may play an important role. Conjugation of D-glucaric acid[724] and of salicylamide[725] has been reported to be decreased in G-6-PD-deficient jaundiced infants, but not in infants with hemolytic disease due to Rh incompatibility.

    2.4.2.6. Favism. Favism is potentially one of the most serious clinical consequences of G-6-PD deficiency. The occurrence of acute hemolysis following ingestion of the beans or inhalation of the pollen of *Vicia fava* (the broad bean) has been recognized since antiquity. Favism is a disorder which occurs most commonly among children between 1 and 5 years of age[726,727] (Fig. 10). In some series,[726] but not in others,[727] it is observed more frequently in males. Even in large general hospitals only isolated cases of favism have been found among adults.[726] Most cases of favism result from the ingestion of fresh beans, and the seasonal incidence (Fig. 11) coincides with the ripening of the beans.[726] Favism also occurs when dry beans are eaten, and the severity of the hemolytic reaction seems to be approximately the same with fresh and dry beans.[726] Favism has been observed in nursing infants whose mothers have ingested fava beans,[726,728,729] and in a child who ingested milk of a goat which

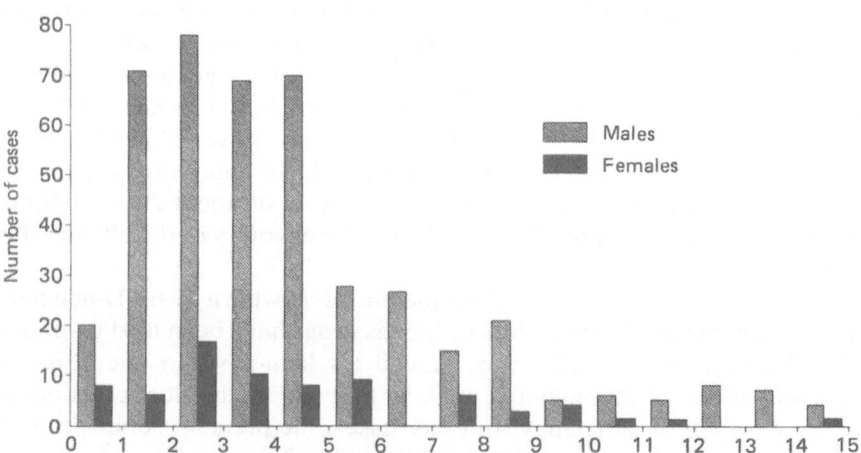

FIGURE 10.   Age and sex distribution in favism. (Redrawn from Kattamis *et al.*,[726] through the courtesy of the authors and the British Medical Association.)

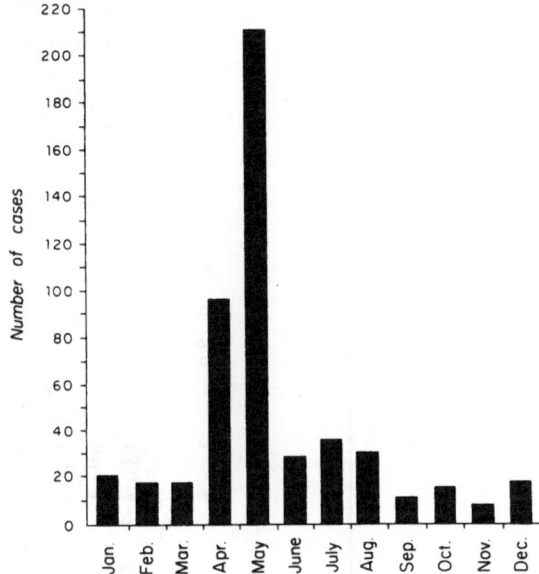

FIGURE 11. Seasonal incidence of favism. (Redrawn from Kattamis *et al.*,[726] through the courtesy of the authors and the British Medical Association.)

had eaten the beans.[730] The quantity required to cause favism may be very small; in one case the characteristic attack was attributed to the intake of a single seed.[730] It has been claimed that favism may occur after inhalation of pollen.[730,731] A 1905 review of 1211 cases is cited as indicating that 38% of the attacks were pollen-induced.[730] In reality, pollen inhalation is probably an uncommon cause of attacks. The development of favism could not be attributed to this cause in any of 506 patients in one series,[726] and the incidence of the disease in March (Fig. 11), when the beans flower, was very low.

According to Luisada,[730] the first symptoms of favism appear within a few seconds after inhalation of pollen to 5 to 24 hr after ingestion of fava beans. The symptoms consist of malaise, headache, dizziness, nausea, vomiting, chills, pallor, lumbar pain, and fever. Hemoglobinuria appears within 5 to 30 hr following exposure to beans, and a few hours later jaundice is observed.[730] Fever and marked leukocytosis may be present.[730] Sometimes the red cells in the peripheral blood are distorted in shape and the hemoglobin may appear to be contracted away from the membrane.[732] It has been claimed that the levels of red cell lipids decline during hemolysis.[468] The typical attack lasts from 2 to 6 days. Fatalities usually occur within the first 2 days and rarely during the third day.[730] Most patients in one series were hospitalized several days after the beans were eaten[726] (Fig. 12). Although favism may be quite mild,[727] in many cases the

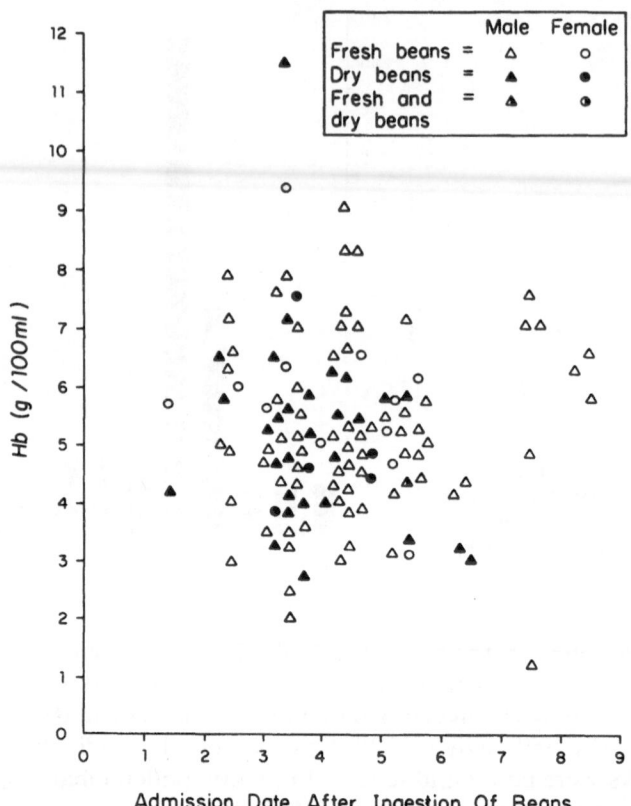

FIGURE 12. Hemoglobin levels on the day of admission in relation to the time since ingestion of fava bean in a group of subjects with favism studied by Kattamis *et al.*[726] (Redrawn with permission of the authors and the British Medical Association.)

anemia is very severe. In Kattamis' series of hospitalized patients[726] the hemoglobin concentration of the blood was below 6 g/100 ml in 81%, and below 4 g/100 ml in 30% of the patients. In one patient a hemoglobin level of less than 1 g/100 ml was recorded. Acute renal failure is apparently not uncommon, at least in adults. Of 62 cases reviewed by Symvoulidis *et al.*,[733] 16 developed this complication, 10 requiring dialysis, and 3 terminating in death. Before transfusions were readily available, fatalities were not uncommon; a mortality rate of 8% was reported in 1905.[730]

   2.4.2.6a. The Predisposition to Favism. Favism has been observed in many different population groups. While it is most common in Italy[731] and in Greece,[726] cases have been documented in English,[734,735] Polish,[736] Portuguese,[737] Thai,[738] Sephardic Jewish,[55,579,739] Algerian,[582] Chinese,[740] but not in African subjects.

In 1956, Crosby noted the similarity between primaquine-induced hemolytic anemia and favism and suggested that these two hemolytic disorders might have a common denominator.[741] Soon thereafter, Sansone and Segni noted that the glutathione levels[742] and stability[199] of the red cells of patients with a history of favism were diminished; similar observations were made independently in Israel by Szeinberg et al.[55,579,739] It soon became apparent that all patients with favism are G-6-PD-deficient,[79,166,446,575,592,649,743] yet many patients with G-6-PD deficiency are able to ingest fava beans without experiencing hemolytic episodes. Indeed, even individuals with favism have usually ingested fava beans several times without untoward effects before experiencing their first hemolytic episode.[726] Furthermore, when ^{51}Cr-labeled G-6-PD-deficient erythrocytes are infused into the circulation of a normal subject who then ingests fava beans, destruction of the labeled cells does not occur[548,734,744] unless the recipient is fava-bean-sensitive.[744]

It is apparent that some factor in addition to G-6-PD deficiency is required for the development of favism. It has been suggested that this factor is inherited as an autosomal gene,[745] but how it functions is as yet unkown. Decreased excretion of D-glucaric acid has been reported to occur in pesons who are susceptible to the hemolytic effect of the fava bean; this finding[746] and that of impaired formation of salicylamide glucuronide[747,748] were interpreted as indicating a defect in glucuronide formation in such persons.[746,748] Although at one time it was regarded very likely that sensitivity to the hemolytic effect of fava beans had an immunologic basis,[730,749] the use of modern immunologic techniques has afforded no support to the importance of immunologic reactions in the etiology of favism.[750]

2.4.2.6b. The Active Factor. Several substances in fava beans have been considered as possible hemolytic principles. It has been shown that the pyrimidine aglycones, vicine and convicine, have the capacity to oxidize the GSH of G-6-PD-deficient[751,752] and even of normal cells.[753] There is no direct evidence, however, that these substances produce hemolytic anemia in subjects with favism, and the relationship of these materials to undefined substances in fava bean extracts which lower red cell GSH levels *in vitro* is unknown.[754-756] Fava beans are a rich source of 3-(3,4-dihydroxyphenyl)-L-alanine (L-dopa), and it has been suggested that this material may be the hemolytic agent,[596] particularly after its oxidation to dopa-quinone.[597] However, the challenge of ^{51}Cr-labeled G-6-PD-deficient cells with L-dopa failed to result in hemolysis.[477,598] Such results cannot be considered to be conclusive, since a challenge of G-6-PD-deficient cells with fava beans in a normal recipient fails to result in their destruction.[548,734,744] Nonetheless, with the widespread use of L-dopa in the treatment of parkinsonism, the absence of reports of hemolytic crises in G-6-PD-deficient subjects militates strongly against L-dopa as the active hemolytic principle. A possible synergistic effect between L-dopa and the pyrimidine derivative, isoumaril, found in fava beans, has been suggested.[752]

2.4.2.7. *Hereditary Nonspherocytic Hemolytic Anemia.* Although the vast majority of G-6-PD-deficient persons go through life without ever knowing that they have inherited a red cell enzyme deficiency or experiencing any untoward effects from G-6-PD deficiency, a few G-6-PD-deficient patients suffer from lifelong nonspherocytic hemolytic anemia. Most patients with hereditary nonspherocytic hemolytic anemia due to G-6-PD deficiency have inherited an unusual variant with characteristics which apparently deprive the red cells of most functional G-6-PD activity. Such variants are listed under class 1 in Table IV. The properties of such variants which may account for their *in vivo* impotence are discussed in Section 2.3.4. In a few instances chronic hemolysis without known inciting cause has been observed in patients with G-6-PD Mediterranean.[307,415,757]

Hereditary nonspherocytic hemolytic anemia due to G-6-PD deficiency may be heralded in the newborn period by severe jaundice requiring exchange transfusion,[296,328,330,533,758] or it may be discovered much later in life.[326,366,464,499] The steady state level of hemoglobin may be normal in patients in which the hemolysis is fully compensated by increased bone marrow activity.[307,313,315,325,499] On the other hand, steady state hemoglobin levels as low as 8.0 g/100 ml have been observed.[759] Marked anemia usually occurs as a response to intercurrent infections[293,296,309,314,316,318,325,503,758] or after the administration of drugs[316,566,759] or fava beans.[314,762] During hemolytic crisis hematocrit levels as low as 9[316] or 11.5%,[767] hemoglobin levels as low as 4[761] or 2.1 g/100 ml,[323] and a red cell count of 660,000[762] have been recorded. Some family members who may be presumed to have had the same defect have died of "anemia" or under unexplained circumstances.[464,763] Abdominal pain has been observed in a number of patients[293,307,326,415,535,764]; its origin has not been clear, but it may have been due either to hemolytic crises or to gallbladder disease which is commonly observed in this disorder.[307,326,380,415,503,533,764–766] Mild jaundice is usually present. Splenomegaly is the rule,[298,300,309,314,316,318,328,366,464,495,503,566,582,759,763,765,767,768] but in some cases the spleen does not seem to be palpably enlarged.[304,313,316,331,464,499,760,761] In a few cases cataracts have been observed[328,533,534] and optic atrophy has been noted.[535] The appearance of the blood film is that of a hemolytic state with macrocytosis, aniso- and poikilocytosis, and occasional stippling.[59,315,318,535,761,764,768] The white count is usually normal[304,307,318,325,331,380,464,499,533,535,566,758–760,762,763,765,768,769] or may be slightly elevated,[415,759] but in a few instances mild leukopenia has been recorded.[304,307,503] The platelet count is normal[304,307,315, 325,331,415,464,499,533,566,758,762,765,767] or slightly increased,[763] the osmotic fragility is normal,[59,299,306,308,309,380,464,503,759,761,764,767] or fragility may be slightly increased.[293,415,533] The results of the autohemolysis test have been variable: in some type I autohemolysis,[533] and in others mixed or atypical patterns[293,415,464] are observed. Autohemolysis may also be normal.[306,464,535] In one case abnormal sideroblasts were present in the bone marrow[304] but usually marrow examination is unremarkable.

In a few instances splenic sequestration studies have been carried out by labeling the patient's cells with ^{51}Cr and counting over the liver and spleen. Liver/spleen ratios of approximately unity have been observed,[331,464,533,535,761,768] but in one patient a 1:3 ratio was measured and splenectomy was successful.[415] In this patient coexistent hereditary spherocytosis may also have been present, however.

Frequently the red cell enzyme activities of heterozygotes for these variants are normal.[59,331,464,769] This is true because the life span of the affected cells is very short, and thus most of the cells remaining in the circulation are normal.[770]

2.5. Diagnosis

The first method to be developed for the diagnosis of what we now recognize to be G-6-PD deficiency consisted of the incubation of red cells with acetylphenylhydrazine for 4 hr, followed by microscopic examination of the erythrocytes (Fig. 4). In this system most normal erythrocytes form only one or two large Heinz bodies; ordinarily less than 30% of the red cells from normal donors form five or more inclusions. In contrast, over 40% of G-6-PD-deficient cells form many small Heinz bodies. This procedure is neither practical nor, by current standards, reliable. Many factors, including the hematocrit and the degree of oxygenation of the blood,[42] influence the results. Furthermore, positive tests may be encountered in defects other than G-6-PD deficiency such as unstable hemoglobins.

The first biochemical method for the detection of G-6-PD deficiency was the GSH stability test.[771] In this procedure whole blood is incubated with acetylphenylhydrazine, and the disappearance of GSH is measured. Although more reliable and technically less capricious than the Heinz body test, this procedure has largely been superseded by more direct measurement of enzyme activity. False positive results may be obtained in the blood of newborns because of the exhaustion of the endogenous supply of glucose,[772] and in patients with hemoglobin E-thalassemia disease.[773] Although much less sensitive to oxygenation than the Heinz body test, GSH instability can be induced in normal samples incubated with acetylphenyldrazine by subjecting them to continuous oxygenation.[51,774] With G-6-PD Aarhus, anomalous GSH stability data have unaccountably been observed when ACD, but not when heparin or EDTA, was used as an anticoagulant.[775]

Many direct assay methods for the measurement of G-6-PD activity have been described. Most of these depend on the increased absorbance at 340 nm which occurs as NADP$^+$ is reduced to NADPH.[61,743,776–780] A colorimetric method in which the reduction of NADPH is linked to dichloroendophenol[781] and fluorometric techniques[782–784] have also been described.

With customary methods for assay of G-6-PD more than 1 mole of NADP$^+$ is reduced for each mole of glucose-6-phosphate oxidized; the 6-phosphogluconate formed in the G-6-PD reaction serves as substrate for 6-phosphogluconate dehydrogenase (6-PGD) in the hemolysate so that additional NADP$^+$ is reduced. The assay results are therefore affected not only by the level of G-6-PD but also by that of 6-PGD. Glock and McLean[776] described two methods for circumventing this source of inaccuracy. In one of these an excess of purified 6-PGD is added to the reaction system. In the second and more commonly used technique, an excess of 6-phosphogluconate is added to both the assay system and the blank. Effects of the 6-PGD reaction, which proceeds at its maximal rate in both cuvettes, are therefore canceled, and the results reflect the activity of G-6-PD alone. Although this procedure theoretically estimates G-6-PD activity more accurately than the usual type of G-6-PD assay, it is not suitable for measurement of G-6-PD activity in deficient samples. This is true because the procedure actually measures the activity of G-6-PD plus 6-PGD minus 6-PGD activity. When the activity of 6-PGD is much higher than that of G-6-PD, minor experimental differences in 6-PGD activity produce exaggerated changes in the calculated G-6-PD activity. Another novel method for the accurate measurement of G-6-PD activity is to inhibit 6-PGD activity with high concentrations of 2,3-DPG.[779]

Many procedures designed to screen for G-6-PD deficiency have been described. The reduction of a number of dyes can be linked to the reduction of NADP$^+$ through NADPH diaphorase, which is normally present in hemolysates. The first such method utilized brilliant cresyl blue as the receptor dye.[785] This relatively simple technique, widely used for many years, has several disadvantages. Brilliant cresyl blue is autooxidizable, and it is therefore necessary to shield the mixture from air by adding mineral oil. Furthermore, the rate of decolorization differs greatly with different lots of dye.[786] Tests utilizing methylene blue,[787,788] dichloroendophenol,[786,789,790] or a tetrazolium derivative[791] have therefore been introduced. Since leukomethylene blue is selectively absorbed by the erythrocyte, the rate of removal of color from the suspending solution[792,793] or the staining of the erythrocytes[794] can form the basis for detection of G-6-PD deficiency.

Linking G-6-PD activity to the reduction of methemoglobin through a dye has also served as a basis for a screening technique for the detection of G-6-PD deficiency. The methemoglobin reduction test is carried out by incubating blood with nitrite, which oxidizes hemoglobin to methemoglobin, and with methylene blue, which catalyzes its reduction to hemoglobin.[795] Normal samples reduce methemoglobin to hemoglobin in such a system; G-6-PD-deficient samples lack this capacity. False positive results are a common problem,[796] particularly if the blood samples have been stored for more than a few hours.

The ascorbate–cyanide test[587,588] depends on the detoxification of hydrogen peroxide by normal red blood cells. In this test catalase is inhibited by cyanide, and the interaction of ascorbate with hemoglobin generates hydrogen peroxide. In the absence of adequate G-6-PD activity peroxide causes the oxidative denaturation of hemoglobin to brownish pigments, while normal samples detoxify the hydrogen peroxide through the glutathione peroxidase pathway. The disadvantages of this system include its lack of specificity and its requirement of relatively large volumes of blood. False positive results are obtained with unstable hemoglobins, glutathione deficiency, and even with abnormalities such as pyruvate kinase deficiency.[797]

A relatively unique method for the detection of G-6-PD deficiency depends on the inhibition of glutathione reductase by chromate.[798] Chromate inhibition of this enzyme depends on the generation of NADPH,[799] and therefore does not occur in G-6-PD-deficient cells.

The most simple, reliable, and specific screening method for the detection of G-6-PD deficiency is the fluorescent spot test.[800] This technique depends on the fact that NADPH fluoresces in long-wave ultraviolet light whereas $NADP^+$ does not. Blood is added to a reaction mixture consisting of saponin to lyse the red cells, glucose-6-phosphate, $NADP^+$, and buffer. After 5 or 10 min of incubation the mixture is spotted on filter paper, allowed to dry, and examined under long-wave ultraviolet light. The sensitivity of the method may be increased by incorporating GSSG into the reaction mixture[801]; when GSSG is present, small amounts of NADPH which may be formed by the residual G-6-PD in mildly deficient

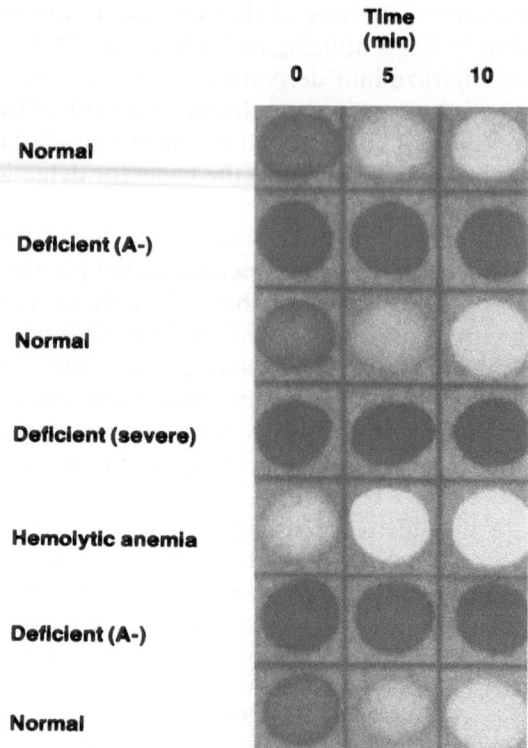

FIGURE 13. The fluorescent spot screening test for G-6-PD deficiency. Ten microliters of blood was added to 100 μl of screening solution[813] and allowed to stand for 5 and 10 min at room temperature before spotting on Whatman #1 filter paper. The paper was photographed under long-wave ultraviolet light through a Tiffin aero #2 yellow filter.

samples are reoxidized by the glutathione reductase reaction. This technique has been extensively used,[546,802–809,814] and has proven highly reliable for the detection of G-6-PD deficiency; it has been automated.[466,784,810,811] The test is very specific, and detection of G-6-PD levels lower than about 50% of normal is consistently achieved without appreciable numbers of false positive or false negative results (Fig. 13). Blood dried on filter paper[804–806,813,814] or stored for several weeks[800] is satisfactory for testing.

The detection of G-6-PD deficiency in normal males poses no problems; in females, however, or in any patient who has recently experienced a hemolytic reaction, serious problems in the detection of G-6-PD deficiency may arise. Heterozygotes for G-6-PD deficiency have two red cell populations, normal red cells and G-6-PD-deficient cells,[51,52] and the proportions of normal and deficient cells may vary greatly.[815,816] Detection methods that depend on the lysis of red cells and the estimation of average red cell G-6-PD activity, either quantitatively or by a screening method, do not have the capacity to identify those subjects who have less than 60% abnormal cells.[797] Detection of such individuals requires reliance upon specially designed techniques. The first of these to be developed[816] depends on measurement of the rate of methemoglobin reduction in the presence of Nile blue sulfate, a dye that catalyzes NADPH-linked methemoglobin reduction but which does not permit interaction to occur between normal and G-6-PD-deficient cells.[427] Combination of this technique with the histochemical detection of red cells containing methemoglobin by the method of Kleihauer and Betke[817] provides another method for the detection of G-6-PD-deficient heterozygotes.[818] The interaction of hemoglobin with the tetrazolium dye MTT can also be used for this purpose.[819,820] A cytochemical method[821] which purported to measure G-6-PD directly using a tetrazolium derivative probably does not measure G-6-PD activity at all, since these dyes react directly with hemoglobin. The ascorbate–cyanide test[587,797] and the chromate inhibition method,[797] which depend on the behavior of each red cell as an independent metabolic unit, appear to be more sensitive than other screening procedures in the detection of heterozygotes for G-6-PD deficiency. It has been proposed that measurement of the ratio of G-6-PD activity to that of 6-phosphogluconate dehydrogenase might be useful in the detection of the heterozygous state.[822] This suggestion assumes that this maneuver corrects for differences in red cell age. There is no reason to suppose, however, that this technique is useful, because the problem of heterozygote detection has little to do with cell age. Moreover, 6-phosphogluconate dehydrogenase is one of the less age-sensitive enzymes.

Hemolysis in persons with G-6-PD A− and some of the other more mildly deficient variants characteristically results in destruction of the older, more enzyme-deficient erythrocytes; remaining in the circulation are the younger red cells which are likely to have normal or near-normal G-6-PD activity. In such instances centrifugation of the blood and the application of screening procedures to the bottom, older layer of cells appear to be very useful.[803,807] Quantitative G-6-PD assays of red cells of such patients usually show that activity is at the lower limits of normal in the presence of a reticulocytosis or when the activity of age-dependent enzymes such as hexokinase or glutamate oxaloacetate transaminase is considerably increased. This finding suggests that the patient is actually G-6-PD-deficient. Family studies may also be quite helpful in patients with hemolysis in whom the existence of G-6-PD deficiency is supected.

2.6. Treatment

G-6-PD-deficient individuals should not be given drugs which precipitate hemolysis. It is doubtful that this can be accomplished by providing the patient with a list of such drugs; in the stressful circumstances which surround illness he is likely to forget admonitions given in the distant past. If a list of drugs is provided, it should at least be a sensible one, and should not include agents such as aspirin, which he knows from his own experience to be harmless. When the patient's own experience has taught him that he can ingest many of the proscribed drugs with impunity, doubt is cast upon the importance of avoiding any of the drugs on the list. Patients belonging to cultures in which fava beans are a common dietary constituent should be warned against eating them. Children who have eaten the beans without harm may have an attack of favism following a later meal. On the other hand, G-6-PD-deficient adults who have eaten fava beans many times without untoward effects may probably continue to enjoy them safely.

Primary responsibility for the avoidance of hemolytic drugs rests with the physician. Many of the potentially most harmful drugs—e.g., nitrofurantoin, primaquine, and sulfapyridine—are obtainable only on prescription, and it is prudent to test patients for G-6-PD deficiency before prescribing them. It is as important for the physician to recognize that some drugs are innocuous as it is that he be cognizant of those that are hemolytic. The G-6-PD-deficient patient should not be deprived of the benefits of therapy with sulfonamides such as Gantrisin, which are not hemolytic. There is no reason to deny the G-6-PD-deficient patient with malaria the advantages of chloroquine therapy. Even primaquine can be given to the individual with G-6-PD A− deficiency, provided the initial dose consists of only 15 mg/day or 45 mg once or twice weekly[628] and the blood count is monitored.

Little can be done to avoid hemolytic episodes incidental to infection. Yet awareness that they are related to G-6-PD deficiency will obviate unnecessary diagnostic measures. When severe jaundice appears in infectious hepatitis, knowledge that a patient is G-6-PD-deficient has significant effect on the physician's appraisal of the prognosis.

When hemolytic episodes are very severe transfusion may be required. The use of blood transfusion has been effective in reducing the high mortality once observed in children with favism. Similarly, hemolysis due to infection or drug ingestion may necessitate transfusion in persons with severe types of G-6-PD deficiency; the need for transfusion should rarely arise in persons with G-6-PD A−. Exchange transfusion may be indicated in infants with severely deficient G-6-PD variants when the serum bilirubin rises to very high levels, since kernicterus may occur (see Section 2.4.2.5). The same criteria which are applied to infants with ABO or Rh incompatibility seem appropriate for the G-6-PD-deficient infant. Care should be taken to use nondeficient blood for exchange purposes. Phenobarbital has been alleged to lessen the degree of hyperbilirubinemia.[823,824] Phototherapy has also been advocated as a treatment modality.[825]

Effective treatment for patients with class 1 variants, those that cause nonspherocytic hemolytic anemia, is not available. Splenectomy occasionally appears to be beneficial. In 1969, a review of over 40 cases of G-6-PD deficiency revealed that in 12 patients in whom splenectomy had been carried out,[415] improvement was observed in only 4 cases. In additional cases which have been reported there has been a possible response in five patients[298,330,333,759,826] and no response in an additional five patients from three families.[307,331] In one case the response was undetermined.[329] An excellent response to splenectomy was observed in one father and son with the Mediterranean type of G-6-PD deficiency. The fact that the red cells of these two patients had a marked increase in osmotic fragility raised the question of whether they also had hereditary spherocytosis, but the overall interpretation of this family is by no means clear.[415] Corticosteroids were administered to four patients with nonspherocytic hemolytic anemia, apparently before the existence of G-6-PD deficiency had been established. None appeared to benefit.[296,325,582,761] One patient was also given 6-mercaptopurine.[296] Folate, which is given in other hemolytic anemias, may be prescribed. Transfusion is rarely needed.

A number of therapies for G-6-PD deficiency have been attempted experimentally, all without success. The possibility that xylitol[827] or isocitrate[828] may be useful as a substrate for $NADP^+$ reduction has been proposed, but the results of clinical studies with xylitol with and without added riboflavin have been discouraging.[169,830] Administration of nicotinic acid increases NAD^+ levels but has little effect on $NADP^+$; the hope that it might stabilize some unstable variants of G-6-PD was not realized.[831] The possibility that EDTA administration might be helpful in the treatment of G-6-PD deficiency has been mentioned,[832] but studies in animal systems provide no encouragement for this approach.[661]

Genetic counseling may be useful in cases of G-6-PD variants associated with hereditary nonspherocytic anemia. The clinical consequences of other variants are sufficiently mild that genetic advice is of little value. Community-wide screening for G-6-PD deficiency is likely to produce more anxiety and harm than good. Blood bank screening for G-6-PD deficiency, advocated by some,[117,435] would be counterproductive[437] (see Section 2.4.1.1).

References

1.   MUEHLENS,P., 1926, DIE BEHANDLUNG DER NATURLICHEN MENSCHLICHEN MALARIA-INFEKTION MIT PLASMOCHIN. NATURWISSENSCHAFTEN 14:1162-1166

2.   CORDES,W., 1926, EXPERIENCES WITH PLASMOCHIN IN MALARIA. UNITED FRUIT CO. (MED. DEPT.) 15TH ANNUAL REPORT, 66-71, BOSTON

3.   CORDES,W., 1927, OBSERVATIONS ON THE TOXIC EFFECT OF PLASMOCHIN. UNITED FRUIT CO. (MED. DEPT.) 16TH ANNUAL REPORT, 62-67, BOSTON

4.   CORDES,W., 1928, ZWISCHENFALLE BEI DER PLASMOCHINBEHANDLUNG. ARCH SCHIFFS UND TROPEN HYG 32:143-148

5.   EISELBERG,K.P., 1927, POISONING (PLASMOCHIN): 2 CASES. WIEN KLIN WOCHENSCHR 40:525

6.   BROSIUS,O.T., 1927, PLASMOCHIN IN MALARIA. UNITED FRUIT CO. (MED. DEPT.) 16TH ANNUAL REPORT, 26-53

7.   BROSIUS,O.T., 1928, PLASMOCHIN IN MALARIA. UNITED FRUIT CO. (MED. DEPT.) 17TH ANNUAL REPORT, 51-70

8.   PALMA,M.D., 1928, PLASMOCHIN THERAPY IN MALARIA. RIFORMA MD 44:753-756

9.   NAMIKAWA,H., 1928, SYMPTOMS OF POISONING IN THE TREATMENT OF MALARIA. TAIWAN IGAKKAI ZASSHI 284:1298-1305

10. MENK,W., 1928, COMBINED QUININE AND PLASMOCHIN TREATMENT FOR MALARIA IN HAITIAN NEGROES. UNITED FRUIT CO. (MED. DEPT.) 16TH ANNUAL REPORT, 78:81

11. ROSKOTT,E.R.A. AND SENO,R., 1928, EXPERIENCE OF PLASMOCHIN. GENESK TIJDSCHR NED INDIE 68:80-98

12. KLIGLER,I.F. AND REITLER,R., 1929, STUDIES IN MALARIA. IV. PROPHYLACTIC USE OF PLASMOCHIN IN A BEDOUIN POPULATION. RIV MALARIOL 8:28-33

13. MANAI,A., 1929, ITTERO DA PLASMOCHINA. POLICLINICO (SEZ PRAT) 36:1215-1217

14. BAERMANN,G. AND SMITS,E., 1929, UEBER PLASMOCHIN. II. MITTEILUNG. ARCH SCHIFFS UND TROPEN HYG 33:24-37

15. FREIMAN,M., 1929, PLASMOQUINE AND PLASMOQUINE COMPOUND IN THE TREATMENT OF MALARIA. J TROP MED HYG 32:165-169

16. MANIFOLD,J.A., 1931, REPORT ON A TRIAL OF PLASMOQUINE AND QUININE IN THE TREATMENT OF BENIGN TERTIAN MALARIA. J ROY ARMY MED CORPS 56:321-338

17. MISSIROLI,A. AND MARINO,P., 1934, ANWENDUNG DES CHINOPLASMIN
     ZUR MALARIASANIERUNG. ARCH SCHIFFS UND TROPEN HYG 38:1-16

18. AMY,A.C., 1934, HEMOGLOBINURIA: A NEW PROBLEM ON THE INDIAN
     FRONTIER. J ROY ARMY MED CORPS 62:178-191, 269-278, 318-
     329

19. FICACCI,L., 1935, EMOGLOBINURIA DA PLASMOCHINA. POLICLINICO
     (SEZ PRAT) 42:136-139

20. SEIN,M., 1937, CASE OF HEMOGLOBINURIA CAUSED BY PLASMOCHIN,
     TAKEN AS PROPHYLACTIC AGAINST MALARIA. INDIAN MED GAZ 72:86-
     87

21. MANN,W.N., 1943, HAEMOGLOBINURIA FOLLOWING THE ADMINISTRATION
     OF PLASMOQUINE. TRANS R SOC TROP MED HYG 37:151-155

22. SMITH,S., 1943, NOTE REGARDING HEMOGLOBINURIA FOLLOWING
     THE ADMINISTRATION OF PLASMOCHIN. TRANS R SOC TROP MED HYG
     37:155-156

23. BRAUN,K. AND DE VRIES,A., 1944, PLASMOCHIN AND QUININE AS
     THE CAUSE OF ACUTE HAEMOLYTIC ANAEMIA. HAREFUAH 27:219-
     221

24. WEST,J.B. AND HENDERSON,A.B., 1944, PLASMOCHIN INTOXICATION.
     BULL US ARMY MED DEPT 82:87

25. SWANTZ,H.E. AND BAYLISS,M., 1945, HEMOGLOBINURIA. REPORT
     OF 10 CASES OF ITS OCCURRENCE IN NEGROES DURING CONVALESCENCE
     FROM MALARIA. WAR MED 7:104-107

26. HARDGROVE,M. AND APPLEBAUM,I.L., 1946, PLASMOCHIN TOXICITY:
     ANALYSIS OF 258 CASES. ANN INTERN MED 25:103-112

27. DIMSON,S.B. AND MC MARTIN,R.B., 1946, PAMAQUINE
     HAEMOGLOBINURIA. Q J MED 15:25-46

28. LOEB,R.F., 1946, ACTIVITY OF A NEW ANTIMALARIAL AGENT,
     PENTAQUINE (SN-13,276). STATEMENT APPROVED BY THE BOARD
     FOR COORDINATION OF MALARIAL STUDIES. JAMA 132:321-323

29. AICHLEY,J.A., YOUNT,E.H., HUSTED,J.R., PULLMAN,T.N.,
     ALVING,A.S. AND EICHELBERGER,L., 1948, REACTIONS OBSERVED
     DURING TREATMENT WITH PENTAQUINE, ADMINISTERED WITH QUINACRINE
     (ATABRINE) METACHLORIDNE (SN-11,437) AND WITH SULFADIAZINE.
     J NATL MALARIA SOC 7:118-124

30. TURCHETTI,A., 1948, FORME POCO FREQUENTI DI EMOGLOBINURIA
     DA FARMACI IN CORSO DI INFEZIONE MALARICA. RIFORMA MD
     62:325-328

31. KENG,K.L., 1948, EEN GEVAL VAN ZWARTWATERKOORTS MET CYANOSE
     (METHAEMOGLOBINAEMIA), WAARSCHIJNLIJK DOOR PLASMOCHINE.
     MED MAANDBL 1:342-347

32. EARLE JR,D.P., BIGELOW,F.S., ZUBRED,C.G. AND KANE,C.A.,
     1948, STUDIES ON THE CHEMOTHERAPY ON THE HUMAN MALARIAS.
     IX. EFFECT OF PRIMAQUINE ON THE BLOOD CELLS OF MAN. J CLIN
     INVEST 27:121-129

33. MER,G., BIRNBAUM,D. AND KLIGLER,I.J., 1940, LYSIS OF BLOOD
OF MALARIA PATIENTS BY BILE OR BILE SALTS. TRANS R SOC TROP
MED HYG 34:373-378

34. COATNEY,G.R., COOPER,W.C., EYLES,D.E., CULWELL,W.V.,
WHITE,W.C. AND LINTS,H.A., 1950, STUDIES IN HUMAN MALARIA.
XXVII. OBSERVATIONS ON THE USE OF PENTAQUINE IN THE PREVENTION
AND TREATMENT OF CHESSON STRAIN VIVAX MALARIA. J NATL
MALARIA SOC 9:222-232

35. FELDMAN,H.A., PACKER,H., MURPHY,F.D. AND WATSON,R.B., 1947,
PAMAQUINE NAPHTHOATE AS A PROPHYLACTIC FOR MALARIAL
INFECTIONS. J CLIN INVEST 26:77-86

36. JONES JR,R., JACKSON,L.S., DI LORENZO,A., MARX,R.L.,
LEVY,B.L., KENNY,E.C., GILBERT,M., JOHNSTON,N.N. AND
ALVING,A.S., 1953, KOREAN VIVAX MALARIA. III. CURATIVE
EFFECT AND TOXICITY OF PRIMAQUINE IN DOSES FROM 10-30 MG/D.
AM J TROP MED HYG 2:977-982

37. ZYLMANN,G., 1944, IN VITRO UND IN VIVO VERSUCHE UEBER DIE
HAEMOLYTISCHEN EIGENSCHAFTEN DER SYNTHETISCHEN MALARIAMITTEL.
DEUT TROPENMED ZTSCHR 48:7-18

38. BIRNBAUM,D., GOLDBLUM,N. AND KLIGLER,I.J., 1946, FURTHER
OBSERVATIONS ON THE ENHANCED FRAGILITY OF RED CELLS IN
MALARIA PATIENTS. ACTA MED ORIENT 5:177-184

39. EDGCOMB,J.H., ARNOLD,J., YOUNT,E.H., ALVING,A.S. AND
EICHELBERGER,L., 1950, PRIMAQUINE, SN 13272, A NEW CURATIVE
AGENT IN VIVAX MALARIA: A PRELIMINARY REPORT. J NATL MALARIA
SOC 9:285-292

40. DERN,R.J., WEINSTEIN,I.M., LE ROY,G.V., TALMAGE,D.W. AND
ALVING,A.S., 1954, THE HEMOLYTIC EFFECT OF PRIMAQUINE. I.
THE LOCALIZATION OF THE DRUG- INDUCED HEMOLYTIC DEFECT IN
PRIMAQUINE-SENSITIVE INDIVIDUALS. J LAB CLIN MED 43:303-
309

41. BEUTLER,E., DERN,R.J. AND ALVING,A.S., 1954, THE HEMOLYTIC
EFFECT OF PRIMAQUINE. III. A STUDY OF PRIMAQUINE-SENSITIVE
ERYTHROCYTES. J LAB CLIN MED 44:177-184

42. BEUTLER,E., DERN,R.J. AND ALVING,A.S., 1955, THE HEMOLYTIC
EFFECT OF PRIMAQUINE. VI. AN IN VITRO TEST FOR SENSITIVITY
OF ERYTHROCYTES TO PRIMAQUINE. J LAB CLIN MED 45:40-50

43. BEUTLER,E., DERN,R.J., FLANAGAN,C.L. AND ALVING,A.S., 1955,
THE HEMOLYTIC EFFECT OF PRIMAQUINE. VII. BIOCHEMICAL STUDIES
OF DRUG-SENSITIVE ERYTHROCYTES. J LAB CLIN MED 45:286-295

44. BEUTLER,E., 1957, THE GLUTATHIONE INSTABILITY OF DRUG-
SENSITIVE RED CELLS. A NEW METHOD FOR THE IN VITRO DETECTION
OF DRUG-SENSITIVITY. J LAB CLIN MED 49:84-94

45. CARSON,P.E., FLANAGAN,C.L., ICKES,C.E. AND ALVING,A.S.,
1956, ENZYMATIC DEFICIENCY IN PRIMAQUINE-SENSITIVE
ERYTHROCYTES. SCIENCE 124:484-485

46. WALLER,H.D., LOEHR,G.W. AND TABATABAI,M., 1957, HAEMOLYSE
    UND FEHLEN VON GLUCOSE-6-PHOSPHAT-DEHYDROGENASE IN ROTEN
    BLUTZELLEN (EINE FERMENTANOMALIE DER ERYTHROCYTEN). KLIN
    WOCHENSCHR 35:1022-1027

47. CHILDS,B., ZINKHAM,W., BROWNE,E.A., KIMBRO,E.L. AND
    TORBERT,J.V., 1958, A GENETIC STUDY OF A DEFECT IN GLUTATHIONE
    METABOLISM OF THE ERYTHROCYTE. JOHNS HOPKINS MED J 102:21-
    37

48. OHNO,S., KAPLAN,W.D. AND KINOSITA,R., 1959, FORMATION OF
    THE SEX CHROMATIN BY A SINGLE X-CHROMOSOME IN LIVER CELLS
    OF RATTUS NORVEGICUS. EXP CELL RES 18:415-418

49. BROWN,S.W., 1966, HETEROCHROMATIN. SCIENCE 151:417-425

50. BEUTLER,E., 1962, BIOCHEMICAL ABNORMALITIES ASSOCIATED WITH
    HEMOLYTIC STATES. MECHANISMS OF ANEMIA IN MAN WEINSTEIN,I.
    AND BEUTLER,E. ED. 195, MC GRAW-HILL, NEW YORK

51. BEUTLER,E., YEH,M. AND FAIRBANKS,V.F., 1962, THE NORMAL
    HUMAN FEMALE AS A MOSAIC OF X-CHROMOSOME ACTIVITY: STUDIES
    USING THE GENE FOR G-6-PD DEFICIENCY AS A MARKER. PROC NATL
    ACAD SCI USA 48:9-16

52. BEUTLER,E. AND BALUDA,M.C., 1964, THE SEPARATION OF GLUCOSE-
    6-PHOSPHATE DEHYDROGENASE-DEFICIENT ERYTHROCYTES FROM THE
    BLOOD OF HETEROZYGOTES FOR GLUCOSE-6-PHOSPHATE DEHYDROGENASE
    DEFICIENCY. LANCET 1:189-192

53. LYON,M.F., 1962, SEX CHROMATIN AND GENE ACTION IN THE
    MAMMALIAN X-CHROMOSOME. AM J HUM GENET 14:135-148

54. SZEINBERG,A., SHEBA,C. AND ADAM,A., 1958, ENZYMATIC
    ABNORMALITY IN ERYTHROCYTES OF A POPULATION SENSITIVE TO
    VICIA FABA OR DRUG INDUCED HEMOLYTIC ANEMIA. NATURE 181:1256

55. SZEINBERG,A., SHEBA,C., HIRSHORN,N. AND BODONYI,E., 1957,
    STUDIES ON ERYTHROCYTES IN CASES WITH PAST HISTORY OF FAVISM
    AND DRUG-INDUCED ACUTE HEMOLYTIC ANEMIA. BLOOD 12:603-613

56. MARKS,P.A. AND GROSS,R.T., 1959, ERYTHROCYTE GLUCOSE-6-
    PHOSPHATE DEHYDROGENASE DEFICIENCY: EVIDENCE OF DIFFERENCES
    BETWEEN NEGROES AND CAUCASIANS WITH RESPECT TO THIS
    GENETICALLY DETERMINED TRAIT. J CLIN INVEST 38:2253-2262

57. BOYER,S.H., PORTER,I.H. AND WEILBACHER,R.G., 1962,
    ELECTROPHORETIC HETEROGENEITY OF GLUCOSE-6-PHOSPHATE
    DEHYDROGENASE AND ITS RELATIONSHIP TO ENZYME DEFICIENCY IN
    MAN. PROC NATL ACAD SCI USA 48:1868-1876

58. KIRKMAN,H.N. AND HENDRICKSON,E.M., 1963, SEX-LINKED
    ELECTROPHORETIC DIFFERENCE IN GLUCOSE-6-PHOSPHATE
    DEHYDROGENASE. AM J HUM GENET 15:241-258

59. NEWTON JR,W.A. AND BASS,J.C., 1958, GLUTATHIONE SENSITIVE
    CHRONIC NON-SPHEROCYTIC HEMOLYTIC ANEMIA. AM J DIS CHILD
    96:501-502

60.   KIRKMAN,H.N., RILEY JR,H.D. AND CROWELL,B.B., 1960, DIFFERENT
      ENZYMIC EXPRESSIONS OF MUTANTS OF HUMAN GLUCOSE-6-PHOSPHATE
      DEHYDROGENASE. PROC NATL ACAD SCI USA 46:938-944

61.   BETKE,K., BEUTLER,E., BREWER,G.J., KIRKMAN,H.N., LUZZATTO,L.,
      MOTULSKY,A.G., RAMOT,B. AND SINISCALCO,M., 1967,
      STANDARDIZATION OF PROCEDURES FOR THE STUDY OF GLUCOSE-6-
      PHOSPHATE DEHYDROGENASE. REPORT OF A WHO SCIENTIFIC GROUP.
      WHO TECH REP SER NO. 366

62.   YOSHIDA,A., 1967, A SINGLE AMINO ACID SUBSTITUTION (ASPARAGINE
      TO ASPARTIC ACID) BETWEEN NORMAL (B+) AND THE COMMON NEGRO
      VARIANT (A+) OF HUMAN GLUCOSE-6-PHOSPHATE DEHYDROGENASE.
      PROC NATL ACAD SCI USA 57:835-840

63.   YOSHIDA,A., 1970, AMINO ACID SUBSTITUTION (HISTIDINE TO
      TYROSINE) IN A GLUCOSE-6-PHOSPHATE DEHYDROGENASE VARIANT
      (G6PD HEKTOEN) ASSOCIATED WITH OVERPRODUCTION. J MOL BIOL
      52:483-490

64.   MARKS,P.A. AND GROSS,R.T., 1959, FURTHER CHARACTERIZATION
      OF THE ENZYMATIC DEFECT IN ERYTHROCYTE GLUCOSE-6-PHOSPHATE
      DEHYDROGENASE DEFICIENCY. A GENETICALLY DETERMINED TRAIT.
      J CLIN INVEST 38:1023-1024

65.   ADAM,A., 1961, LINKAGE BETWEEN DEFICIENCY OF GLUCOSE-6-
      PHOSPHATE DEHYDROGENASE AND COLOUR-BLINDNESS. NATURE 189:686

66.   KALMUS,H., 1962, DISTANCE AND SEQUENCE OF THE LOCI FOR
      PROTAN AND DEUTAN DEFECTS AND FOR GLUCOSE-6-PHOSPHATE
      DEHYDROGENASE DEFICIENCY. NATURE 194:214-215

67.   SINISCALCO,M. AND FILIPPI,G., 1964, RECOMBINATION BETWEEN
      PROTAN AND DEUTAN GENES; DATA ON THEIR RELATIVE POSITIONS
      IN RESPECT OF THE G6PD LOCUS. NATURE 204:1062-1064

68.   PORTER,I.H., SCHULZE,J. AND MC KUSICK,V.A., 1962, GENETICAL
      LINKAGE BETWEEN THE LOCI FOR GLUCOSE-6-PHOSPHATE DEHYDROGENASE
      DEFICIENCY AND COLOUR-BLINDNESS IN AMERICAN NEGROES. ANN
      HUM GENET 26:107-122

69.   MC KUSICK,V.A. AND RUDDLE,F.H., 1977, THE STATUS OF THE
      GENE MAP OF THE HUMAN CHROMOSOMES. SCIENCE 196:390-405

70.   PRASAD,A.S., TRANCHIDA,L., KONNO,E.T., BERMAN,L., ALBERT,S.,
      SING,C. AND BREWER,G.J., 1968, HEREDITARY SIDEROBLASTIC
      ANEMIA AND GLUCOSE-6-PHOSPHATE DEHYDROGENASE DEFICIENCY IN
      A NEGRO FAMILY. J CLIN INVEST 47:1415-1424

71.   ADAM,A., SHEBA,C., RACE,R.R., SANGER,R., TIPPETT,P.,
      HAMPER,J. AND GAVIN,J., 1962, LINKAGE RELATIONS OF THE X-
      BORNE GENES RESPONSIBLE FOR GLUCOSE-6-PHOSPHATE DEHYDROGENASE
      AND FOR THE XG BLOOD-GROUPS. LANCET 1:1188-1189

72.   SINISCALCO,M., FILIPPI,G., LATTE,B., PIOMELLI,S., RATTAZZI,M.,
      GAVIN,J., SANGER,R. AND RACE,R.R., 1966, FAILURE TO DETECT
      LINKAGE BETWEEN XG AND OTHER X-BORNE LOCI IN SARDINIANS.
      ANN HUM GENET 29:231-252

73. ZATZ,M., ITSKAN,S.B., SANGER,R., FROTA-PRESSOA,O. AND
SALDANHA,P.H., 1974, NEW LINKAGE DATA FOR THE X-LINKED
TYPES OF MUSCULAR DYSTROPHY AND G6PD VARIANTS, COLOUR
BLINDNESS, AND XG BLOOD GROUPS. J MED GENET 11:321-327

74. ADAM,A., SHEBA,C., SANGER,R. AND RACE,R.R., 1966, THE
LINKAGE RELATION OF G6PD TO XG. AM J HUM GENET 18:110
(LETTERS TO THE EDITOR)

75. RACE,R.R. AND SANGER,R., 1975, XG AND X-CHROMOSOME MAPPING.
BLOOD GROUPS IN MAN CHAPTER 29:594-618, BLACKWELL SCIENTIFIC,
OXFORD, LONDON

76. FRANCKE,U., BAKAY,B., CONNOR,J.D., COLDWELL,J.G. AND
NYHAN,W.L., 1974, LINKAGE RELATIONSHIPS OF X-LINKED ENZYMES
GLUCOSE-6-PHOSPHATE DEHYDROGENASE AND HYPOXANTHINE GUANINE
PHOSPHORIBOSYLTRANSFERASE: RECOMBINATION IN FEMALE OFFSPRING
OF COMPOUND HETEROZYGOTES. AM J HUM GENET 26:512-522

77. TRUJILLO,J., FAIRBANKS,V.F., OHNO,S. AND BEUTLER,E., 1961,
CHROMOSOMAL CONSTITUTION IN GLUCOSE-6-PHOSPHATE-DEHYDROGENASE
DEFICIENCY. LANCET 2:1454-1455

78. MC GOVERN,J.J., ISSELBACHER,K., ROSE,P.J. AND GROSSMAN,M.S.,
1958, OBSERVATIONS ON THE GLUTATHIONE (GSH) STABILITY OF
RED BLOOD CELLS. AM J DIS CHILD 96:502

79. GROSS,R.T., HURWITZ,R.E. AND MARKS,P.A., 1958, AN HEREDITARY
ENZYMATIC DEFECT IN ERYTHROCYTE METABOLISM: GLUCOSE-6-
PHOSPHATE DEHYDROGENASE DEFICIENCY. J CLIN INVEST 37:1176-
1184

80. GARTLER,S.M., LISKAY,R.M., CAMPBELL,B.K., SPARKES,R. AND
GANT,N., 1972, EVIDENCE FOR TWO FUNCTIONAL X CHROMOSOMES
IN HUMAN OOCYTES. CELL DIFFERENTIATION 1:215-218

81. BREWER,G.J., GALL,J.C., HONEYMAN,M., GERSHOWITZ,H.,
SCHREFFLER,D.C., DERN,R.J. AND HAMES,C., 1967, INHERITANCE
OF QUANTITATIVE EXPRESSION OF ERYTHROCYTE GLUCOSE-6-PHOSPHATE
DEHYDROGENASE ACTIVITY IN THE NEGRO - A TWIN STUDY. BIOCHEM
GENET 1:41-53

82. GARTLER,S.M. AND LINDER,D., 1964, DEVELOPMENTAL AND
EVOLUTIONARY IMPLICATIONS OF THE MOSAIC NATURE OF THE G-6-
PD SYSTEM. COLD SPRING HARBOR SYMP QUANT BIOL 29:253-260

83. GARTLER,S.M. AND SPARKES,R.S., 1963, THE LYON-BEUTLER
HYPOTHESIS AND ISOCHROMOSOME X PATIENTS WITH THE TURNER
SYNDROME. LANCET 2:411

84. BEUTLER,E., 1964, THE DISTRIBUTION OF GENE PRODUCTS AMONG
POPULATIONS OF CELLS IN HETEROZYGOUS HUMANS. COLD SPRING
HARBOR SYMP QUANT BIOL 29:261-271

85. NYHAN,W.L., BAKAY,B., CONNOR,J.D., MARKS,J.F. AND KEELE,D.K.,
1970, HEMIZYGOUS EXPRESSION OF GLUCOSE-6-PHOSPHATE
DEHYDROGENASE IN ERYTHROCYTES OF HETEROZYGOTES FOR THE
LESCH-NYHAN SYNDROME. PROC NATL ACAD SCI USA 65:214-218

86. BEUTLER,E., COLLINS,Z. AND IRWIN,L., 1967, VALUE OF GENETIC
     VARIANTS OF GLUCOSE-6-PHOSPHATE DEHYDROGENASE IN TRACING
     THE ORIGIN OF MALIGNANT TUMORS. N ENGL J MED 276:389-391

87. DAVIDSON,R.G., NITOWSKY,H.M. AND CHILDS,B., 1963,
     DEMONSTRATION OF TWO POPULATIONS OF CELLS IN THE HUMAN
     FEMALE HETEROZYGOUS FOR GLUCOSE-6-PHOSPHATE DEHYDROGENASE
     VARIANTS. PROC NATL ACAD SCI USA 50:481-485

88. FIALKOW,P.J., 1976, CLONAL ORIGIN OF HUMAN TUMORS. BIOCHIM
     BIOPHYS ACTA 458:283-321

89. FIALKOW,P.J., 1974, THE ORIGIN AND DEVELOPMENT OF HUMAN
     TUMORS STUDIED WITH CELL MARKERS. NEW ENGL J MED 291:26-35

90. FIALKOW,P.J., 1972, USE OF GENETIC MARKERS TO STUDY CELLULAR
     ORIGIN AND DEVELOPMENT OF TUMORS IN HUMAN FEMALES. ADV
     CANCER RES 15:191-226

91. GARTLER,S.M., ZIPRKOWSKI,L., KRAKOWSKI,A., EZRA,R.,
     SZEINBERG,A. AND ADAM,A., 1966, G-6-PD MOSAICISM AS A TRACER
     IN THE STUDY OF HEREDITARY MULTIPLE TRICHOEPITHELIOMA. AM
     J HUM GENET 18:282-287

92. FIALKOW,P.J., GARTLER,S.M. AND YOSHIDA,A., 1967, CLONAL
     ORIGIN OF CHRONIC MYELOCYTIC LEUKEMIA IN MAN. PROC NATL
     ACAD SCI USA 58:1468-1471

93. ONI,S.B., OSUNKOYA,B.O. AND LUZZATTO,L., 1970, PAROXYSMAL
     NOCTURNAL HEMOGLOBINURIA: EVIDENCE FOR MONOCLONAL ORIGIN
     OF ABNORMAL RED CELLS. BLOOD 36:145-152

94. BENDITT,E.P. AND BENDITT,J.M., 1973, EVIDENCE FOR A MONOCLONAL
     ORIGIN OF HUMAN ATHEROSCLEROTIC PLAQUES. PROC NATL ACAD
     SCI USA 70:1753-1756

95. PEARSON,T.A., WANG,A., SOLEZ,K. AND HEPTINSTALL,R.H., 1975,
     CLONAL CHARACTERISTICS OF FIBROUS PLAQUES AND FATTY STREAKS
     FROM HUMAN AORTAS. AM J PATHOL 81:379-387

96. COMINGS,D.E., 1966, THE INACTIVE X CHROMOSOME. LANCET
     2:1137-1138

97. SINISCALCO,M., KLINGER,H.P., EAGLE,H., KOPROWSKI,H.,
     FUJIMOTO,W.Y. AND SEEGMILLER,J.E., 1969, EVIDENCE FOR
     INTERGENIC COMPLEMENTATION IN HYBRID CELLS DERIVED FROM
     TWO HUMAN DIPLOID STRAINS EACH CARRYING AN X-LINKED MUTATION.
     PROC NATL ACAD SCI USA 62:793-799

98. DEOL,M.S. AND WHITTEN,W.K., 1972, X-CHROMOSOME INACTIVATION.
     DOES IT OCCUR AT THE SAME TIME IN ALL CELLS OF THE EMBRYO?.
     NATURE (NEW BIOL) 240:277-278

99. HITZEROTH,H.W., BENDER,K., ROPERS,H.H. AND GEERTHSEN,J.M.P.,
     1977, TENTATIVE EVIDENCE FOR 3-4 HAEMATOPOIETIC STEM CELLS
     IN MAN. HUM GENET 35:175-183

100. VERHORST,D., 1973, POLYMORPHISM IN GLUCOSE-6-PHOSPHATE
     DEHYDROGENASE IN THE GERMAN LARGE-WHITE. ANIM BLOOD GROUPS
     BIOCHEM GENET 4:65-68

101. SMITH,J.E., RYER,K. AND WALLACE,L., 1976, GLUCOSE-6-PHOSPHATE DEHYDROGENASE DEFICIENCY IN A DOG. ENZYME 21:379-382

102. WERTH,G. AND MUELLER,G., 1967, VERERBBARER GLUCOSE-6-PHOSPHATDEHYDROGENASEMANGEL IN DEN ERYTHROCYTEN VON RATTEN. KLIN WOCHENSCHR 45:265-269

103. CHEUN,L.H., 1966, GLUCOSE-6-PHOSPHATE DEHYDROGENASE ACTIVITY IN ERYTHROCYTES OF EXPERIMENTAL ANIMALS. J CLIN PATHOL 19:614-616

104. SMITH,J.E., 1968, LOW ERYTHROCYTE GLUCOSE-6-PHOSPHATE DEHYDROGENASE ACTIVITY AND PRIMAQUINE INSENSITIVITY IN SHEEP. J LAB CLIN MED 71:826-833

105. NAIK,S.N. AND ANDERSON,D.E., 1971, GLUCOSE-6-PHOSPHATE DEHYDROGENASE AND HEMOGLOBIN TYPES IN CATTLE. J ANIM SCI 32:132-136

106. PANIKER,N.V. AND BEUTLER,E., 1972, GLUCOSE-6-PHOSPHATE DEHYDROGENASE AND NADPH DIAPHORASE IN CATTLE ERYTHROCYTES. J ANIM SCI 34:75-76

107. ARENDS,T., 1971, HEMOGLOBINOPATHIES AND ENZYME DEFICIENCIES IN LATIN AMERICAN POPULATIONS. THE ONGOING EVOLUTION OF LATIN AMERICAN POPULATIONS CHS. C. THOMAS, SPRINGFIELD, ILL

108. VERGNES,H. AND LARROUY,G., 1967, LES DEFICITS EN G6PD DANS LES POPULATIONS DES ANDES BOLIVIENNES. SOC FRANC D'HEMAT 7:124-128

109. NANCE,W.E., 1964, GENETIC TESTS WITH A SEX-LINKED MARKER: G-6-PD. COLD SPRING HARBOR SYMP QUANT BIOL 29:415-425

110. LEWGOY,F. AND SALZANO,F.M., 1964, CITED BY ARENDS, T. REFERENCE 107.

111. SALDANHA,P.H., NOBREGA,F.G. AND MAIA,J.C.C., 1969, DISTRIBUTION AND HEREDTARY OF ERYTHROCYTE G6PD ACTIVITY AND ELECTROPHORETIC VARIANTS AMONG DIFFERENT RACIAL GROUPS AT SAO PAULO, BRAZIL. J MED GENET 6:48-54

112. GRAY,G.R. AND MARION,R.B., 1971, THALASSEMIA AND G-6-PD DEFICIENCY IN CHINESE-CANADIANS: ADMISSION SCREENING OF A HOSPITAL POPULATION. CAN MED ASSOC J 105:283-286

113. SZATHMARY,E.J.E., COX,D.W., GERSHOWITZ,H., RUCKNAGEL,D.L. AND SCHANFIELD,M.S., 1974, THE NORTHERN AND SOUTHEASTERN OJIBWA: SERUM PROTEINS AND RED CELL ENZYME SYSTEMS. AM J PHYS ANTHROPOL 40:49-66

114. RESTREPO M,A. AND GUTIERREZ,E., 1968, THE FREQUENCY OF GLUCOSE-6-PHOSPHATE DEHYDROGENASE DEFICIENCY IN COLOMBIA. AM J HUM GENET 20:82-85

115. GONZALEZ,R., BALLESTER,J.M., ESTRADA,M., LIMA,F., MARTINEZ,G., WADE,M., COLOMBO,B. AND VENTO,R., 1976, A STUDY OF THE GENETICAL STRUCTURE OF THE CUBAN POPULATION: RED CELL AND SERUM BIOCHEMICAL MARKERS. AM J HUM GENET 28:585-596

116. GONZALEZ,R., ESTRADA,M. AND COLOMBO,B., 1975, G-6-PD
     POLYMORPHISM AND RACIAL ADMIXTURE IN THE CUBAN POPULATION.
     HUMANGENETIK 26:75-78

117. VAN DER SAR,A., SCHOUTEN,H. AND STRUYKER BOUDIER,A.M.,
     1964, GLUCOSE-6-PHOSPHATE DEHYDROGENASE DEFICIENCY IN RED
     CELLS. INCIDENCE IN THE CURACAO POPULATION, ITS CLINICAL
     AND GENETIC ASPECTS. ENZYME 27:289-310

118. PIK,C., LOOS,J.A., JONXIS,J.H.P. AND PRINS,H.K., 1965,
     CITED BY ARENDS, T. REFERENCE 107.

119. SMINK,D.A. AND PRINS,H.K., 1965, HEREDITARY AND ACQUIRED
     BLOOD FACTORS IN THE NEGROID POPULATION OF SURINAM. V.
     ELECTROPHORETIC HETEROGENEITY OF G-6-PD. TROP GEOGR MED
     17:236-242

120. GIBBS,W.N., OTTEY,F. AND DYER,H., 1972, DISTRIBUTION OF
     GLUCOSE-6-PHOSPHATE DEHYDROGENASE PHENOTYPES IN JAMAICA.
     AM J HUM GENET 24:18-23

121. LISKER,R., PEREZ BRICENO,R., SOSA,R. AND SHEIN,M., 1976,
     ASPECTOS HEREDITARIOS Y EPIDEMIOLOGICOS DE LA DEFICIENCIA
     DE GLUCOSA-6- DESHIDROGENASA ERITHROCITICA EN MEXICO. GAC
     MED MEX 111:454-458

122. ALVAR LORIA,Q.B.P., 1963, ESTUDIOS SOBRE ALGUNAS
     CARACTERISTACAS HEMATOLOGICAS HEREDITARIAS EN LA POBLACION
     MEXICANA. III. DEFICIENCIA EN LA GLUCOSA 6-FOSFATO
     DESHIDROGENASA ERITROCITICA EN 7 GRUPOS INDIGENAS Y ALGUNOS
     MESTIZOS. GAC MED MEX 93:299-303

123. LISKER,R., 1965, CARACTERISTICAS GENETICAS HEMATOLOGICAS
     DE LA POBLACION MEXICANA. GAC MED MEX 95:1027-1036

124. LISKER,R., LORIA,A. AND CORDOVA,M.S., 1965, STUDIES ON
     SEVERAL GENETIC HEMATOLOGICAL TRAITS OF THE MEXICAN
     POPULATION. VIII. HEMOGLOBIN S, GLUCOSE-6-PHOSPHATE
     DEHYDROGENASE DEFICIENCY, AND OTHER CHARACTERISTICS IN A
     MALARIAL REGION. AM J HUM GENET 17:179-187

125. LISKER,R., LORIA,A., LLAVEN,J.G., GUTTMAN,R. AND REYES,G.R.,
     1962, NOTE PRELIMINAIRE SUR LA FREQUENCE DES HEMOGLOBULINES
     ANORMALES ET DE LA DEFICIENCE EN G-6-PD DANS LA POPULATION
     MEXICAINE. REV FRANC ETUDE CLIN BIOL 7:76-78

126. HELMS,M.W., 1964, CITED BY ARENDS, T. REFERENCE 107.

127. BEST,W.R., 1959, ABSENCE OF ERYTHROCYTE GLUCOSE-6-PHOSPHATE
     DEHYDROGENASE DEFICIENCY IN CERTAIN PERUVIAN INDIANS. J
     LAB CLIN MED 54:791

128. MODIANO,G., BERNINI,L., CARTER,N.D., SANTACHIARA,B.,
     DETTER,J.C., BAUR,E.W., PAOLUCCI,A.M., GIGLIANI,F.,
     MORPURGO,G., SANTOLAMAZZA,C., SCOZZARI,R., TERRENATO,L.,
     MERRA KHAN,P., NIJENHUIS,L.E. AND KANASHIRO,V.K., 1972,
     SURVEY OF SEVERAL RED CELL AND SERUM GENETIC MARKERS IN A
     PERUVIAN POPULATION. AM J HUM GENET 24:111-123

129. SUTTON,R.N.P., 1963, ERYTHROCYTE GLUCOSE-6-PHOSPHATE-
DEHYDROGENASE DEFICIENCY IN TRINIDAD. LANCET 1:855

130. DOEBLIN,T.D., INGALL,G.B., PINKERTON,P.H., DRONAMRAJU,K.R.
AND BANNERMAN,R.M., 1968, GENETIC STUDIES OF THE SENECA
IDIANS: HAPTOGLOBINS, TRANSFERRINS, G-6-PD DEFICIENCY,
HEMOGLOBINOPATHY, COLOR BLINDNESS, MORPHOLOGICAL TRAITS
AND DERMATOGLYPHICS. ACTA GENET 18:251-260

131. BEUTLER,E., JOHNSON,C., POWARS,D. AND WEST,C., 1974,
PREVALENCE OF GLUCOSE-6-PHOSPHATE DEHYDROGENASE DEFICIENCY
IN SICKLE CELL DISEASE. N ENGL J MED 290:826-828

132. KRAUS,A.P., NEELY,C.L., CAREY,F.T. AND KRAUS,L.M., 1962,
DETECTION OF DEFICIENT ERYTHROCYTE REGENERATION OF REDUCED
TRIPHOSPHOPYRIDINE NUCLEOTIDE FROM GLUCOSE-6-PHOSPHATE.
EVALUATION OF A RAPID SCREENING TEST. ANN INTERN MED 56:765-
773

133. FRISCHER,H., BOWMAN,J.E., CARSON,P.E., PIECKMANN,K.H.,
WILLERSON JR,D. AND COLWELL,E.J., 1973, ERYTHROCYTIC
GLUTATHIONE REDUCTASE, GLUCOSE-6-PHOSPHATE DEHYDROGENASE,
AND 6-PHOSPHOGLUCONIC DEHYDROGENASE DEFICIENCIES IN
POPULATIONS OF THE UNITED STATES, SOUTH VIETNAM, IRAN, AND
ETHIOPIA. J LAB CLIN MED 81:603-612

134. UDDIN,D.E., DICKSON,L.G. AND BRODINE,C.E., 1974, GLUCOSE-
6-PHOSPHATE DEHYDROGENASE DEFICIENCY IN MILITARY RECRUITS.
JAMA 227:1408-1409

135. O FLYNN,M.E.D. AND HSIA,D.Y., 1963, SERUM BILIRUBIN LEVELS
AND GLUCOSE-6-PHOSPHATE DEHYDROGENASE DEFICIENCY IN NEWBORN
AMERICAN NEGROES. J PEDIATR 63:160-161

136. PORTER,I.H., BOYER,S.H., WATSON-WILLIAMS,E.J., ADAM,A.,
SZEINBERG,A. AND SINISCALCO,M., 1964, VARIATION OF GLUCOSE-
6-PHOSPHATE DEHYDROGENASE IN DIFFERENT POPULATIONS. LANCET
1:895-899

137. WEITKAMP,L. AND NEEL,J.V., 1970, GENE FREQUENCIES AND
MICRODIFFERENTIATION AMONG THE MAKIRITARE INDIANS. 3. NINE
ERYTHROCYTE ENZYME SYSTEMS. AM J HUM GENET 22:533-537

138. BOADA,J., 1963, CITED BY ARENDS, T. REFERENCE 107.

139. ACQUATELLA,G.C., 1967, CITED BY ARENDS, T. REFERENCE 107.

140. SONNET,J. AND MICHAUX,J.L., 1960, GLUCOSE-6-PHOSPHATE
DEHYDROGENASE DEFICIENCY , HAPTOGLOBIN GROUPS, BLOOD GROUPS
AND SICKLE-CELL TRAIT IN THE BANTUS OF WEST BELGIAN CONGO.
NATURE 188:504-505

141. HASCHEMIAN,G. AND MENNE,F., 1972, BEOBACHTUNGEN EINER
FAMILIE MIT GALAKTOSAEMIE UND, DUARTE-VARIANTE. HUMANGENETIK
15:223-226

142. MOTULSKY,A.G., VANDEPITTE,J. AND FRASER,G.R., 1966, POPULATION
GENETIC STUDIES IN THE CONGO. I. GLUCOSE-6-PHOSPHATE
DEHYDROGENASE DEFICIENCY, HEMOGLOBIN S, AND MALARIA. AM J
HUM GENET 18:514-537

143. LUTTRELL,V. AND LEA,C., 1965, G 6 PD DEFICIENCY IN E
      AFRICANS. EAST AFR MED J 42:313-315

144. ALLISON,A.C., 1960, GLUCOSE 6-PHOSPHATE DEHYDROGENASE
      DEFICIENCY IN RED BLOOD CELLS OF EAST AFRICANS. NATURE
      186:531-532

145. VERGNES,H., GHERARDI,M. AND BOULOUX,C., 1975, ERYTHROCYTE
      GLUCOSE-6-PHOSPHATE DEHYDROGENASE IN THE NIOKOLONKO (MALINKE
      OF THE NIOKOLO) OF EASTERN SENEGAL. IDENTIFICATION OF A
      SLOW VARIANT WITH NORMAL ACTIVITY (TACOMA-LIKE). HUM HERED
      25:80-87

146. RAGAB,A.H., EL-ALFI,O.S. AND ABBOUD,M.A., 1966, INCIDENCE
      OF GLUCOSE-6-PHOSPHATE DEHYDROGENASE DEFICIENCY IN EGYPT.
      AM J HUM GENET 18:21-25

147. SZEINBERG,A., 1963, G6PD DEFICIENCY AMONG JEWS--GENETIC
      AND ANTHROPOLOGICAL CONSIDERATIONS. THE GENETICS OF MIGRANT
      AND ISOLATE POPULATIONS GOLDSCHMIDT,E. ED. 69-72 WILLIAMS
      AND WILKINS

148. SHEBA,C. AND ADAM,A., 1962, A SURVEY OF SOME GENETICAL
      CHARACTERS IN ETHIOPIAN TRIBES. AM J PHYS ANTHROPOL 20:167

149. ALLISON,A.C., CHARLES,L.J. AND MC GREGOR,I.A., 1961,
      ERYTHROCYTE GLUCOSE-6-PHOSPHATE DEHYDROGENASE DEFICIENCY
      IN WEST AFRICA. NATURE 190:1198 (LETTER TO EDITOR)

150. KNOX,E.G. AND MC GREGOR,I.A., 1965, G 6 PD DEFICIENCY IN
      A GAMBIAN VILLAGE. TRANS R SOC TROP MED HYG 59:46-58

151. OWUSU,S.K. AND OPARE MANTE,A., 1972, ELECTROPHORETIC
      CHARACTERISATION OF GLUCOSE-6-PHOSPHATE DEHYDROGENASE IN
      GHANA. LANCET 2:44 (LETTER TO THE EDITOR)

152. OWUSU,S.K., FOLI,A.K., KONOTEY-AHULU,F.I.D. AND JANOSI,M.,
      1972, FREQUENCY OF GLUCOSE-6-PHOSPHATE DEHYDROGENASE
      DEFICIENCY IN TYPHOID FEVER IN GHANA. LANCET 1:320

153. ACQUAYE,C.T.A. AND OLDHAM,J.H., 1973, VARIANTS OF HAEMOGLOBIN
      AND GLUCOSE-6-PHOSPHATE DEHYDROGENASE 1. DISTRIBUTION IN
      SOUTHERN GHANA. GHANA MED J 12:412-418

154. HAILES,A.M. AND ROBERTS,D.F., 1962, G 6 PD DEFICIENCY
      SCREENING IN MADEIRA. HUM BIOL 34:206-213

155. DODIN,A., 1965, DEFICIT EN GLUCOSE 6 PHOSPHATE DESHYDROGENASE.
      ARCH INST PASTEUR MADAGASCAR 33:233-237

156. LUZZATTO,L. AND ALLAN,N.C., 1968, RELATIONSHIP BETWEEN THE
      GENES FOR GLUCOSE-6-PHOSPHATE DEHYDROGENASE AND FOR HEMOGLOBIN
      IN A NIGERIAN POPULATION. NATURE 219:1041-1042

157. HARRIS,R. AND GILLES,H.M., 1961, GLUCOSE-6-PHOSPHATE
      DEHYDROGENASE DEFICIENCY IN THE PEOPLES OF THE NIGER DELTA.
      ANN HUM GENET 25:199-206

158. CAPPS,F.P.A., GILLES,H.M., JOLLY,H. AND WORLLEDGE,S.M.,
      1963, GLUCOSE-6-PHOSHATE DEHYDROGENASE DEFICIENCY AND
      NEONATAL JAUNDICE IN NIGERIA. THEIR RELATION TO USE OF
      PROPHYLACTIC VITAMIN K. LANCET 2:379-383

159. BERNSTEIN,R.E., 1963, OCCURRENCE AND CLINICAL IMPLICATIONS OF RED-CELL GLUCOSE-6-PHOSPHATE DEHYDROGENASE DEFICIENCY IN SOUTH AFRICAN RACIAL GROUPS. S AFR MED J 37:447-451

160. MARTI,H.R., SCHOEPF,K. AND GSELL,O.R., 1965, FREQUENCY OF HAEMOGLOBIN S AND G-6-PD DEFICIENCY IN SOUTHERN TANZANIA. BR MED J 1:1476

161. LOTHE,F., 1967, ERYTHROCYTE GLUCOSE-6-PHOSPHATE DEHYDROGENASE DEFICIENCY IN UGANDA. NATURE 215:299-300

162. PAPIHA,S.S., ROBERTS,D.F., ALI,S.G.M. AND ISLAM,M.M., 1975, SOME HEREDITARY BLOOD FACTORS OF THE BENGALI MUSLIM OF BANGLADESH (RED CELL ENZYMES, HAEMOGLOBINS, AND SERUM PROTEINS). HUMANGENETIK 28:285-293

163. ENG,L.L. AND GIOK,P.H., 1964, GLUCOSE-6-PHOSPHATE DEHYDROGENASE DEFICIENCY IN INDONESIA. NATURE 204:88-89

164. BEUTLER,E., YEH,M.K.Y. AND NECHELES,T., 1959, INCIDENCE OF THE ERYTHROCYTIC DEFECT ASSOCIATED WITH DRUG SENSITIVITY AMONG ORIENTAL SUBJECTS. NATURE 183:684-685

165. CHAN,T.K., TODD,D. AND WONG,C.C., 1964, ERYTHROCYTE GLUCOSE-6-PHOSPHATE DEHYDROGENASE DEFICIENCY IN CHINESE. BR MED J 2:102

166. VELLA,F., 1959, FAVISM IN ASIA. MED J AUST 2:196-197

167. HOSKOVA,A., CECH,M. AND NOLL,A., 1965, O MOZNOSTI DEFEKTU GLUKOZO-6-FOSFATDEHYDROGENAZY U NAS. CAS LEK CESK 104:262

168. PLATO,C.C., RUCKNAGEL,D.L. AND GERSHOWITZ,H., 1964, STUDIES ON THE DISTRIBUTION OF GLUCOSE-6-PHOSPHATE DEHYDROGENASE DEFICIENCY, THALASSEMIA, AND OTHER GENETIC TRAITS IN THE COASTAL AND MOUNTAIN VILLAGES OF CYPRUS. AM J HUM GENET 16:267-283

169. BUCHANAN,J.G., WILSON,F.S. AND NIXON,A.D., 1973, SURVEY FOR ERYTHROCYTE GLUCOSE-6-PHOSPHATE DEHYDROGENASE DEFICIENCY IN FIJI. AM J HUM GENET 25:36-41

170. ERODOHAZI,M. AND HIGHMAN,W.J., 1962, GLUCOSE-6-PHOSPHATE-DEHYDROGENASE DEFICIENCY IN BRITAIN. LANCET 2:1274

171. CHAN,T.K., 1966, G-6-PD IN WEST SCOTLAND. LANCET 2:752

172. ZANNOS-MARIOLEA,L. AND KATTAMIS,C., 1961, GLUCOSE-6-PHOSPHATE DEHYDROGENASE IN GREECE. BLOOD 18:34-47

173. STAMATOYANNOPOULOS,G., PANAYOTOPOULOS,A. AND MOTULSKY,A.G., 1966, THE DISTRIBUTION OF G-6-PD DEFICIENCY IN GREECE. AM J HUM GENET 18:296-308

174. VALAES,T., KARAKLIS,A., STRAVRAKAKIS,D., BAVELA-STRAVRAKAKIS,K., PERAKIS,A. AND DOXIADIS,S.A., 1969, INCIDENCE AND MECHANISM OF NEONATAL JAUNDICE RELATED TO GLUCOSE-6-PHOSPHATE DEHYDROGENASE DEFICIENCY. PEDIATR RES 3:448-458

175.   ALLISON,A.C., ASKONAS,B.A., BARNICOT,N.A., BLUMBERG,B.S.
       AND KRIMBAS,C., 1963, DEFICIENCY OF ERYTHROCYTE GLUCOSE-6-
       PHOSPHATE DEHYDROGENASE IN GREEK POPULATIONS. ANN HUM GENET
       26:237-242

176.   STAMATOYANNOPOULOS,G. AND FESSAS,P., 1964, THALASSEMIA,
       GLUCOSE-6-PHOSPHATE DEHYDROGENASE DEFICIENCY, SICKLING AND
       MALARIAL ENDEMICITY IN GREECE: A STUDY OF FIVE AREAS. BR
       MED J 1:875-879

177.   DOXIADIS,S.A., FESSAS,P., VALAES,T. AND MASTROKALOS,N.,
       1961, GLUCOSE-6-PHOSPHATE DEHYDROGENASE DEFICIENCY. LANCET
       1:297-301

178.   KIRIMLIDIS,S., POLITIS,E., DROSSOS,C., SCALOUMBAKAS,N.,
       PAPAIOANNOU,M. AND PHILLIPPIDIS,P., 1965, GLUCOSE-6-PHOSPHATE-
       DEHYDROGENASE DEFICIENCY IN GREECE. STUDY BY USING A
       MODIFICATION OF BEUTLER AND FAIRBANKS SPOT TEST. HELV
       PAEDIATR ACTA 20:490-496

179.   CHOREMIS,C., ZANNOS-MARIOLEA,L. AND KATTAMIS,M.D.C., 1962,
       FREQUENCY OF GLUCOSE-6-PHOSPHATE-DEHYDROGENASE DEFICIENCY
       IN CERTAIN HIGHLY MALARIOUS AREA OF GREECE. LANCET 1:17-18

180.   CHOREMIS,C., KATTAMIS,C., ZANNOS-MARIOLEA,L., FESSAS,P.,
       STAMATOYANNOPOULOS,G., KARAKLIS,A. AND BELIOS,G., 1963,
       THREE INHERITED RED-CELL ABNORMALITIES IN A DISTRICT OF
       GREECE. LANCET 1:907-909

181.   FRASER,G.R., DEFARANAS,B., KATTAMIS,C.A., RACE,R.R.,
       SANGER,R. AND STAMATOYANNOPOULOS,G., 1964, GLUCOSE-6-
       PHOSPHATE DEHYDROGENASE, COLOUR VISION AND XG BLOOD GROUPS
       IN GREECE: LINKAGE AND POPULATION DATA. ANN HUM GENET
       27:395-403

182.   FESSAS,P., DOXIADIS,S.A. AND VALAES,T., 1962, NEONATAL
       JAUNDICE IN GLUCOSE-6-PHOSPHATE DEHYDROGENASE DEFICIENT
       INFANTS. BR MED J 2:1359-1362

183.   PLATO,C.C., CRUZ,M.T. AND KURLAND,L.T., 1964, FREQUENCY OF
       GLUCOSE-6-PHOSPHATE DEHYDROGENASE DEFICIENCY, RED-GREEN
       COLOUR BLINDNESS AND XGA BLOOD-GROUP AMONG CHAMORROS. NATURE
       202:728

184.   JIM,R.T.S., 1967, SURVEY FOR ERYTHROCYTE GLUCOSE-6-PHOSPHATE
       DEHYDROGENASE DEFICIENCY IN HAWAII. ACTA HAEMATOL 37:94-99

185.   YUE,P.C.K. AND STRICKLAND,M., 1965, GLUCOSE-6-PHOSPHATE-
       DEHYDROGENASE DEFICIENCY AND NEONATAL JAUNDICE IN CHINESE
       MALE INFANTS IN HONG KONG. LANCET 1:350-351

186.   WALTER,H., NEUMANN,S. AND NEMESKERI,J., 1965,
       POPULATIONGENETISCHE UNTERSUCHUNGEN UEBER DIE VERTEILUNG
       VON HAEMOGLOBIN S UND GLUCOSE-6-PHOSPHAT-DEHYDROGENASEMANGEL
       IM BODROGKOEZ (NORDOSTUNGARN). HUMANGENETIK 1:651-657

187.   BAXI,A.J., BALAKRISHNAN,V., UNDEVIA,J.V. AND SANGHVI,L.D.,
       1963, GLUCOSE-6-PHOSPHATE DEHYDROGENASE DEFICIENCY IN THE
       PARSEE COMMUNITY, BOMBAY. INDIAN J MED SCI 17:493-500

188. BAXI,A.J., BALAKRISHNAN,V. AND SANGHVI,L.D., 1961, DEFICIENCY
     OF GLUCOSE-6-PHOSPHATE DEHYDROGENASE-OBSERVATIONS ON A
     SAMPLE FROM BOMBAY. CURR SCI 30:16-17

189. DESHMUKH,V.V. AND SHARMA,K.D., 1968, DEFICIENCY OF ERYTHROCYTE
     GLUCOSE-6-PHOSPHATE DEHYDROGENASE AND SICKLE SELL TRAIT:
     A SURVEY OF MAHAR STUDENTS AT AURANGABAD, MAHARASHTRA.
     INDIAN J MED RES 56:821-825

190. SAHA,N., KIRK,R.L., SHANBHAG,S., JOSHI,S.R. AND BHATIA,H.M.,
     1976, POPULATION GENETIC STUDIES IN KERALA AND THE NILGIRIS
     (SOUTH WEST INDIA). HUM HERED 26:175-197

191. BAXI,A.J., 1974, GLUCOSE-6-PHOSPHATE DEHYDROGENASE DEFICIENCY-
     A NOTE ON THE DISTRIBUTION OF GENE FREQUENCY IN INDIA. PROC
     1ST CONF OF THE IND SOC OF HUM GEN (HUMAN POPULATION GENETICS
     IN INDIA) 1:60-66

192. BOWMAN,J.E. AND WALKER,D.G., 1961, THE ORIGIN OF GLUCOSE-
     6-PHOSPHATE DEHYDROGENASE DEFICIENCY IN IRAN: THEORETICAL
     CONSIDERATIONS. PROC 2ND INTL CONGRESS OF HUM GENET 583-
     586

193. BOWMAN,J.E. AND WALKER,D.G., 1961, VIRTUAL ABSENCE OF
     GLUTATHIONE INSTABILITY OF THE ERYTHROCYTES AMONG ARMENIANS
     IN IRAN. NATURE 191:221-223

194. WALKER,D.G. AND BOWMAN,J.E., 1959, GLUTATHIONE STABILITY
     OF THE ERYTHROCYTES IN IRANIANS. NATURE 184:1325

195. MILBAUER,B., PELED,N. AND SVIRSKY,S., 1973, NEONATAL
     HYPERBILIRUBINEMIA AND GLUCOSE-6-PHOSPHATE DEHYDROGENASE
     DEFICIENCY. ISR J MED SCI 9:1547-1552

196. ZAIDMAN,J.L., LEIBA,H., SCHARF,S. AND STEINMAN,I., 1976,
     RED CELL GLUCOSE-6-PHOSPHATE DEHYDROGENASE DEFICIENCY IN
     ETHNIC GROUPS IN ISRAEL. CLIN GENET 9:131-133

197. BRUNETTI,P., 1965, INCIDENCA DEL DIFETTO DI G-6-PD NELL'
     ITALIA CENTRALE. HAEMATOLOGICA (PAVIA) 50:203-219

198. SINISCALCO,M., BERNINI,L., FILIPPI,G., LATTE,B., MEERA
     KHAN,P., PIOMELLI,S. AND RATTAZZI,M., 1966, POPULATION
     GENETICS OF HAEMOGLOBIN VARIANTS, THALASSAEMIA AND G-6-PD
     DEFICIENCY, WITH PARTICULAR REFERENCE TO THE MALARIA
     HYPOTHESIS. BULL WHO 34:379-393

199. SANSONE,G., SEGNI,G. AND DE CECCO,C., 1958, IL DIFETTO
     BIOCHIMICO ERITROCITARIO PREDISPONENTE ALL'EMOLISI FAVICA.
     PRIME RICERCHE SULLA POPOLAZIONE LIGURE E SU QUELLA SARDA.
     BOLL SOC ITAL BIOL SPER 34:1558-1561

200. MODIANO,G., BENERECETTI-SANTACHIARA,A.S., GONANO,F., ZEI,G.,
     CAPALDO,A. AND CAVALLI-SFORZA,L.L., 1965, AN ANALYSIS OF
     ABO, MN, RH, HP, TF AND G-6-PD TYPES IN A SAMPLE FROM THE
     HUMAN POPULATION OF THE LECCE PROVINCE. ANN HUM GENET 29:19-
     31

201. SINISCALCO,M., BERNINI,L., LATTE,B. AND MOTULSKY,A.G.,
     1961, FAVISM AND THALASSAEMIA IN SARDINIA AND THEIR
     RELATIONSHIP TO MALARIA. NATURE 190:1179-1181

202.   MIWA,S., TERAMURA,K., IRISAWA,K. AND OYAMA,H., 1965, GLUCOSE-
       6-PHOSPHATE DEHYROGENASE (G-6-PD) DEFICIENCY. II. INCIDENCE
       OF G-6-PD DEFICIENCY IN JAPANESE. ACTA HAEMATOL JAP 28:590-
       592

203.   BLACKWELL,R.Q., RO,I.H. AND YEN,L., 1968, LOW INCIDENCE OF
       ERYTHROCYTE G-6-PD DEFICIENCY IN KOREANS. VOX SANG 14:299-
       303

204.   RUFFIE,J. AND TALEB,N., 1965, ETUDE HEMOTYPOLOGIQUE DES
       ETHNIES LIBANAISES HERMANN, PARIS

205.   TALEB,N., LOISELET,J., GHORRA,F. AND SFEIR,H., 1964, SUR
       LA DEFICIENCE EN GLUCOSE-6-PHOSPHATE-DESHYDROGENASE DANS
       LES POPULATIONS AUTOCHTONES DU LIBAN. C R ACAD SCI (PARIS)
       258:5749-5751

206.   ENG,L.L. AND CHIN,J., 1964, ABNORMAL HAEMOGLOBIN AND GLUCOSE-
       6-PHOSPHATE DEHYDROGENASE DEFICIENCY IN MALAYAN ABORIGINES.
       NATURE 204:291-292

207.   ENG,L.L., CHIN,J. AND TI,T.S., 1964, GLUCOSE-6-PHOSPHATE
       DEHYDROGENASE DEFICIENCY IN BRUNEI, SABAH AND SARAWAK. ANN
       HUM GENET 28:173-176

208.   ENG,L.L. AND TI,T.S., 1964, GLUCOSE-6-PHOSPHATE DEHYDROGENASE
       DEFICIENCY IN MALAYANS. TRANS R SOC TROP MED HYG 58:500-
       502

209.   GANESAN,J.,.ENG,L.-.I. AND POON,O.B., 1975, ABNORMAL
       HEMOGLOBINS, GLUCOSE-6-PHOSPHATE DEHYDROGENASE DEFICIENCY
       AND HEREDITARY OVALOCYTOSIS IN THE DAYAKS OF SARAWAK. HUM
       HERED 25:258-262

210.   VELLA,F., 1961, THE INCIDENCE OF GLUCOSE-6-PHOSPHATE
       DEHYROGENASE DEFICIENCY IN SINGAPORE. EXPERIENTIA 17:181-
       182

211.   SAHA,N. AND BANERJEE,B., 1971, ERYTHROCYTE G-6-PD DEFICIENCY
       AMONG CHINESE AND MALAYS OF SINGAPORE. TROP GEOGR MED
       23:141-144

212.   GRECH,J.L. AND VICATOU,M., 1973, GLUCOSE-6-PHOSPHATE
       DEHYDROGENASE DEFICIENCY IN MALTESE NEWBORN INFANTS. BR J
       HAEMATOL 25:261-269

213.   CAUCHI,M.N., 1970, THE INCIDENCE OF GLUCOSE-6-PHOSPHATE
       DEHYDROGENASE DEFICIENCY AND THALASSEMIA IN MALTA. BR J
       HAEMATOL 18:101-106

214.   NITOWSKY,H.M., SODERMAN,D.D. AND HERZ,F., 1965, GLUCOSE-6-
       PHOSPHATE-DEHYDROGENASE DEFICIENCY IN FILIPINOS. LANCET
       1:917

215.   MOTULSKY,A.G., STRANSKY,E. AND FRASER,G.R., 1964, GLUCOSE-
       6-PHOSPHATE DEHYDROGENASE (G6PD) DEFICIENCY, THALASSAEMIA,
       AND ABNORMAL HAEMOGLOBINS IN THE PHILIPPINES. J MED GENET
       1:102-106

216. SCHNEER,J.H., 1968, A SURVEY FOR ERYTHROCYTE GLUCOSE-6-
      PHOSPHATE DEHYDROGENASE DEFICIENCY IN RUMANIA. ACTA HAEMATOL
      40:44-47

217. GELPI,A.P., 1965, GLUCOSE-6-PHOSPHATE DEHYDROGENASE DEFICIENCY
      IN SAUDI ARABIA: A SURVEY. BLOOD 25:486-493

218. PELLICER,A. AND CASADO,A., 1970, FREQUENCY OF THALASSEMIA
      AND G-6-PD DEFICIENCY IN FIVE PROVINCES OF SPAIN. AM J HUM
      GENET 22:298-303

219. FLATZ,G. AND DUEREN,R., 1967, GLUCOSE-6-PHOSPHATE
      DEHYDROGENASE DEFICIENCY IN SPAIN. HUMANGENETIK 4:81-83

220. ABEYARATNE,K.P., PREMAWANSA,S., RAJAPAKSE,L., ROBERTS,D.F.
      AND PAPIHA,S.S., 1976, A SURVEY OF GLUCOSE-6-PHOSPHATE-
      DEHYDROGENASE DEFICIENCY IN THE NORTH CENTRAL PROVINCE OF
      SRI LANKA (FORMERLY CEYLON). AM J PHYS ANTHROPOL 44:135-
      138

221. MOTULSKY,A.G., LEE,T.C. AND FRASER,G.R., 1965, GLUCOSE-6-
      PHOSPHATE DEHYDROGENASE (G6PD) DEFICIENCY, THALASSAEMIA,
      AND ABNORMAL HAEMOGLOBINS IN TAIWAN. J MED GENET 2:18-20

222. LEE,T.C., SHIH,L.Y., HUANG,P.C., LIN,C.C., BLACKWELL,B.N.,
      BLACKWELL,R.Q. AND HSIA,D.Y., 1963, GLUCOSE-6-PHOSPHATE
      DEHYDROGENASE DEFICIENCY IN TAIWAN. AM J HUM GENET 15:126-
      132

223. FLATZ,G., THANANGKUL,O., SIMARAK,S. AND MANMONTRI,M., 1964,
      GLUCOSE-6-PHOSPHATE DEHYDROGENASE DEFICIENCY AND JAUNDICE
      IN NEWBORN INFANTS IN NORTHERN THAILAND. ANN PAEDIAT 203:39-
      45

224. KRUATRACHUE,M., CHOROENLARP,P. AND CHONGSUPHAJAISIDDHI,T.,
      1962, ERYTHROCYTE GLUCOSE-6-PHOSPHATE DEHYDROGENASE AND
      MALARIA IN THAILAND. LANCET 2:1183-1186

225. TUCHINDA,S., RUCKNAGEL,D.L., NA-NAKORN,S. AND WASI,P.,
      1968, THE THAI VARIANT AND THE DISTRIBUTION OF ALLELES OF
      6-PHOSPHOGLUCONATE DEHYDROGENASE AND THE DISTRIBUTION OF
      GLUCOSE-6-PHOSPHATE DEHYDROGENASE DEFICIENCY IN THAILAND.
      BIOCHEM GENET 2:253-264

226. WASI,P., NA-NAKORN,S. AND SUINGDUMRONG,A., 1967, STUDIES
      OF THE DISTRIBUTION OF HAEMOGLOBIN E, THALASSAEMIAS AND
      GLUCOSE-6-PHOSPHATE DEHYDROGENASE DEFICIENCY IN NORTH-
      EASTERN THAILAND. NATURE 214:501-502

227. SAY,B., OZAND,P., BERKEL,I. AND CEVIK,N., 1965, ERYTHROCYTE
      GLUCOSE-6-PHOSPHATE DEHYDROGENASE DEFICIENCY IN TURKEY.
      ACTA PAEDIATR SCAND 54:319-324

228. ERMILCHENKO,G.V. AND SOLOVIEVA,N.P., 1973, A STUDY OF THE
      INCIDENCE OF DEFICIENCY OF THE ACTIVITY OF GLUCOSO-6-
      PHOSPHORIC DEHYDROGENASE IN THE BLOOD OF PERSONS RESIDING
      IN THE ARKHANGELSK REGION. PROBL GEMATOL PERELIV KROVI
      18:23-26

229. YOUEL,D.B., STRICKLAND,G.T., BINH,B.A., CLARKSON,R. AND
      BLACKWELL,R.Q., 1971, LOW INCIDENCE OF ERYTHROCYTE G-6-P
      D DEFICIENCY IN VIETNAMESE AND MONTAGNARDS OF SOUTH VIETNAM.
      VOX SANG 20:555-558

230. CHAT,L.X., QUANG,L.S., HUMBERT,C. AND GIAO,C.Q., 1968, LE
      DEFICIT EN GLUCOSE-6-PHOSPHATE DEHYDROGENASE AU VIET-NAM.
      NOUV REV FR HEMATOL 8:878-884

231. FRASER,G.R., GRUNWALD,P. AND STAMATOYANNOPOULOS,G., 1966,
      GLUCOSE-6-PHOSPHATE DEHYDROGENASE (G6PD) DEFICIENCY, ABNORMAL
      HAEMOGLOBINS, AND THALASSAEMIA IN YUGOSLAVIA. J MED GENET
      3:35-41

232. KIDSON,C. AND GORMAN,J.G., 1962, A CHALLENGE TO THE CONCEPT
      OF SELECTION BY MALARIA IN GLUCOSE-6-PHOSPHATE DEHYDROGENASE
      DEFICIENCY. NATURE 196:49-51

233. BUDTZ-OLSEN,O., 1961, ABSENCE OF RED CELL ENZYME DEFICIENCY
      IN AUSTRALIAN ABORIGINES. NATURE 192:765

234. KIDSON,C. AND GAJDUSEK,D.C., 1962, GLUCOSE-6-PHOSPHATE
      DEHYDROGENASE DEFICIENCY IN MICRONESIAN PEOPLES. AUST J
      SCI 25:61-62

235. PARSONS,I.C. AND RYAN,P.K., 1962, OBSERVATIONS ON GLUCOSE-
      6-PHOSPHATE DEHYDROGENASE DEFICIENCY IN PAPUANS. MED J AUST
      2:585-587

236. KIDSON,C. AND GAJDUSEK,D.C., 1962, CONGENITAL DEFECTS OF
      THE CENTRAL NERVOUS SYSTEM ASSOCIATED WITH HYPERENDEMIC
      GOITER IN A NEOLITHIC HIGHLAND SOCIETY OF NETHERLANDS NEW
      GUINEA. II. GLUCOSE-6-PHOSPHATE DEHYDROGENASE IN THE MULIA
      POPULATION. PEDIATRICS 29:364-368

237. PRINS,H.K., LOOS,J.A. AND MEUWISSEN,J.H.E., 1963, G 6 PD
      DEFICIENCY IN WEST NEW GUINEA. TROP GEOGR MED 15:361-370

238. KIDSON,C., 1961, DEFICIENCY OF G 6 PD: SOME ASPECTS OF THE
      TRAIT IN PEOPLE OF PAPUA-NEW GUINEA. MED J AUST 48:506-509

239. NIXON,A.D. AND BUCHANAN,J.G., 1969, SURVEY FOR ERYTHROCYTE
      GLUCOSE-6-PHOSPHATE DEHYDROGENASE DEFICIENCY IN POLYNESIANS.
      AM J HUM GENET 21:305-309

240. MC CURDY,P.R., KAMEL,K. AND SELIM,O., 1974, HETEROGENEITY
      OF RED CELL GLUCOSE-6-PHOSPHATE DEHYDROGENASE (G-6-PD)
      DEFICIENCY IN EGYPT. J LAB CLIN MED 84:673-680

241. STAMATOYANNOPOULOS,G., YOSHIDA,A., BACOPOULOS,C. AND
      MOTULSKY,A., 1967, ATHENS VARIANT OF GLUCOSE-6-PHOSPHATE
      DEHYDROGENASE. SCIENCE 157:831-833

242. KIRKMAN,H.N., DOXIADIS,S.A., VALAES,T., TASSOPOULOS,N. AND
      BRINSON,A.G., 1965, DIVERSE CHARACTERISTICS OF GLUCOSE-6-
      PHOSPHATE DEHYDROGENASE FROM GREEK CHILDREN. J LAB CLIN
      MED 65:212-221

243. GHERARDI,M., BIERME,R., CORBERAND,J., PRIS,J. AND VERGNES,H.,
      1976, DISTRIBUTION OF G6PD TYPES IN THE POPULATION OF
      SOUTHWEST FRANCE: COMMON VARIANTS AND NEW VARIANTS. HUM
      HERED 26:279-289

244. ALLISON,A.C., 1961, GENETIC FACTORS IN RESISTANCE TO MALARIA. ANN NY ACAD SCI 91:710-729

245. ALLISON,A.C. AND CLYDE,D.F., 1961, MALARIA AND GLUCOSE-6-PHOSPHATE DEHYDROGENASE. BR MED J 1:1358 (CORRESPONDENCE)

246. MOTULSKY,A.G., 1961, GLUCOSE-6-PHOSPHATE DEHYDROGENASE DEFICIENCY HAEMOLYTIC DISEASE OF THE NEWBORN, AND MALARIA. LANCET 1:1168-1169

247. BUTLER,T., 1973, G-6-PD DEFICIENCY AND MALARIA IN BLACK AMERICANS IN VIETNAM. MILIT MED 138:153-155

248. KRUATRACHUE,M., SADUDEE,N. AND SRIRIPANICH,B., 1970, GLUCOSE-6-PHOSPHATE-DEHYDROGENASE-DEFICIENCY AND MALARIA IN THAILAND: THE COMPARISON OF PARASITE DENSITIES AND MORTALITY RATES. ANN TROP MED PARASITOL 64:11-14

249. HUHEEY,J.E. AND MARTIN,D.L., 1975, MALARIA, FAVISM AND GLUCOSE-6-PHOSPHATE DEHYDROGENASE DEFICIENCY. EXPERIENTIA 31:1145-1147

250. LUZZATTO,L., USANGA,E.A. AND REDDY,S., 1969, GLUCOSE 6-PHOSPHATE DEHYDROGENASE DEFICIENT RED CELLS: RESISTANCE TO INFECTION BY MALARIAL PARASITES. SCIENCE 164:839-842

251. MARKS,P.A., SZEINBERG,A. AND BANKS,J., 1961, ERYTHROCYTE GLUCOSE-6-PHOSPHATE DEHYDROGENASE OF NORMAL AND MUTANT HUMAN SUBJECTS: PROPERTIES OF THE PURIFIED ENZYME. J BIOL CHEM 236:10-17

252. BALINSKY,D. AND BERNSTEIN,R.E., 1963, THE PURIFICATION AND PROPERTIES OF GLUCOSE-6-PHOSPHATE DEHYDROGENASE FROM HUMAN ERYTHROCYTES. BIOCHIM BIOPHYS ACTA 67:313-315

253. KIRKMAN,H.N., 1962, GLUCOSE-6-PHOSPHATE DEHYDROGENASE FROM HUMAN ERYTHROCYTES. I. FURTHER PURIFICATION AND CHARACTERIZATION. J BIOL CHEM 237:2364-2370

254. CHUNG,A.E. AND LANGDON,R.G., 1963, HUMAN ERYTHROCYTE GLUCOSE-6-PHOSPHATE DEHYDROGENASE I. ISOLATION AND PROPERTIES OF THE ENZYME. J BIOL CHEM 238:2309-2316

255. YOSHIDA,A., 1966, GLUCOSE-6-PHOSPHATE DEHYDROGENASE OF HUMAN ERYTHROCYTES. I. PURIFICATION AND CHARACTERIZATION OF NORMAL (B+) ENZYME. J BIOL CHEM 241:4966-4976

256. RATTAZZI,M.C., 1969, ISOLATION AND PURIFICATION OF HUMAN ERYTHROCYTE GLUCOSE-6-PHOSPHATE DEHYDROGENASE FROM SMALL AMOUNTS OF BLOOD. BIOCHIM BIOPHYS ACTA 181:1-11

257. KAHN,A. AND DREYFUS,J.C., 1974, PURIFICATION OF GLUCOSE-6-PHOSPHATE DEHYDROGENASE FROM RED BLOOD CELLS AND FROM HUMAN LEUKOCYTES. BIOCHIM BIOPHYS ACTA 334:257-265

258. YOSHIDA,A., 1970, ENZYME PURIFICATION BY SELECTIVE ELUTION WITH SUBSTRATE ANALOG FROM ION-EXCHANGE COLUMNS: APPLICATION TO GLUCOSE-6-PHOSPHATE DEHYDROGENASE, PSEUDOCHOLINESTERASE, LACTATE DEHYDROGENASE, AND ALANINE DEHYDROGENASE. ANAL BIOCHEM 37:357-367

259.   DE FLORA,A., GIULIANO,F. AND MORELLI,A., 1973, RAPID
       PURIFICATION OF GLUCOSE 6-PHOSPHATE DEHYDROGENASE FROM
       HUMAN ERYTHROCYTES BY MEANS OF AFFINITY CHROMATOGRAPHY.
       ITAL J BIOCHEM 22:258-270

260.   YOSHIDA,A., 1975, PURIFICATION OF HUMAN RED CELL GLUCOSE
       6-PHOSPHATE DEHYDROGENASE BY AFFINITY CHROMATOGRAPHY. J
       CHROMATOGR 114:321-327

261.   DE FLORA,A., MORELLI,A., BENATTI,U. AND GIULIANO,F., 1975,
       AN IMPROVED PROCEDURE FOR RAPID ISOLATION OF GLUCOSE 6-
       PHOSPHATE DEHYDROGENASE FROM HUMAN ERYTHROCYTES. ARCH
       BIOCHEM BIOPHYS 169:362-363

262.   CHUNG,A.E. AND LANGDON,R.G., 1963, HUMAN ERYTHROCYTE GLUCOSE
       6-PHOSPHATE DEHYDROGENASE. II. ENZYME-COENZYME
       INTERRELATIONSHIP. J BIOL CHEM 238:2317-2324

263.   KIRKMAN,H.N. AND HENDRICKSON,E.M., 1962, GLUCOSE-6-PHOSPHATE
       DEHYDROGENASE FROM HUMAN ERYTHROCYTES. II. SUBACTIVE STATES
       OF THE ENZYME FROM NORMAL PERSONS. J BIOL CHEM 237:2371-
       2376

264.   COHEN,P. AND ROSEMEYER,M.A., 1969, SUBUNIT INTERACTIONS OF
       GLUCOSE-6-PHOSPHATE DEHYDROGENASE FROM HUMAN ERYTHROCYTES.
       EUR J BIOCHEM 8:8-15

265.   YOSHIDA,A., 1968, SUBUNIT STRUCTURE OF HUMAN GLUCOSE-6-
       PHOSPHATE DEHYDROGENASE AND ITS GENETIC IMPLICATION. BIOCHEM
       GENET 2:237-243

266.   RATTAZZI,M.C., 1968, GLUCOSE-6-PHOSPHATE DEHYDROGENASE FROM
       HUMAN ERYTHROCYTES: MOLECULAR WEIGHT DETERMINATION BY GEL
       FILTRATION. BIOCHEM BIOPHYS RES COMMUN 31:16-24

267.   BONSIGNORE,A., CANCEDDA,R., NICOLINI,A., DAMIANI,G. AND DE
       FLORA,A., 1971, METABOLISM OF HUMAN ERYTHROCYTE GLUCOSE-6-
       PHOSPHATE DEHYDROGENASE VI. INTERCONVERSION OF MULTIPLE
       MOLECULAR FORMS. ARCH BIOCHEM BIOPHYS 147:493-501

268.   BABALOLA,A.O.G., BEETLESTONE,J.G. AND LUZZATTO,L., 1976,
       GENETIC VARIANTS OF HUMAN ERYTHROCYTE GLUCOSE-6-PHOSPHATE
       DEHYDROGENASE. J BIOL CHEM 251:2993-3002

269.   WRIGLEY,N.G., HEATHER,J.V., BONSIGNORE,A. AND DE FLORA,A.,
       1972, HUMAN ERYTHROCYTE GLUCOSE 6-PHOSPHATE DEHYDROGENASE:
       ELECTRON MICROSCOPE STUDIES ON STRUCTURE AND INTERCONVERSION
       OF TETRAMERS, DIMERS AND MONOMERS. J MOL BIOL 68:483-499

270.   BEUTLER,E. AND COLLINS,Z., 1965, HYBRIDIZATION OF GLUCOSE-
       6-PHOSPHATE DEHYDROGENASE FROM RAT AND HUMAN ERYTHROCYTES.
       SCIENCE 150:1306-1307

271.   ROSA,R. AND DREYFUS,J.C., 1969, HYBRIDATION DE LA GLUCOSE-
       6-PHOSPHATE DESHYDROGENASE DES GLOBULES ROUGES ET DES
       GLOBULES BLANCS HUMAINS AVEC L' ENZYME DE DIFFERENTS TISSUS
       DE RAT. CLIN CHIM ACTA 24:199-202

272.   BEUTLER,E. AND COLLINS,Z., 1966, HYBRIDIZATION STUDIES IN
       THE FURTHER CHARACTERIZATION OF ERYTHROCYTE GLUCOSE-6-
       PHOSPHATE DEHYDROGENASE. EXPERIENTIA 22:827-828

273. YOSHIDA,A., STEINMANN,L. AND HARBERT,P., 1967, IN VITRO
HYBRIDIZATION OF NORMAL AND VARIANT HUMAN GLUCOSE-6-PHOSPHATE
DEHYDROGENASE. NATURE 216:275-276

274. AFOLAYAN,A. AND LUZZATTO,L., 1971, GENETIC VARIANTS OF
HUMAN ERYTHROCYTE GLUCOSE-6-PHOSPHATE DEHYDROGENASE. I.
REGULATION OF ACTIVITY BY OXIDIZED AND REDUCED NICOTINAMIDE
ADENINE DINUCLEOTIDE PHOSPHATE. BIOCHEMISTRY 10:415-419

275. LUZZATTO,L., 1967, REGULATION OF THE ACTIVITY OF GLUCOSE-
6-PHOSPHATE DEHYDROGENASE BY NADP+ AND NADPH. BIOCHIM
BIOPHYS ACTA 146:18-25

276. BEUTLER,E., 1975, UNPUBLISHED

277. YOSHIDA,A., 1967, HUMAN GLUCOSE-6-PHOSPHATE DEHYDROGENASE:
PURIFICATION AND CHARACTERIZATION OF NEGRO TYPE VARIANT
(A+) AND COMPARISON WITH NORMAL ENZYME (B+). BIOCHEM GENET
1:81-99

278. SMITH,E. AND BEUTLER,E., 1966, ANOMERIC SPECIFICITY OF
HUMAN ERYTHROCYTE GLUCOSE-6-PHOSPHATE DEHYDROGENASE. PROC
SOC EXP BIOL MED 122:671-673

279. YOSHIDA,A., STAMATOYANNOPOULOS,G. AND MOTULSKY,A.G., 1968,
BIOCHEMICAL GENETICS OF GLUCOSE-6-PHOSPHATE DEHYDROGENASE
VARIATION. ANN NY ACAD SCI 155:868-879

280. KISSIN,C. AND BEUTLER,E., 1968, THE UTILIZATION OF GLUCOSE
BY NORMAL GLUCOSE-6-PHOSPHATE DEHYDROGENASE AND BY GLUCOSE-
6-PHOSPHATE DEHYDROGENASE MEDITERRANEAN. PROC SOC EXP BIOL
MED 128:595-601

281. LUZZATTO,L. AND AFOLAYAN,A., 1971, GENETIC VARIANTS OF
HUMAN ERYTHROCYTE GLUCOSE-6-PHOSPHATE DEHYDROGENASE. II.
IN VITRO AND IN VIVO FUNCTION OF THE A- VARIANT. BIOCHEMISTRY
10:420-423

282. YOSHIDA,A., 1973, HEMOLYTIC ANEMIA AND G-6-PD DEFICIENCY.
SCIENCE 179:532-537

283. AVIGAD,G., 1966, INHIBITION OF GLUCOSE-6-PHOSPHATE
DEHYDROGENASE BY ADENOSINE- 5-TRIPHOSPHATE. PROC NATL ACAD
SCI USA 56:1543-1547

284. SMITH,J.E. AND ANWER,M.S., 1971, STUDIES ON GLUCOSE-6-
PHOSPHATE DEHYDROGENASE:VARIABILITY IN ATP INHIBITION.
EXPERIENTIA 27:835-836

285. BEN-BASSAT,I. AND BEUTLER,E., 1973, INHIBITION BY ATP OF
ERYTHROCYTE GLUCOSE-6-PHOSPHATE DEHYDROGENASE VARIANTS.
PROC SOC EXP BIOL MED 142:410-411

286. YOSHIDA,A. AND LIN,M., 1973, REGULATION OF GLUCOSE-6-
PHOSPHATE DEHYDROGENASE ACTIVITY IN RED BLOOD CELLS FROM
HEMOLYTIC AND NONHEMOLYTIC VARIANT SUBJECTS. BLOOD 41:877-
891

287. LUZZATTO,L. AND AFOLAYAN,A., 1968, DIFFERENT TYPES OF HUMAN
ERYTHROCYTE GLUCOSE-6-PHOSPHATE DEHYDROGENASE, WITH
CHARACTERIZATION OF TWO NEW GENETIC VARIANTS. J CLIN INVEST
47:1833-1842

288. MARKS,P.A. AND BANKS,J., 1960, INHIBITION OF MAMMALIAN
      GLUCOSE-6-PHOSPHATE DEHYDROGENASE BY STEROIDS. PROC NATL
      ACAD SCI USA 46:447-452

289. OERTEL,G.W. AND RUBELEIN,I., 1969, EFFECTS OF
      DEHYDROEPIANDROSTERONE AND ITS CONJUGATES UPON THE ACTIVITY
      OF GLUCOSE-6-PHOSPHATE DEHYDROGENASE IN HUMAN ERYTHROCYTES.
      BIOCHIM BIOPHYS ACTA 184:459-460

290. OERTEL,G.W. AND BENES,P., 1973, INHIBITION OF GLUCOSE-6-
      PHOSPHATE DEHYDROGENASE BY SYNTHETIC STEROIDS AND STEROID
      CONJUGATES. ACTA ENDOCRINOL (SUPPL) (KBH) 173:114 (ABSTRACT)

291. KIRKMAN,H.N., 1963, GENETIC CONTROL OF HUMAN ENZYMES.
      PEDIATR CLIN NORTH AM 10:299-318

292. BATTISTUZZI,G., ESAN,G.J.F., FASUAN,F.A., MODIANO,G. AND
      LUZZATTO,L., 1977, COMPARISON OF GDA AND GDB ACTIVITIES IN
      NIGERIANS. A STUDY OF THE VARIATION OF THE G6PD ACTIVITY.
      AM J HUM GENET 29:31-36

293. KAHN,A., BOULARD,M., HAKIM,J., SCHAISON,G., BOIVIN,P. AND
      BERNARD,J., 1974, ANEMIE HEMOLYTIQUE CONGENITALE NON
      SPHEROCYTAIRE PAR DEFICIT EN GLUCOSE-6-PHOSPHATE-
      DESHYDROGENASE ERYTHROCYTAIRE. DESCRIPTION DE DEUX NOUVELLES
      VARIANTES:GD (-) SAINT LOUIS (PARIS) ET GD (-) HAYEM. NOUV
      REV FR HEMATOL 14:587-600

294. JUNIEN,C., KAPLAN,J.-.C., MEIENHOFER,M.C., MAIGRET,P. AND
      SENDER,A., 1974, G 6 PD BAUDELOCQUE: A NEW UNSTABLE VARIANT
      CHARACTERIZED IN CULTURED FIBROBLASTS. ENZYME 18:48-59

295. PINTO,P.V.C., NEWTON JR,W.A. AND RICHARDSON,K.E., 1966,
      EVIDENCE FOR FOUR TYPES OF ERYTHROCYTE GLUCOSE-6-PHOSPHATE
      DEHYDROGENASE FROM G-6-PD DEFICIENT HUMAN SUBJECTS. J CLIN
      INVEST 45:823-831

296. BEUTLER,E., GROOMS,A.M., MORGAN,S.K. AND TRINIDAD,F., 1972,
      CHRONIC SEVERE HEMOLYTIC ANEMIA DUE TO G-6-PD CHARLESTON:
      A NEW DEFICIENT VARIANT. J PEDIATR 80:1005-1009

297. HABACON,E.A., HONIG,G.R., VIDA,L.N. AND BEUTLER,E., 1978,
      G-6-PD LINCOLN PARK: A NEW VARIANT ASSOCIATED WITH CHRONIC
      HEMOLYTIC ANEMIA. UNPUBLISHED

298. CEDERBAUM,A.I. AND BEUTLER,E., 1975, NONSPHEROCYTIC HEMOLYTIC
      ANEMIA DUE TO G-6-PD GRAND PRAIRIE. IRCS 3:579

299. GROSSMAN,A., RAMANATHAN,K., JUSTICE,P., GORDON,J.,
      SHAHIDI,N.T. AND HSIA,D., 1966, CONGENITAL NONSPHEROCYTIC
      HEMOLYTIC ANEMIA ASSOCIATED WITH ERYTHROCYTE G-6-PD DEFICIENCY
      IN A NEGRO FAMILY. PEDIATRICS 37:624-629

300. FELDMAN,R., GROMISCH,D.S., LUHBY,A.L. AND BEUTLER,E., 1977,
      CONGENITAL NONSPHEROCYTIC HEMOLYTIC ANEMIA DUE TO GLUCOSE-
      6-PHOSPHATE DEHYDROGENASE EAST HARLEM: A NEW DEFICIENT
      VARIANT. J PEDIATR 90:89-91

301. TANAKA,K.R. AND BEUTLER,E., 1969, HEREDITARY HEMOLYTIC
      ANEMIA DUE TO GLUCOSE-6-PHOSPHATE DEHYDROGENASE TORRANCE:
      A NEW VARIANT. J LAB CLIN MED 73:657-667

302. NAKAI,T. AND YOSHIDA,A., 1974, G6PD HEIAN, A GLUCOSE-6-
PHOSPHATE DEHYDROGENASE VARIANT ASSOCIATED WITH HEMOLYTIC
ANEMIA FOUND IN JAPAN. CLIN CHIM ACTA 51:199-203

303. HOWELL,E.B., NELSON,A.J. AND JONES,O.W., 1972, A NEW G-6-
PD VARIANT ASSOCIATED WITH CHRONIC NON-SPHEROCYTIC HAEMOLYTIC
ANAEMIA IN A NEGRO FAMILY. J MED GENET 9:160-164

304. THIGPEN,J.T., STEINBERG,M.H., BEUTLER,E., GILLESPIE JR,G.T.,
DREILING,B.J. AND MORRISON,F.S., 1974, GLUCOSE-6-PHOSPHATE
DEHYDROGENASE JACKSON. A NEW VARIANT ASSOCIATED WITH
HEMOLYTIC ANEMIA. ACTA HAEMATOL 51:310-314

305. CHAN,T.K. AND LAI,M.C.S., 1972, GLUCOSE 6-PHOSPHATE
DEHYDROGENASE: IDENTITY OF ERYTHROCYTE AND LEUKOCYTE ENZYME
WITH REPORT OF A NEW VARIANT IN CHINESE. BIOCHEM GENET
6:119-124

306. RAMOT,B., BEN-BASSAT,I. AND SHCHORY,M., 1969, NEW GLUCOSE-
6-PHOSPHATE DEHYDROGENASE VARIANTS OBSERVED IN ISRAEL AND
THEIR ASSOCIATION WITH CONGENITAL NONSPHEROCYTIC HEMOLYTIC
DISEASE. J LAB CLIN MED 74:895-901

307. BEUTLER,E., MATHAI,C.K. AND SMITH,J.E., 1968, BIOCHEMICAL
VARIANTS OF GLUCOSE-6-PHOSPHATE DEHYDROGENASE GIVING RISE
TO CONGENITAL NONSPHEROCYTIC HEMOLYTIC DISEASE. BLOOD
31:131-150

308. TALALAK,P. AND BEUTLER,E., 1969, G-6-PD BANGKOK:A NEW
VARIANT FOUND IN CONGENITAL NONSPHEROCYTIC HEMOLYTIC DISEASE
(CNHD). BLOOD 33:772-776

309. KIRKMAN,H.N. AND RILEY JR,H.D., 1961, CONGENITAL
NONSPHEROCYTIC HEMOLYTIC ANEMIA. AM J DIS CHILD 102:313-
320

310. NANCE,W.E., 1964, TURNER'S SYNDROME, TWINNING, AND AN
UNUSUAL VARIANT OF GLUCOSE-6-PHOSPHATE DEHYDROGENASE. AM
J HUM GENET 16:380-392

311. WONG,P.W.K., SHIH,L.-.Y. AND HSIA,D.Y.Y., 1965,
CHARACTERIZATION OF GLUCOSE-6-PHOSPHATE DEHYDROGENASE AMONG
CHINESE. NATURE 208:1323-1324

312. KIRKMAN,H.N., ROSENTHAL,I.M., SIMON,E.R., CARSON,P.E. AND
BRINSON,A.G., 1964, "CHICAGO I" VARIANT OF GLUCOSE-6-
PHOSPHATE DEHYDROGENASE IN CONGENITAL HEMOLYTIC DISEASE.
J LAB CLIN MED 63:715-725

313. NECHELES,T.F., SNYDER,L.M. AND STRAUSS,W., 1971, GLUCOSE-
6-PHOSPHATE DEHYDROGENASE BOSTON. A NEW VARIANT ASSOCIATED
WITH CONGENITAL NONSPHEROCYTIC HEMOLYTIC DISEASE. HUMANGENETIK
13:218-221

314. RATTAZZI,M.C., CORASH,L.M., VAN ZANEN,G.E., JAFFE,E.R. AND
PIOMELLI,S., 1971, G6PD DEFICIENCY AND CHRONIC HEMOLYSIS:
FOUR NEW MUTANTS--RELATIONSHIPS BETWEEN CLINICAL SYNDROME
AND ENZYME KINETICS. BLOOD 38:205-218

315.   MILLER,D.R. AND WOLLMAN,M.R., 1974, A NEW VARIANT OF GLUCOSE-
       6-PHOSPHATE DEHYDROGENASE DEFICIENCY HEREDITARY HEMOLYTIC
       ANEMIA, G6PD CORNELL: ERYTHROCYTE, LEUKOCYTE, AND PLATELET
       STUDIES. BLOOD 44:323-331

316.   MIWA,S., ONO,J., NAKASHIMA,K., ABE,S., KAGEOKA,T.,
       SHINOHARA,K., ISOBE,J. AND YAMAGUCHI,H., 1976, TWO NEW
       GLUCOSE 6-PHOSPHATE DEHYDROGENASE VARIANTS ASSOCIATED WITH
       CONGENITAL NONSPHEROCYTIC HEMOLYTIC ANEMIA FOUND IN JAPAN:
       GD(-) TOKUSHIMA AND GD(-) TOKYO. AM J HEMATOL 1:433-442

317.   BEUTLER,E. AND MATSUMOTO,F., 1975, UNPUBLISHED

318.   WILSON,W.W., 1976, CONGENITAL HEMOLYTIC ANEMIA DUE TO
       DEFICIENCY OF GLUCOSE-6-PHOSPHATE DEHYDROGENASE. ROCKY MT
       MED J 73:160-162

319.   GAHR,M., SCHROETER,W., STURZENEGGER,M., BORNHALM,D. AND
       MARTI,H.R., 1976, GLUCOSE-6-PHOSPHATE DEHYDROGENASE (G-6-
       PD) DEFICIENCY IN SWITZERLAND. HELV PAEDIATR ACTA 31:159-
       166

320.   VUOPIO,P., HARKONEN,R., JOHNSSON,R. AND NUUTINEN,M., 1973,
       RED CELL GLUCOSE-6-PHOSPHATE DEHYDROGENASE DEFICIENCY IN
       FINLAND. ANN CLIN RES 5:168-173

321.   HARKONEN,M. AND VUOPIO,P., 1974, RED CELL GLUCOSE-6-PHOSPHATE
       DEHYDROGENASE DEFICIENCY IN FINLAND. ANN CLIN RES 6:187-
       197

322.   SHATSKAYA,T.L., KRASNOPOLSKAYA,K.D. AND IDELSON,L.I., 1976,
       THE NEW FORM OF GLUCOSE-6-PHOSPHATE DEHYDROGENASE (G6PD
       "KALUGA") FROM ERYTHROCYTES OF A PATIENT WITH CHRONIC NON-
       SPHEROCYTIC HEMOLYTIC ANEMIA. VOPR MED KHIM 22:764-768

323.   JOHNSON,G.J., KAPLAN,M.E. AND BEUTLER,E., 1977, G-6-PD LONG
       PRAIRIE: A NEW MUTANT EXHIBITING NORMAL SENSITIVITY TO
       INHIBITION BY NADPH AND ACCOMPANIED BY NONSPHEROCYTIC
       HEMOLYTIC ANEMIA. BLOOD 49:247-251

324.   BEUTLER,E., MATSUMOTO,F. AND DAIBER,A., 1974, NONSPHEROCYTIC
       HEMOLYTIC ANEMIA DUE TO G-6-PD PANAMA. IRCS 2:1389

325.   BEUTLER,E. AND ROSEN,R., 1970, NONSPHEROCYTIC CONGENITAL
       HEMOLYTIC ANEMIA DUE TO A NEW G-6-PD VARIANT: G-6-PD
       ALHAMBRA. PEDIATRICS 45:230-235

326.   BEUTLER,E., KELLER,J.W. AND MATSUMOTO,F., 1976, A NEW
       GLUCOSE-6-P DEHYDROGENASE (G-6-PD) VARIANT ASSOCIATED WITH
       NONSPHEROCYTIC HEMOLYTIC ANEMIA: G-6-PD ATLANTA. IRCS
       4:579

327.   CHAN,T.K. AND TODD,D., 1972, CHARACTERISTICS AND DISTRIBUTION
       OF GLUCOSE-6-PHOSPHATE DEHYDROGENASE-DEFICIENT VARIANTS IN
       SOUTH CHINA. AM J HUM GENET 24:475-484

328.   WESTRING,D.W. AND PISCIOTTA,A.V., 1966, ANEMIA, CATARACTS,
       AND SEIZURES IN PATIENT WITH GLUCOSE-6-PHOSPHATE DEHYDROGENASE
       DEFICIENCY. ARCH INTERN MED 118:385-390

329. MILNER,G., DELAMORE,I.W. AND YOSHIDA,A., 1974, G-6-PD MANCHESTER: A NEW VARIANT ASSOCIATED WITH CHRONIC NONSPHEROCYTIC HEMOLYTIC ANEMIA. BLOOD 43:271-276

330. SNYDER,L.M., NECHELES,T.F. AND REDDY,W.J., 1970, G-6-PD WORCESTER: A NEW VARIANT, ASSOCIATED WITH X-LINKED OPTIC ATROPHY. AM J MED 49:125-132

331. WEINREICH,J., BUSCH,D., GOTTSTEIN,U., SCHAEFER,J. AND ROHR,J., 1968, UEBER ZWEI NEUE FAELLE VON HEREDITAERER NICHTSPHAEROCYTAERER HAEMOLYTISCHER ANAEMIE BEI GLUCOSE-6-PHOSPHAT-DEHYDROGENASE-DEFEKT IN EINER NORD DEUTSCHEN FAMILIE. KLIN WOCHENSCHR 46:146-149

332. BUSCH,D. AND BOIE,K., 1970, GLUCOSE-6-PHOSPHATE-DEHYDROGENASE-DEFECT IN DEUTSCHLAND II. EIGENSCHAFTEN DES ENZYMS (TYP FREIBURG). KLIN WOCHENSCHR 48:74-78

333. BALINSKY,D., GOMPERTS,E., CAYANIS,E., JENKINS,T., BRYER,D., BERSOHN,I. AND METZ,J., 1973, GLUCOSE-6-PHOSPHATE DEHYDROGENASE JOHANNESBURG: A NEW VARIANT WITH REDUCED ACTIVITY IN A PATIENT WITH CONGENITAL NON-SPHEROCYTIC HAEMOLYTIC ANAEMIA. BR J HAEMATOL 25:385-391

334. MC CURDY,P.R., 1975, UNPUBLISHED

335. CASTRO,G.A.M. AND SNYDER,L.M., 1974, G6PD SAN JOSE: A NEW VARIANT CHARACTERIZED BY NADPH INHIBITION STUDIES. HUMANGENETIK 21:361-363

336. MC CURDY,P.R., MALDONADO,N., DILLON,D.E. AND CONRAD,M.E., 1973, VARIANTS OF GLUCOSE-6-PHOSPHATE DEHYDROGENASE (G-6-PD) ASSOCIATED WITH G-6-PD DEFICIENCY IN PUERTO RICANS. J LAB CLIN MED 82:432-437

337. KAHN,A., NORTH,M.L., MESSER,J. AND BOIVIN,P., 1975, G-6-PD "ANKARA", A NEW G-6PD VARIANT WITH DEFICIENCY FOUND IN A TURKISH FAMILY. HUMANGENETIK 27:247-250

338. NORTH,M.L., KAHN,A., MESSER,J., WILLARD,D. AND BOIVIN,P., 1975, ICTERE NEO-NATAL ET DEFICIT EN G-6-PD ANKARA, UNE NOUVELLE VARIANTE ENZYMATIQUE DECOUVERTE DANS UNE FAMILLE TURQUE. NOUV REV FR HEMATOL 15:454-459

339. PAWLAK,A.L., ZAGORSKI,Z., ROZYNKOWA,D. AND HORST,A., 1970, POLISH VARIANT OF GLUCOSE-6-PHOSPHATE DEHYDROGENASE (G-6-PD LUBLIN). HUMANGENETIK 10:340-343

340. YOSHIDA,A., BAUR,E.W. AND MOTULSKY,A.G., 1970, A PHILIPPINO GLUCOSE-6-PHOSPHATE DEHYDROGENASE VARIANT (G6PD UNION) WITH ENZYME DEFICIENCY AND ALTERED SUBSTRATE SPECIFICITY. BLOOD 35:506-513

341. KIRKMAN,H.N., KIDSON,C. AND KENNEDY,M., 1968, VARIANTS OF HUMAN GLUCOSE-6-PHOSPHATE DEHYDROGENASE. STUDIES OF SAMPLES FROM NEW GUINEA. HEREDITARY DISORDERS OF ERYTHROCYTE METABOLISM BEUTLER,E. ED. 126-145, CITY OF HOPE SYMP. SERIES, VOL. I, GRUNE & STRATTON, N.Y.

342.   MC CURDY,P.R., BLACKWELL,P.Q., TODD,D., TSO,S.C. AND
       TUCHINDA,S., 1970, FURTHER STUDIES ON GLUCOSE-6-PHOSPHATE
       DEHYDROGENASE DEFICIENCY IN CHINESE SUBJECTS. J LAB CLIN
       MED 75:788-797

343.   CARANDINA,G., MORETTO,E., ZECCHI,G. AND CONIGHI,C., 1976,
       GLUCOSE-6-PHOSPHATE DEHYDROGENASE FERRARA. A NEW VARIANT
       OF G-6-PD IDENTIFIED IN NORTHERN ITALY. ACTA HAEMATOL
       56:116-122

344.   KIRKMAN,H.N. AND LUAN ENG,L.-.I., 1969, VARIANTS OF GLUCOSE
       6 PHOSPHATE DEHYDROGENASE IN INDONESIA. NATURE 221:959

345.   MC CURDY,P.R. AND MAHMOOD,L., 1970, RED CELL GLUCOSE-6-
       PHOSPHATE DEHYDROGENASE DEFICIENCY IN PAKISTAN. J LAB CLIN
       MED 76:943-948

346.   KIRKMAN,H.N., SCHETTINI,F. AND PICKARD,B.M., 1964,
       MEDITERRANEAN VARIANT OF GLUCOSE-6-PHOSPHATE DEHYDROGENASE.
       J LAB CLIN MED 63:726-735

347.   RAMOT,B., BAUMINGER,S., BROK,F., GAFNI,D. AND SHWARTZ,J.,
       1964, CHARACTERIZATION OF GLUCOSE-6-PHOSPHATE DEHYDROGENASE
       IN JEWISH MUTANTS. J LAB CLIN MED 64:895-904

348.   YOSHIDA,A., 1975, UNPUBLISHED

349.   PANICH,V., SUNGNATE,T., WASI,P. AND NA NAKORN,S., 1972, G-
       6-PD MAHIDOL. THE MOST COMMON GLUCOSE-6-PHOSPHATE
       DEHYDROGENASE VARIANT IN THAILAND. J MED ASSOC THAI 55:576-
       585

350.   GEERDINK,R.A., HORST,R. AND STAAL,G.E.J., 1973, AN IRAQI
       JEWISH FAMILY WITH A NEW RED CELL GLUCOSE-6-PHOSPHATE
       DEHYDROGENASE VARIANT (GD-BAGDAD) AND KERNICTERUS. ISR J
       MED SCI 9:1040-1043

351.   STAAL,G.E.J., 1974, PERSONAL COMMUNICATION

352.   KAHN,A., HAKIM,J., COTTREAU,D. AND BOIVIN,P., 1975, GD (-
) MATAM, AN AFRICAN GLUCOSE-6-PHOSPHATE DEHYDROGENASE
       VARIANT WITH ENZYME DEFICIENCY. BIOCHEMICAL AND IMMUNOLOGICAL
       PROPERTIES IN VARIOUS HEMOPOIETIC TISSUES. CLIN CHIM ACTA
       59:183-190

353.   KAHN,A., BERNARD,J.-.F., COTTREAU,D., MARIE,J. AND BOIVIN,P.,
       1975, GD(-)ABRAMI. A DEFICIENT G-6PD VARIANT WITH HEMIZYGOUS
       EXPRESSION IN BLOOD CELLS OF A WOMAN WITH PRIMARY
       MYELOFIBROSIS. HUMANGENETIK 30:41-46

354.   SHATSKAYA,T.L., KRASNOPOLSKAYA,K.D. AND IDELSON,L.J., 1976,
       MUTANT FORMS OF ERYTHROCYTE GLUCOSE-6-PHOSPHATE DEHYDROGENASE
       IN ASHKENAZI. DESCRIPTION OF TWO NEW VARIANTS: G6PD KIROVOGRAD
       AND G6PD ZHITOMIR. HUM GENET 33:175-178

355.   GAHR,M., BORNHALM,D. AND SCHROETER,W., 1976, HAEMOLYTIC
       ANAEMIA DUE TO GLUCOSE-6-PHOSPHATE DEHYDROGENASE (G6PD)
       DEFICIENCY: DEMONSTRATION OF TWO NEW BIOCHEMICAL VARIANTS,
       G6PD HAMM AND G6PD TARSUS. BR J HAEMATOL 33:363-370

356. PANICH,V., SUNGNATE,T. AND NA NAKORN,S., 1972, ACUTE INTRAVASCULAR HEMOLYSIS AND RENAL FAILURE IN A NEW GLUCOSE-6- PHOSPHATE DEHYDROGENASE VARIANT: G-6-PD SIRIRAJ. J MED ASSOC THAI 55:726-731

357. LISKER,R., BRICENO,R.P., ZAVALA,C., NAVARRETE,J.I., WESSELS,M. AND YOSHIDA,A., 1977, A GLUCOSE 6-PHOSPHATE DEHYDROGENASE GD (-) CASTILLA VARIANT CHARACTERIZED BY MILD DEFICIENCY ASSOCIATED WITH DRUG INDUCED HEMOLYTIC ANEMIA. J LAB CLIN MED 90:754-759

358. STAMATOYANNOPOULOS,G., VOIGTLANDER,V., KOTSAKIS,P. AND AKRIVAKIS,A., 1971, GENETIC DIVERSITY OF THE "MEDITERRANEAN" GLUCOSE-6-PHOSPHATE DEHYDROGENASE DEFICIENCY PHENOTYPE. J CLIN INVEST 50:1253-1261

359. BEUTLER,E., 1975, GLUCOSE-6-PHOSPHATE DEHYDROGENASE DEFICIENCY: A NEW INDIAN VARIANT. G 6 PD JAMMU. TRENDS IN HAEMATOLOGY SEN,N.N. AND BASU,A.K. ED. 279-283, N.N. SEN, CALCUTTA INDIA

360. PANICH,V., 1974, G-6-PD INTANON. A NEW GLUCOSE-6-PHOSPHATE DEHYDROGENASE VARIANT. HUMANGENETIK 21:203-205

361. VERGNES,H., YOSHIDA,A., GOURDIN,D., GHERARDI,M., BIERME,R. AND RUFFIE,J., 1974, GLUCOSE-6-PHOSPHATE DEHYDROGENASE TOULOUSE. A NEW VARIANT WITH MARKED INSTABILITY AND SEVERE DEFICIENCY DISCOVERED IN A FAMILY OF MEDITERRANEAN ANCESTRY. ACTA HAEMATOL 51:240-249

362. FERNANDEZ,M. AND FAIRBANKS,V.F., 1968, GLUCOSE-6-PHOSPHATE DEHYDROGENASE DEFICIENCY IN THE PHILLIPINES: REPORT OF A NEW VARIANT-- G 6 PD PANAY. MAYO CLIN PROC 43:645-660

363. NAKASHIMA,K., 1976, UNPUBLISHED

364. PAWLAK,A.L., MAZURKIEWICZ,C.A., ORDYNSKI,J., ROZYNKOWA,D. AND HORST,A., 1975, G-6-PD POZNAN, VARIANT WITH SEVERE ENZYME DEFICIENCY. HUMANGENETIK 28:163-165

365. KAHN,A., ESTERS,A. AND HABEDANK,M., 1976, GD(-)AACHEN, A NEW VARIANT OF DEFICIENT GLUCOSE-6-PHOSPHATE DEHYDROGENASE. HUM GENET 32:171-180

366. SIEGEL,N.H. AND BEUTLER,E., 1971, HEMOLYTIC ANEMIA CAUSED BY G-6-PD CARSWELL, A NEW VARIANT. ANN INTERN MED 75:437-439

367. MARKS,P.A., BANKS,J. AND GROSS,R., 1962, GENETIC HETEROGENEITY OF GLUCOSE-6-PHOSPHATE DEHYDROGENASE DEFICIENCY. NATURE 194:454-456

368. YOSHIDA,A., STAMATOYANNOPOULOS,G. AND MOTULSKY,A., 1967, NEGRO VARIANT OF GLUCOSE-6-PHOSPHATE DEHYDROGENASE DEFICIENCY (A-) IN MAN. SCIENCE 155:97-99

369. KIRKMAN,H.N., MC CURDY,P.R. AND NAIMAN,J.L., 1964, FUNCTIONALLY ABNORMAL GLUCOSE-6-PHOSPHATE DEHYDROGENASES. COLD SPRING HARBOR SYMP QUANT BIOL 29:391-398

370. HURWIC,M., 1970, DZIEDZICZNY NIEDOBOR DEHYDROGENAZY GLUKOZO-
      6-FOSFORANOWEJ W KRWINCE CZERWONEJ. POSTEPY HIG MED DOSW
      24:497-522

371. KISSIN,C. AND COTTE,J., 1970, ETUDE D'UN VARIANT DE GLUCOSE-
      6-PHOSPHATE DESHYDROGENASE: LE TYPE CONSTANTINE. ENZYME
      11:277-284

372. SANSONE,G., PERRONI,L. AND YOSHIDA,A., 1975, GLUCOSE-6-
      PHOSPHATE DEHYDROGENASE VARIANTS FROM ITALIAN SUBJECTS
      ASSOCIATED WITH SEVERE NEONATAL JAUNDICE. BR J HAEMATOL
      31:159-165

373. VERGNES,H., GHERARDI,M. AND YOSHIDA,A., 1976, G6PD LOZERE
      AND TRINACRIA-LIKE. SEGREGATION OF TWO NON HEMOLYTIC VARIANTS
      IN A FRENCH FAMILY. HUM GENET 34:293-298

374. CROOKSTON,J.H., YOSHIDA,A., LIN,M. AND BOOSER,D.J., 1973,
      G 6 PD TORONTO. BIOCHEM J 8:259-265

375. NAKASHIMA,K., ONO,J., ABE,S., MIWA,S. AND YOSHIDA,A., 1977,
      G6PD UBE, A GLUCOSE-6-PHOSPHATE DEHYDROGENASE VARIANT FOUND
      IN FOUR UNRELATED JAPANESE FAMILIES. AM J HUM GENET 29:24-
      30

376. REYS,L., MANSO,C. AND STAMATOYANNOPOULOS,G., 1970, GENETIC
      STUDIES ON SOUTHEASTERN BANTU OF MOZAMBIQUE. I. VARIANTS
      OF GLUCOSE-6-PHOSPHATE DEHYDROGENASE. AM J HUM GENET 22:203-
      215

377. STAMATOYANNOPOULOS,G., 1975, UNPUBLISHED

378. MC CURDY,P.R., KIRKMAN,H.N., NAIMAN,J.L., JIM,R.T.S. AND
      PICKARD,B.M., 1966, A CHINESE VARIANT OF GLUCOSE-6-PHOSPHATE
      DEHYDROGENASE. J LAB CLIN MED 67:374-385

379. KAPLAN,J.C., ROSA,R., SERINGE,P. AND HOEFFEL,J.C., 1967,
      LE POLYORPHISME GENETIQUE DE LA GLUCOSE-6-PHOSPHATE
      DESHYDROGENASE ERYTHROCYTAIRE CHEZ L'HOMME. ENZYME 8:332-
      340

380. MANDELLI,F., AMADORI,S., DE LAURENZI,A., KAHN,A., ISACCHI,G.
      AND PAPA,G., 1977, GLUCOSE-6-PHOSPHATE DEHYDROGENASE
      VELLETRI. ACTA HAEMATOL 57:121-126

381. PANICH,V. AND SUNGNATE,T., 1973, CHARACTERIZATION OF GLUCOSE-
      6-PHOSPHATE DEHYDROGENASE IN THAILAND. HUMANGENETIK 18:39-
      46

382. MIWA,S., NAKASHIMA,K., ONO,J., FUJII,H. AND SUZUKI,E.,
      1977, THREE GLUCOSE 6-PHOSPHATE DEHYDROGENASE VARIANTS
      FOUND IN JAPAN. HUM GENET 36:327-334

383. BEUTLER,E. AND MATSUMOTO,F., 1977, A NEW GLUCOSE-6-PHOSPHATE
      DEHYDROGENASE VARIANT: G-6-PD (-) LOS ANGELES. IRCS 5:89

384. SANSONE,G., PERRONI,L., YOSHIDA,A. AND DAVE,V., 1977, A
      NEW GLUCOSE-6-PHOSPHATE DEHYDROGENASE VARIANT (GD TRINACRIA)
      IN TWO UNRELATED FAMILIES OF SICILIAN ANCESTRY. ITAL J
      BIOCH 26:44-50

385. KAPLAN,J.C., HANZLICKOVA LEROUX,A., NICHOLAS,A.M., ROSA,R., WEILER,C. AND LEPERCQ,G., 1970, A NEW GLUCOSE-6-PHOSPHATE DEHYDROGENASE VARIANT (G6PD PORT-ROYAL). ENZYME 12:25-32

386. KIRKMAN,H.N., SIMON,E.R. AND PICKARD,B.M., 1965, SEATTLE VARIANT OF GLUCOSE-6-PHOSPHATE DEHYDROGENASE. J LAB CLIN MED 66:834-840

387. AZEVEDO,E., KIRKMAN,H.N., MORROW,A.C. AND MOTULSKY,A.G., 1968, VARIANTS OF RED CELL GLUCOSE-6-PHOSPHATE DEHYDROGENASE AMONG ASIATIC INDIANS. ANN HUM GENET 31:373-379

388. NURSE,G.T. AND BALINSKY,D., 1975, UNPUBLISHED

389. YOSHIDA,A., BAUR,E. AND VOIGTLANDER,B., 1975, UNPUBLISHED

390. VERGNES,H., GHERARDI,M., QUILICI,J.C., YOSHIDA,A. AND GIACARDY,R., 1973, G-6-PD LUZ-SAINT-SAUVEUR: A NEW VARIANT WITH ABNORMAL ELECTROPHORETIC MOBILITY MILD ENZYME DEFICIENCY AND ABSENCE OF HAEMATOLOGICAL DISORDERS. IRCS (73-7) 3-1-14 (ABSTRACT)

391. STAMATOYANNOPOULOS,G., KOTSAKIS,P., VOIGTLANDER,V. AND MOTULSKY,A.G., 1970, ELECTROPHORETIC DIVERSITY OF GLUCOSE-6-PHOSPHATE DEHYDROGENASE AMONG GREEKS. AM J HUM GENET 22:587-596

392. STAMATOYANNOPOULOS,G., VOIGTLAENDER,V. AND AKRIVAKIS,A., 1970, THESSALY VARIANT OF GLUCOSE-6-PHOSPHATE DEHYDROGENASE. HUMANGENETIK 9:23-25

393. YOSHIDA,A. AND BAUR,E., 1975, UNPUBLISHED

394. LONG,W.K., KIRKMAN,H.N. AND SUTTON,H.E., 1965, ELECTROPHORETICALLY SLOW VARIANTS OF GLUCOSE-6-PHOSPHATE DEHYDROGENASE FROM RED CELLS OF NEGROES. J LAB CLIN MED 65:81-87

395. HOOK,E.B., STAMATOYANNOPOULOS,G., YOSHIDA,A. AND MOTULSKY,A.G., 1968, GLUCOSE-6-PHOSPHATE DEHYDROGENASE MADRONA:A SLOW ELECTROPHORETIC GLUCOSE-6-PHOSPHATE DEHYDROGENASE VARIANT WITH KINETIC CHARACTERISTICS SIMILAR TO THOSE OF NORMAL TYPE. J LAB CLIN MED 72:404-409

396. NIESSNER,H. AND BEUTLER,E., 1973, CONTAMINATION OF COMMERCIALLY AVAILABLE INTERMEDIATES OF THE GLYCOLYTIC PATHWAY. EXPERIENTIA 29:268-270

397. AZEVEDO,E.S. AND YOSHIDA,A., 1969, BRAZILIAN VARIANT OF GLUCOSE-6-PHOSPHATE DEHYDROGENASE (GD MINAS GERAIS). NATURE 222:380-382

398. DERN,R.J., MC CURDY,P.R. AND YOSHIDA,A., 1969, A NEW STRUCTURAL VARIANT OF GLUCOSE-6-PHOSPHATE DEHYDROGENASE WITH A HIGH PRODUCTION RATE (G6PD). J LAB CLIN MED 73:283-290

399. RATTAZZI,M.C., BERNINI,L.F., FIORELLI,G. AND MANNUCCI,P.M., 1967, ELECTROPHORESIS OF GLUCOSE-6-PHOSPHATE DEHYDROGENASE: A NEW TECHNIQUE. NATURE 213:79-80

400. SPARKES,R.S., BALUDA,M.C. AND TOWNSEND,D.E., 1969, CELLULOSE
      ACETATE ELECTROPHORESIS OF HUMAN GLUCOSE-6-PHOSPHATE
      DEHYDROGENASE. J LAB CLIN MED 73:531-534

401. PETERSON JR,W.D., STULBERG,C.S., SWANBORG,N.K. AND
      ROBINSON,A.R., 1968, GLUCOSE-6-PHOSPHATE DEHYDROGENASE
      ISOENZYMES IN HUMAN CELL CULTURES DETERMINED BY SUCROSE-
      AGAR GEL AND CELLULOSE ACETATE ZYMOGRAMS. PROC SOC EXP BIOL
      MED 128:772-776

402. ELLIS,N. AND ALPERIN,J.B., 1972, LABORATORY SUGGESTIONS:
      A RAPID METHOD FOR ELECTROPHORESIS OF ERYTHROCYTE GLUCOSE-
      6-PHOSPHATE DEHYDROGENASE ON CELLULOSE ACETATE PLATES. AM
      J CLIN PATHOL 57:534-536

403. HAYWOOD,B., STARKWEATHER,W., SPENCER,H. AND ZARAFONETIS,C.,
      1968, ELECTROPHORETIC SEPARATION OF GLUCOSE-6-PHOSPHATE
      DEHYDROGENASE FROM HUMAN ERYTHROCYTES WITH AGAR GELS. J
      LAB CLIN MED 71:324-327

404. LOUDERBACK,A., BEUTLER,E., NATLAND,M. AND TEMIANKA,D.,
      1969, AGAR GEL ELECTROPHORESIS OF G-6-PD ISOENZYMES. CLINICAL
      RESEARCH 17:149 (ABSTRACT)

405. BAKAY,B., NYHAN,W.L. AND ST J MONKUS,E., 1972, CHANGE IN
      ELECTROPHORETIC MOBILITY OF GLUCOSE-6-PHOSPHATE DEHYDROGENASE
      WITH AGING OF ERTHROCYTES. PEDIATR RES 6:705-712

406. PILLER,G., RAINER,H., MAUPER,L. AND MOSER,K., 1976,
      SAEULENCHROMATOGRAPHISCHE ANREICHERUNG DER "GLUKOSE-6-
      PHOSPHATDEHYDROGENASE WIEN". WIEN KLIN WOCHENSCHR 88:6-9

407. LUZZATTO,L. AND ALLAN,N.C., 1965, DIFFERENT PROPERTIES OF
      GLUCOSE-6-PHOSPHATE DEHYDROGENASE FROM HUMAN ERYTHROCYTES
      WITH NORMAL AND ABNORMAL ENZYME LEVELS. BIOCHEM BIOPHYS
      RES COMMUN 21:547-554

408. LUZZATTO,L. AND OKOYE,V.C.N., 1967, RESOLUTION OF GENETIC
      VARIANTS OF HUMAN ERYTHROCYTE GLUCOSE-6-PHOSPHATE
      DEHYDROGENASE BY THIN LAYER CHROMATOGRAPHY. BIOCHEM BIOPHYS
      RES COMMUN 29:705-709

409. MARKS,P.A. AND TSUTSUI,E.A., 1963, HUMAN GLUCOSE-6-P
      DEHYDROGENASE; STUDIES ON THE RELATION BETWEEN ANTIGENICITY
      AND CATALYTIC ACTIVITY-THE ROLE OF TPN. ANN NY ACAD SCI
      103:903-914

410. KAHN,A., COTTREAU,D. AND BOIVIN,P., 1974, MOLECULAR MECHANISM
      OF GLUCOSE-6-PHOSPHATE DEHYDROGENASE DEFICIENCY. HUMANGENETIK
      25:101-109

411. ROSA,R., ALEXANDRE,Y., KAPLAN,J.C. AND DREYFUS,J.C., 1970,
      COMPORTEMENT IMMUNOLOGIQUE DE LA GLUCOSE-6-PHOSPHATE-
      DESHYDROGENASE ERYTHROCYTAIRE CHEZ DES MUTANTS DEFICIENTS.
      CLIN CHIM ACTA 29:209-214

412. NAKASHIMA,K. AND YOSHIDA,A., 1977, PROBLEMS OF INDIRECT
      IMMUNOLOGIC ASSAY OF SPECIFIC ENZYME ACTIVITY. J LAB CLIN
      MED 89:446-454

413. CARSON,P.E., 1960, GLUCOSE-6-PHOSPHATE DEHYDROGENASE DEFICIENCY IN HEMOLYTIC ANEMIA. FED PROC 19:995-1006

414. BEN-ISHAY,D. AND IZAK,G., 1964, CHRONIC HEMOLYSIS ASSOCIATED WITH GLUCOSE-6-PHOSPHATE DEFICIENCY. J LAB CLIN MED 63:1002-1009

415. BEN-BASSAT,J. AND BEN-ISHAY,D., 1969, HEREDITARY HEMOLYTIC ANEMIA ASSOCIATED WITH GLUCOSE-6-PHOSPHATE DEHYDROGENASE DEFICIENCY (MEDITERRANEAN TYPE). ISR J MED SCI 5:1053-1059

416. MARKS,P.A. AND JOHNSON,A.B., 1958, RELATIONSHIP BETWEEN THE AGE OF HUMAN ERYTHROCYTES AND THEIR OSMOTIC RESISTANCE: A BASIS FOR SEPARATING YOUNG AND OLD ERYTHROCYTES. J CLIN INVEST 37:1542-1548

417. BONSIGNORE,A., FORANINI,A., FANTONI,A., LEONCINI,G. AND SEGNI,P., 1964, RELATIONSHIP BETWEEN AGE AND ENZYMATIC ACTIVITIES IN HUMAN ERYTHROCYTES FROM NORMAL AND FAVA-BEAN-SENSITIVE SUBJECTS. J CLIN INVEST 43:834-842

418. PIOMELLI,S., CORASH,L.M., DAVENPORT,D.D., MIRAGLIA,J. AND AMOROSI,E.L., 1968, IN VIVO LABILITY OF GLUCOSE-6-PHOSHATE DEHYDROGENASE IN GDA- AND GD MEDITERRANEAN DEFICIENCY. J CLIN INVEST 47:940-948

419. SRIVASTAVA,S.K. AND BEUTLER,E., 1968, OXIDIZED GLUTATHIONE LEVELS IN ERYTHROCYTES OF GLUCOSE-6-PHOSPHATE DEHYDROGENASE-DEFICIENT SUBJECTS. LANCET 2:23-24

420. BEUTLER,E. AND SRIVASTAVA,S.K., 1968, THE EFFLUX OF GSSG FROM HUMAN ERYTHROCYTES. METABOLISM AND MEMBRANE PERMEABILITY OF ERYTHROCYTES AND THROMBOCYTES DEUTSCH,E., GERLACH,E. AND MOSER,K. ED. 91-95, GEORG THIEME, STUTTGART

421. SRIVASTAVA,S.K. AND BEUTLER,E., 1969, THE TRANSPORT OF OXIDIZED GLUTATHIONE FROM HUMAN ERYTHROCYTES. J BIOL CHEM 244:9-16

422. SMITH,J.E., 1974, RELATIONSHIP OF IN VIVO ERYTHROCYTE GLUTATHIONE FLUX TO THE OXIDIZED GLUTATHIONE TRANSPORT SYSTEM. J LAB CLIN MED 83:444-450

423. PRCHAL,J., SRIVASTAVA,S.K. AND BEUTLER,E., 1975, ACTIVE TRANSPORT OF GSSG FROM RECONSTITUTED ERYTHROCYTE GHOSTS. BLOOD 46:111-117

424. KELLERMEYER,R.W., CARSON,P.E., SCHRIER,S.L., TARLOV,A.R. AND ALVING,A.S., 1961, THE HEMOLYTIC EFFECT OF PRIMAQUINE. XIV. PENTOSE METABOLISM IN PRIMAQUINE-SENSITIVE ERYTHROCYTES. J LAB CLIN MED 58:715-724

425. DAVIDSON,W.D. AND TANAKA,K.R., 1972, FACTORS AFFECTING PENTOSE PHOSPHATE PATHWAY ACTIVITY IN HUMAN RED CELLS. BR J HAEMATOL 23:371-385

426. KIRKMAN,H.N., GAETANI,G.D., CLEMONS,E.H. AND MARENI,C., 1975, RED CELL NADP+ AND NADPH IN GLUCOSE-6-PHOSPHATE DEHYDROGENASE DEFICIENCY. J CLIN INVEST 55:875-878

427. BEUTLER,E. AND BALUDA,M.C., 1963, METHEMOGLOBIN REDUCTION.
      STUDIES OF THE INTERACTION BETWEEN CELL POPULATIONS AND OF
      THE ROLE OF METHYLENE BLUE. BLOOD 22:323-333

428. MARENI,C. AND GAETANI,G.F.D., 1976, NADP+ AND NADPH IN
      GLUCOSE-6-PHOSPHATE DEHYDROGENASE-DEFICIENT ERYTHROCYTES
      UNDER OXIDATIVE STIMULATION. BIOCHIM BIOPHYS ACTA 430:395-
      398

429. GAETANI,G.D., PARKER,J.C. AND KIRKMAN,H.N., 1974,
      INTRACELLULAR RESTRAINT: A NEW BASIS FOR THE LIMITATION IN
      RESPONSE TO OXIDATIVE STRESS IN HUMAN ERYTHROCYTES CONTAINING
      LOW-ACTIVITY VARIANTS OF GLUCOSE-6-PHOSPHATE DEHYDROGENASE.
      PROC NATL ACAD SCI USA 71:3584-3587

430. NEIMANN,N., DREYFUS,J.C., PIERSON,M., DUCAS,J. AND
      STOESSEL,J.M., 1963, LE METHEMOGLOBINEMIE CONGENITALE ET
      RECESSIVE. SON ASSOCIATION AVEC LE DEFICIT EN GLUCOSE 6
      PHOSPHATE DESHYDROGENASE ET LA THALASSEMIE MINEURE. REV
      FRANC ETUDES CLIN ET BIOL 8:757-764

431. BENSINGER,T.A., 1976, PROLONGED MAINTENANCE OF 2,3
      DIPHOSPHOGLYCERATE (2,3-DPG) IN GLUCOSE-6-P DEHYDROGENASE
      (G6PD) DEFICIENT STORED BLOOD. CLINICAL RESEARCH 24:107A

432. BENSINGER,T.A. AND MEDINA,F., 1976, EXCESSIVE PYRUVATE
      ACCUMULATION IN G-6-PD DEFICIENT (G-6-PD-DEF) ERYTHROCYTES
      DURING LIQUID STORAGE. BLOOD 48:993 (ABSTRACT)

433. ORLINA,A.R., JOSEPHSON,A.M. AND MC DONALD,B.J., 1970, THE
      POSTSTORAGE VIABILITY OF GLUCOSE-6-PHOSPHATE DENYDROGENASE-
      DEFICIENT ERYTHROCYTES. J LAB CLIN MED 75:930-936

434. STUCKEY JR,W.J., 1966, HEMOLYTIC ANEMIA AND ERYTHROCYTE
      GLUCOSE-6-PHOSPHATE DEHYDROGENASE DEFICIENCY. AM J MED SCI
      251:104-115

435. TIZIANELLO,A., PANNACCIULLI,I., SALVIDIO,E. AND GAY,A.,
      1963, ERYTHROCYTIC GLUCOSE-6-PHOSPHATE DEHYDROGENASE
      DEFICIENCY AS A PROBLEM IN THE SELECTION OF BLOOD DONORS.
      VOX SANG 8:47-50

436. SALVIDIO,E., PANNACCIULLI,I., STANGONI,A., AJMAR,F.,
      PARAVIDINO,G., GAETANI,G. AND MAROGNA,G., 1969, I DIFETTI
      ENZYMATICI ERITROCITARI NELLA PRATICA TRASFUSIONALE. LA
      TRASFUSIONE DEL SANGUE 14:175-199

437. MC CURDY,P.R. AND MORSE,E.E., 1975, GLUCOSE-6-PHOSPHATE
      DEHYDROGENASE DEFICIENCY AND BLOOD TRANSFUSION. VOX SANG
      28:230-237

438. JAFFE,E.R., 1963, THE REDUCTION OF METHEMOGLOBIN IN
      ERYTHROCYTES OF A PATIENT WITH CONGENITAL METHEMOGLOBINEMIA,
      SUBJECTS WITH ERYTHROCYTE GLUCOSE-6-PHOSPHATE DEHYDROGENASE
      DEFICIENCY, AND NORMAL INDIVIDUALS. BLOOD 21:561-572

439. BONSIGNORE,A., FORNAINI,G., SEGNI,G. AND FANTONI,F., 1960,
      GLUTATHIONE-REDUCTASE AND METHAEMOGLOBIN-REDUCTASE IN
      ERYTHROCYTES OF HUMAN SUBJECTS WITH A CASE HISTORY OF
      FAVISM. ITAL J BIOCHEM 9:345-353

440. SCHRIER,S.L., KELLERMEYER,R.W., CARSON,P.E., ICKES,C.E.
AND ALVING,A.S., 1958, THE HEMOLYTIC EFFECT OF PRIMAQUINE
(IX. ENZYMATIC ABNORMALITIES IN PRIMAQUINE-SENSITIVE
ERYTHROCYTES). J LAB CLIN MED 52:109-117

441. FLATZ,G. AND SIMMERSBACH,F., 1970, FLAVIN ADENINE DINUCLEOTIDE
CONCENTRATION IN ERYTHROCYTES WITH NORMAL AND DEFICIENT
GLUCOSE-6-PHOSPHATE DEHYDROGENASE. KLIN WOCHENSCHR 48:1071-
1072

442. BIENZLE,U., EFFIONG,C.E., AIMAKU,V.E. AND LUZZATTO,L.,
1976, ERYTHROCYTE ENZYMES IN NEONATAL JAUNDICE. ACTA HAEMATOL
55:10-20

443. GAETANI,G.F., GARRE,C.S., AJMAR,F. AND BIANCHI,G.L., 1973,
INFLUENCE OF RIBOFLAVIN AND OF ERYTHROCYTE STROMA ON
GLUTATHIONE REDUCTASE ACTIVITY IN NORMAL, GLUCOSE 6 PHOSPHATE
DEHYDROGENASE DEFICIENT AND LOW GLUTATHIONE REDUCTASE
INDIVIDUALS. BIOMEDICINE 19:469-474

444. FLATZ,G., 1970, ENHANCED BINDING OF FAD TO GLUTATHIONE
REDUCTASE IN G-6-PD DEFICIENCY. NATURE 226:755

445. BEUTLER,E., 1977, GLUCOSE-6-PHOSPHATE DEHYDROGENASE DEFICIENCY
AND RED CELL GLUTATHIONE PEROXIDASE. BLOOD 49:467-469

446. LARIZZA,P., BRUNETTI,P., GRIGNANI,F. AND VENTURA,S., 1958,
L'INDIVIDUALITA BIO-ENZIMATICA DELL'ERITROCITO "FABICO"
SOPRA ALCUNE ANOMALIE BIOCHIMICHE ED ENZIMATICHE DELLE
EMAZIE NEI PAZIENTI AFFETTI DA FAVISMO E NEI LORO FAMILIARI.
HAEMATOLOGICA (PAVIA) 43:205-250

447. LOEHR,G.W. AND WALLER,H.D., 1958, HAEMOLYTISCHE
ERYTHROCYTOPATHIE DURCH FEHLEN VON GLUKOSE-6-PHOSPHAT-
DEHYDROGENASE IN ROTEN BLUTZELLEN ALS DOMINANT VERERBLICHE
KRANKHEIT. KLIN WOCHENSCHR 36:865-869

448. BONSIGNORE,A., FORNAINI,G., SEGNI,G. AND SEITUN,A., 1961,
TRANSKETOLASE AND TRANSALDOLASE REACTIONS IN THE ERYTHROCYTES
OF HUMAN SUBJECTS WITH FAVISM HISTORY. BIOCHEM BIOPHYS RES
COMMUN 4:147-150

449. SCHRIER,S.L., KELLERMEYER,R.W., CARSON,P.E., ALVING,A.S.
AND ICKES,C.E., 1959, THE HEMOLYTIC EFFECT OF PRIMAQUINE.
IX. ENZYMATIC ABNORMALITIES IN PRIMAQUINE-SENSITIVE
ERYTHROCYTES. J LAB CLIN MED 54:232-240

450. BREWER,G.J., POWELL,R.D., SWANSON,S.H. AND ALVING,A.S.,
1964, HEMOLYTIC EFFECT OF PRIMAQUINE. XVII. HEXOKINASE
ACTIVITY OF GLUCOSE-6-PHOSPHATE DEHYDROGENASE-DEFICIENT
AND NORMAL ERYTHROCYTES. J LAB CLIN MED 64:601-612

451. TARLOV,A. AND KELLERMEYER,R.W., 1961, THE HEMOLYTIC EFFECT
OF PRIMAQUINE. XI. DECREASED CATALASE ACTIVITY IN PRIMAQUINE-
SENSITIVE ERYTHROCYTES. J LAB CLIN MED 58:204-216

452. RUSSO,G., SCHILIRO,G. AND GALLONE,G., 1968, L'ATTIVITA
CATALASICA DI GLOBULI ROSSI CARENTI IN GLUCOSIO-6-FOSFATO
DEIDROGENASI. PEDIATRIA (NAPOLI) 76:169-177

453. EZRA,R., SZEINBERG,A. AND SHEBA,C., 1965, CATALASE ACTIVITY
      IN NORMAL AND GLUCOSE-6-PHOSPHATE DEHYDROGENASE DEFICIENT
      RED CELLS. ISR J MED SCI 1:847-849

454. JOHNSON,A.B. AND MARKS,P.A., 1958, GLUCOSE METABOLISM AND
      OXYGEN CONSUMPTION IN NORMAL AND GLUCOSE-6- PHOSPHATE
      DEHYDROGENASE DEFICIENT HUMAN ERYTHROCYTES. CLINICAL RESEARCH
      6:187-188 (ABSTRACT)

455. HELLER,P. AND WEINSTEIN,H., 1959, ALDOLASE, ISOCITRIC
      DEHYDROGENASE AND MALIC DEHYDROGENASE IN GLUCOSE-6- PHOSPHATE
      DEHYDROGENASE DEFICIENT ERYTHROCYTES. J LAB CLIN MED 54:824-
      825

456. HARTZ,J., EL MAGHRABI,R., NAMEN,A., GABR,M., BOWMAN,J.,
      CARSON,P., AJMAR,F. AND KAMEL,K., 1973, ENZYME STUDIES IN
      G-6-PD DEFICIENT ERYTHROCYTES FROM EGYPTIANS, ITALIANS,
      AND AMERICAN NEGROES (PYROPHOSPHATASE, 6-PGD, GLUTAMIC-
      OXALACETIC TRANSAMINASE, ACID PHOSPHATASE, CATALASE AND
      SUPEROXIDE DISMUTASE ASSAYS). CLIN CHIM ACTA 48:117-126

457. OSKI,F.A., SHAHIDI,N.T. AND DIAMOND,L.K., 1963, ERYTHROCYTE
      ACID PHOSPHOMONESTERASE AND GLUCOSE-6-PHOSPHATE DEHYDROGENASE
      DEFICIENCY IN CAUCASIANS. SCIENCE 139:409-410

458. LU,T.C. AND WEI,H., 1967, ERYTHROCYTE ACID PHOSPHOMONOESTERASE
      ACTIVITY IN NEWLY BORN CHINESE DEFICIENT IN GLUCOSE-6-
      PHOSPHATE DEHYDROGENASE. NATURE 213:707-708

459. BOTTINI,E., LUCARELLI,P., AGOSTINO,R., PALMARINO,R.,
      BOSINCO,L. AND ANTOGNONI,G., 1971, FAVISM: ASSOCIATION WITH
      ERYTHROCYTE ACID PHOSPHATASE PHENOTYPE. SCIENCE 171:409-
      411

460. BRUNETTI,P., GRIGNANI,F. AND ERNISLI,G., 1962, BEHAVIOUR
      OF THE ERYTHROCYTE PYROPHOSPHATASE ACTIVITY IN THE ENZYME-
      DEFICENCY HAEMOLYTIC ANAEMIAS. II. A NEW TEST FOR THE
      DETECTION OF THE ENZYME DEFECT. ACTA HAEMATOL 27:246-250

461. RAPOPORT,S. AND SCHEUCH,D., 1960, GLUTATHIONE STABILITY
      AND PYROPHOSPHATASE ACTIVITY IN RETICULOCYTES: DIRECT
      EVIDENCE FOR THE IMPORTANCE OF GLUTATHIONE FOR THE ENZYME
      STATUS IN INTACT CELLS. NATURE 186:967-968

462. SZEINBERG,A. AND CLEJAN,L., 1964, SULFHYDRYL GROUPS IN THE
      RED CELLS OF NORMAL AND GLUCOSE-6-PHOSPHATE DEHYDROGENASE-
      DEFICIENT SUBJECTS. BIOCHIM BIOPHYS ACTA 93:564-572

463. SHAFER,A.W., 1965, THE CARBOHYDRATE INTERMEDIATES OF
      ERYTHROCYTES DEFICIENT IN GLUCOSE-6-PHOSPHATE DEHYDROGENASE.
      BLOOD 26:82-90

464. MOHLER,D.N. AND CROCKETT JR,C.L., 1964, HEREDITARY HEMOLYTIC
      DISEASE SECONDARY TO GLUCOSE-6-PHOSPHATE DEHYDROGENASE
      DEFICIENCY: REPORT OF THREE CASES WITH SPECIAL EMPHASIS ON
      ATP METABOLISM. BLOOD 23:427-444

465. MOHLER,D.N. AND WILLIAMS,W.J., 1961, THE EFFECT OF
      PHENYLHYDRAZINE ON THE ADENOSINE TRIPHOSPHATE CONTENT OF
      NORMAL AND GLUCOSE-6-PHOSPHATE DEHYDROGENASE-DEFICIENT
      HUMAN BLOOD. J CLIN INVEST 40:1735-1742

466. TARLOV,A.R., BREWER,G.J., CARSON,P.E. AND ALVING,A.S., 1962, PRIMAQUINE SENSITIVITY. GLUCOSE-6-PHOSPHATE DEHYDROGENASE DEFICIENCY: AN INBORN ERROR OF METABOLISM OF MEDICAL AND BIOLOGICAL SIGNIFICANCE. ARCH INTERN MED 109:209-234

467. SZEINBERG,A., ZAIDMAN,J. AND CLEJAN,L., 1965, INVESTIGATION OF THE LIPID CONTENT OF NORMAL AND GLUCOSE-6-PHOSPHATE DEHYDROGENASE DEFICIENT RED CELLS. BIOCHIM BIOPHYS ACTA 98:598-606

468. KHALIL,M., AZIZ,Y., TANIOUS,A., MAHMOUD,S. AND GHARIB,B., 1975, STUDY OF RED CELL MEMBRANE LIPIDS IN GLUCOSE-6-PHOSPHATE DEHYDROGENASE DEFICIENCY ANEMIA. GAZETTE OF THE EGYPTIAN PAEDIATRIC ASSOCIATION 23:281-289

469. SZEINBERG,A., ZAIDMAN,J. AND CLEJAN,L., 1965, INVESTIGATION OF THE LIPID CONTENT OF NORMAL AND GLUCOSE-6-PHOSPHATE DEHYDROGENASE DEFICIENT RED CELLS. ISR J MED SCI 1:833-835

470. DANON,D., SHEBA,C. AND RAMOT,B., 1961, THE MORPHOLOGY OF GLUCOSE 6 PHOSPHATE DEHYDROGENASE DEFICIENT ERYTHROCYTES: ELECTRON-MICROSCOPIC STUDIES. BLOOD 17:229-234

471. TILLMANN,W., LABITZKE,N. AND SCHROETER,W., 1977, GUENSTIGE RHEOLOGISCHE EIGENSCHAFTEN DER ERYTHROZYTEN BEIM GLUCOSE-6- PHOSPHATDEHYDROGENASE-MANGEL. KLIN WOCHENSCHR 55:385-391

472. ERSLEV,A.J., 1977, ERYTHROKINETICS. HEMATOLOGY WILLIAMS,W.J., BEUTLER,E., ERSLEV,A.J. AND RUNDLES,R.W. ED. CHAPTER A 19, 2ND EDITION, PP. 1620-1626, MC GRAW-HILL, NEW YORK

473. BREWER,G.J., TARLOV,A.R. AND KELLERMEYER,R.W., 1961, THE HEMOLYTIC EFFECT OF PRIMAQUINE. XII. SHORTENED ERYTHROCYTE LIFE SPAN IN PRIMAQUINE-SENSITIVE MALE NEGROES IN THE ABSENCE OF DRUG ADMINISTRATION. J LAB CLIN MED 58:217-224

474. BERNINI,L., LATTE,B., SINISCALCO,M., PIOMELLI,S., SPADA,U., ADINOLFI,M. AND MOLLISON,P.L., 1964, SURVIVAL OF 51 CR-LABELLED RED CELLS IN SUBJECTS WITH THALASSEMIA-TRAIT OR G6PD DEFICIENCY OR BOTH ABNORMALITIES. BR J HAEMATOL 10:171-180

475. MC CAFFREY,R.P., HALSTED,C.H., WAHAB,M.F.A. AND ROBERTSON,R.P., 1971, CHLORAMPHENICOL-INDUCED HEMOLYSIS IN CAUCASIAN GLUCOSE-6-PHOSPHATE DEHYDROGENASE DEFICIENCY. ANN INTERN MED 74:722-726

476. MUSUMECI,S. AND MAZZONE,D., 1970, STUDIO DELLA SOPRAVVIVENZA ERITROCITARIA IN BAMBINI SICILIANI PORTATORI DI CARENZA DI G6PD. PEDIATRIA (NAPOLI) 78:868-878

477. CHAN,T.K., TODD,D. AND TSO,S.C., 1974, RED CELL SURVIVAL STUDIES IN GLUCOSE-6-PHOSPHATE DEHYDROGENASE DEFICIENCY. BULL HONG KONG MEDICAL ASSOCIATION 26:41-48

478. STAAL,G.E.J., PUNT,K., GEERDINK,R.A., BOS,C.C. AND BARTSTRA,H., 1970, A POSSIBLE NEW VARIANT OF G-6-PD WITH DECREASED ACTIVITY (G-6-PD UTRECHT) IN A DUTCH FAMILY WITH HEREDITARY SPHEROCYTOSIS. SCAND J HAEMATOL 7:401-403

479. RUBINS,J. AND YOUNG,L.E., 1977, HEREDITARY SPHEROCYTOSIS
      AND GLUCOSE-6-PHOSPHATE DEHYDROGENASE DEFICIENCY. DOUBLE
      HEMOLYTIC JEOPARDY. JAMA 237:797-798

480. SANPITAK,N., SUPALERT,Y., CHAYUTIMONKUL,L. AND FLATZ,G.,
      1973, COMBINED ERYTHROCYTE PHOSPHOHEXOSE ISOMERASE AND
      GLUCOSE-6-PHOSPHATE DEHYDROGENASE DEFICIENCY. HUM HERED
      23:83-87

481. SCHROETER,W., BRITTINGER,G., ZIMMERSCHMITT,E., KOENIG,E.
      AND SCHRADER,D., 1971, COMBINED GLUCOSEPHOSPHATE ISOMERASE
      AND GLUCOSE-6-PHOSPHATE DEHYDROGENASE DEFICIENCY OF THE
      ERYTHROCYTES: A NEW HAEMOLYTIC SYNDROME. BR J HAEMATOL
      20:249-261

482. OSKI,F.A., NATHAN,D.G., SIDEL,V.W. AND DIAMOND,L.K., 1964,
      EXTREME HEMOLYSIS AND RED-CELL DISTORTION IN ERYTHROCYTE
      PYRUVATE KINASE DEFICIENCY. N ENGL J MED 270:1023-1030

483. MOSKOWITZ,R.M., 1970, AUTOIMMUNE HEMOLYTIC ANEMIA IN A
      PATIENT WITH A DEFICIENCY OF RED CELL GLUCOSE-6-PHOSPHATE
      DEHYDROGENASE ACTIVITY. JOHNS HOPKINS MED J 126:139-145

484. TCHERNIA,G., NAJEAN,Y., SCHAISON,G., BOIVIN,P., SCIALOM,C.,
      RULLIER,J. AND BERNARD,J., 1968, DEFICIT COMPLET EN GLUCOSE-
      6-PHOSPHATE-DESHYDROGENASE ASSOCIE A UNE CHOLEMIE FAMILIALE
      DE GILBERT. ARCH FR PEDIATR 25:621-637

485. PRYOR,D.S. AND PITNEY,W.R., 1967, HEREDITARY ELLIPTOCYTOSIS:
      A REPORT OF TWO FAMILIES FROM NEW GUINEA. BR J HAEMATOL
      13:126-134

486. OEZER,L. AND MILLS,G.C., 1964, ELLIPTOCYTOSIS WITH HAEMOLYTIC
      ANEMIA. BR J HAEMATOL 10:468-476

487. JUSTICE,P., SHIH,L.Y., GORDON,J., GROSSMAN,A. AND HSIA,D.,
      1966, CHARACTERIZATION OF LEUKOCYTE GLUCOSE-6-PHOSPHATE
      DEHYDROGENASE IN NORMAL AND MUTANT HUMAN SUBJECTS. J LAB
      CLIN MED 68:552-559

488. BONSIGNORE,A., FORNAINI,G., LEONCINI,G., FANTONI,A. AND
      SEGNI,P., 1966, CHARACTERIZATION OF LEUKOCYTE GLUCOSE 6-
      PHOSPHATE DEHYDROGENASE IN SARDINIAN MUTANTS. J CLIN INVEST
      45:1865-1874

489. SCHILIRO,G., RUSSO,A., MAURO,L., PIZZARELLI,G. AND MARINO,S.,
      1976, LEUKOCYTE FUNCTION AND CHARACTERIZATON OF LEUKOCYTE
      GLUCOSE-6-PHOSPHATE DEHYDROGENASE IN SICILIAN MUTANTS.
      PEDIATR RES 10:739-742

490. KAHN,A., BERTRAND,O., COTTREAU,D., BOIVIN,P. AND
      DREYFUS,J.-.C., 1976, STUDIES ON THE NATURE OF DIFFERENT
      MOLECULAR FORMS OF GLUCOSE-6-PHOSPHATE DEHYDROGENASE PURIFIED
      FROM HUMAN LEUKOCYTES. BIOCHIM BIOPHYS ACTA 445:537-548

491. KAHN,A., HAKIM,J., BOIVIN,P., BOUCHEROT,J., DURAND,D. AND
      TROUBE,H., 1974, LEUCOCYTES ET DEFICITS EN G-6-PD
      ERYTHROCYTAIRE. NOUV REV FR HEMATOL 14:291-298

492. SABINE,J.C., JUNG,E.D., FISH,M.B., PESTANER,L.C. AND
RANKIN,R.E., 1963, OBSERVATIONS ON THE INHERITANCE OF
GLUCOSE-6-PHOSPHATE DEHYDROGENASE DEFICIENCY IN ERYTHROCYTES
AND IN LEUCOCYTES. BR J HAEMATOL 9:164-171

493. RAMOT,B., FISHER,S., SZEINBERG,A., ADAM,A., SHEBA,C. AND
GANNI,D., 1959, A STUDY OF SUBJECTS WITH ERYTHROCYTE GLUCOSE-
6-PHOSPHATE DEHYDROGENASE DEFICIENCY. II. INVESTIGATION OF
LEUKOCYTE ENZYMES. J CLIN INVEST 38:2234-2237

494. CHAN,T.K., TODD,D. AND WONG,C.C., 1965, TISSUE ENZYME LEVELS
IN ERYTHROCYTE GLUCOSE-6-PHOSPHATE DEHYDROGENASE DEFICIENCY.
J LAB CLIN MED 66:937-941

495. KAHN,A., LEGER,J., BOIVIN,P., HOLLARD,D. AND HAKIM,J.,
1973, ANEMIE HEMOLYTIQUE CONGENITALE NON SPHEROCYTAIRE PAR
DEFICIT EN G 6 PD: ETUDE PHYSIOLOGIQUE ET BIOCHEIMIQUE
D'UNE VARIANTE INHABITUELLE. RAPPORT AVEC LA G-6-PD
"BENEVENTO". BIOCHIMIE 55:1121-1128

496. COOPER,M.R., DE CHATELET,L.R., MC CALL,C.E., LA VIA,J.F.,
SPURR,C.L. AND BAEHNER,R.L., 1972, COMPLETE DEFICIENCY OF
LEUKOCYTE GLUCOSE-6-PHOSPHATE DEHYDROGENASE WITH DEFECTIVE
BACTERICIDAL ACTIVITY. J CLIN INVEST 51:769-778

497. GRAY,G.R., KLEBANOFF,S.J., STAMATOYANNOPOULOS,G., AUSTIN,T.,
NAIMAN,S.C., YOSHIDA,A., KLIMAN,M.R. AND ROBINSON,G.C.F.,
1973, NEUTROPHIL DYSFUNCTION, CHRONIC GRANULOMATOUS DISEASE,
AND NONSPHEROCYTIC HAEMOLYTIC ANAEMIA CAUSED BY COMPLETE
DEFICIENCY OF GLUCOSE-6-PHOSPHATE DEHYDROGENASE. LANCET
2:530-534

498. GRAY,G.R., NAIMAN,S.C. AND ROBINSON,G.C.F., 1974, PLATELET
FUNCTION AND G-6-PD DEFICIENCY. LANCET 1:997 (LETTER)

499. WALLER,H.D., LOEHR,G.W. AND GAYER,J., 1966, HEREDITAERE
NICHTSPHAEROCYTAERE HAEMOLYTISCHE ANAEMIE DURCH GLUCOSE-
6-PHOSPHATDEHYDROGENASE-MANGEL. (BILDUNG EINES ENZYMPROTEINS
MIT VERAENDERTEN EIGENSCHAFTEN IN DEN BLUTZELLEN EINER
DEUTSCHEN FAMILIE). KLIN WOCHENSCHR 44:122-128

500. SCHLEGEL,R.J. AND BELLANTI,J.A., 1970, LEUCOCYTE G-6-PD
DEFICIENCY AND BACTERICIDAL ACTIVITY. LANCET 1:677

501. BELLANTI,J.A., CANTZ,B.E. AND SCHLEGEL,R.J., 1970, ACCELERATED
DECAY OF GLUCOSE-6-PHOSPHATE DEHYDROGENASE ACTIVITY IN
CHRONIC GRANULOMATOUS DISEASE. PEDIATR RES 4:405-411

502. ERICKSON,R.P., STITES,D.P., FUDENBERG,H.H. AND EPSTEIN,C.J.,
1972, ALTERED LEVELS OF GLUCOSE-6-PHOSPHATE DEHYDROGENASE
STABILIZING FACTORS IN X-LINKED CHRONIC GRANULOMATOUS
DISEASE. J LAB CLIN MED 80:664-653

503. CLOUTIER,M.D. AND BURGERT,E.O., 1966, CONGENITAL
NONSPHEROCYTIC HEMOLYTIC DISEASE SECONDARY TO G-6-PD
DEFICIENCY: REPORT OF 3 CASES. MAYO CLIN PROC 41:316-325

504. WURZEL,H., MC CREARY,T., BAKER,L. AND GUMERMAN,L., 1961,
GLUCOSE-6-PHOSPHATE DEHYDROGENASE ACTIVITY IN PLATELETS.
BLOOD 17:314-318

505. RAMOT,B., SZEINBERG,A., ADAM,A., SHEBA,C. AND GAFNI,D.,
     1959, A STUDY OF SUBJECTS WITH ERYTHROCYTE GLUCOSE-6-
     PHOSPHATE DEHYDROGENASE DEFICIENCY: I. INVESTIGATION OF
     PLATELET ENZYMES. J CLIN INVEST 38:1659-1661

506. DOERY,J.C.G., HIRSH,J. AND DE GRUCHY,G.C., 1969, ERYTHROCYTE
     AND PLATELET GLUCOSE 6-PHOSPHATE DEHYDROGENASE IN NORMAL
     AND MUTANT CAUCASIANS. SCAND J HAEMATOL 6:5-9

507. SCHWARTZ,J.P., COOPERBERG,A.A. AND ROSENBERG,A., 1974,
     PLATELET-FUNCTION STUDIES IN PATIENTS WITH GLUCOSE-6-
     PHOSPHATE DEHYDROGENASE DEFICIENCY. BR J HAEMATOL 27:273-
     280

508. GARTLER,S.M., GANDINI,E. AND CEPPELLINI,R., 1962, GLUCOSE-
     6-PHOSPHATE DEHYDROGENASE DEFICIENT MUTANT IN HUMAN CELL
     CULTURE. NATURE 193:602-603

509. MARKS,P.A., GROSS,R.T. AND HURWITZ,R.E., 1959, GENE ACTION
     IN ERYTHROCYTE DEFICIENCY OF GLUCOSE-6-PHOSPHATE
     DEHYDROGENASE: TISSUE ENZYME-LEVELS. NATURE 183:1266:1267

510. BRUNETTI,P., ROSSETTI,R. AND BROCCIA,G., 1960, NEW FINDINGS
     ON THE BIO-ENZYMOLOGY OF ICTERIC HEMOGLOBINURIC FAVISM.
     III.THE ACTIVITY OF GLUCOSE-6-PHOSPHATE DEHYDROGENASE IN
     THE LIVER PARENCHYMA. CLIN TER 32:338-350

511. CAYANIS,E., GOMPERTS,E.D., BALINSKY,D., DISLER,P. AND
     MYERS,A., 1975, G6PD HILLBROW: A NEW VARIANT OF GLUCOSE-
     6-PHOSPHATE DEHYDROGENASE ASSOCIATED WITH DRUG-INDUCED
     HAEMOLYTIC ANAEMIA. BR J HAEMATOL 30:343-350

512. ZINKHAM,W.H., 1960, ENZYME STUDIES ON LENSES FROM PERSONS
     WITH PRIMAQUINE-SENSITIVE ERYTHROCYTES. AM J DIS CHILD
     100:525-526

513. ORZALESI,N., SORCINELLI,R. AND BINAGHI,F., 1976, GLUCOSE-
     6-PHOSPHATE DEHYDROGENASE IN CATARACTS OF SUBJECTS SUFFERING
     FROM FAVISM. OPHTHAL RES 8:192-194

514. RAMOT,B., SHEBA,C., ADAM,A. AND ASHKENASI,I., 1960,
     ERYTHROCYTE GLUCOSE-6-PHOSPHATE DEHYDROGENASE DEFICIENT
     SUBJECTS: ENZYME-LEVEL IN SALIVA. NATURE 185:931

515. SKLAVUNU-ZURUKZOGLU,S., MAMELETZIS,C. AND KATRIU,D., 1965,
     OBSERVATIONS ON THE GLUCOSE-6-PHOSPHATE DEHYDROGENASE OF
     THE BREAST MILK. HELV PAEDIATR ACTA 20:193-196

516. ROMEO,G., RINALDI,A., URBANO,F. AND FILIPPI,G., 1976, HAIR
     ROOT VERSUS RED CELL INDIVIDUAL PHENOTYPE IN SARDINIAN
     HETEROZYGOTES FOR G6PD DEFICIENCY (MEDITERRANEAN TYPE). AM
     J HUM GENET 28:506-513

517. WIESENFELD,S.L., PETRAKIS,N.L., SAMS,B.J., COLLEN,M.F. AND
     CUTLER,J.L., 1970, ELEVATED BLOOD PRESSURE, PULSE RATE AND
     SERUM CREATININE IN NEGRO MALES DEFICIENT IN GLUCOSE-6-
     PHOSPHATE DEHYDROGENASE. N ENGL J MED 282:1001-1002

518. PETRAKIS,N.L., WIESENFELD,S.L., SAMS,B.J., COLLEN,M.F.,
     CUTLER,J.L. AND SIEGELAUB,A.B., 1970, PREVALENCE OF SICKLE-
     CELL TRAIT AND GLUCOSE-6-PHOSPHATE DEHYDROGENASE DEFICIENCY.
     N ENGL J MED 282:767-770

519. PETRAKIS,N.L., PETRAKIS,S.J., WIESENFELD,S.L. AND SPANIDOU,E.,
     1974, POSSIBLE INCOMPATIBILITY OF GLUCOSE-6-PHOSPHATE
     DEHYDROGENASE DEFICIENCY AND CHAMPIONSHIP ATHLETIC
     PERFORMANCE. MED SCI SPORTS 6:191-192

520. LONG,W.K., WILSON,S.W. AND FRENKEL,E.P., 1967, ASSOCIATIONS
     BETWEEN RED CELL GLUCOSE-6-PHOSPHATE DEHYDROGENASE VARIANTS
     AND VASCULAR DISEASES. AM J HUM GENET 19:35-53

521. CHANMUGAM,D. AND FRUMIN,A.M., 1964, ABNORMAL ORAL GLUCOSE
     TOLERANCE RESPONSE IN ERYTHROCYTE GLUCOSE-6-PHOSPHATE
     DEHYDROGENASE DEFICIENCY. N ENGL J MED 271:1202-1204

522. EPPES,R., BREWER,G., DE GOWIN,R., MC NAMARA,J., FLANAGAN,C.,
     SCHRIER,S., TARLOV,A., POWELL,R. AND CARSON,P., 1966, ORAL
     GLUCOSE TOLERANCE IN NEGRO MEN DEFICIENT IN G-6-PD. N ENGL
     J MED 275:855-861

523. REED,T.E., 1969, CAUCASIAN GENES IN AMERICAN NEGROES.
     SCIENCE 165:762-768

524. PIOMELLI,S., REINDORF,C.A., ARZANIAN,M.T. AND CORASH,L.M.,
     1972, CLINICAL AND BIOCHEMICAL INTERACTIONS OF GLUCOSE-6-
     PHOSPHATE DEHYDROGENASE DEFICIENCY AND SICKLE-CELL ANEMIA.
     N ENGL J MED 287:213-217

525. STEINBERG,M.H. AND DREILING,B.J., 1974, GLUCOSE-6-PHOSPHATE
     DEHYDROGENASE DEFICIENCY IN SICKLE CELL ANEMIA. ANN INTERN
     MED 80:217-220

526. BIENZLE,U., SODEINDE,O., EFFIONG,C.E. AND LUZZATTO,L.,
     1975, GLUCOSE 6-PHOSPHATE DEHYDROGENASE DEFICIENCY AND
     SICKLE CELL ANEMIA: FREQUENCY AND FEATURES OF THE ASSOCIATION
     IN AN AFRICAN COMMUNITY. BLOOD 46:591-597

527. LEWIS,R.A. AND HATHORN,M., 1965, CORRELATION OF S HEMOGLOBIN
     WITH GLUCOSE-6-PHOSPHATE DEHYDROGENASE DEFICIENCY AND ITS
     SIGNIFICANCE. BLOOD 26:176-180

528. SMITS,H.L., OSKI,F.A. AND BRODY,J.I., 1969, THE HEMOLYTIC
     CRISIS OF SICKLE CELL DISEASE: THE ROLE OF GLUCOSE-6-
     PHOSPHATE DEHYDROGENASE DEFICIENCY. J PEDIATR 75:544-551

529. ELIAN,M., 1970, EPILEPSY AND G-6-PD DEFICIENCY. LANCET
     1:364

530. DERN,R.J., GLYNN,M.F. AND BREWER,G.J., 1963, STUDIES ON
     THE CORRELATION OF THE GENETICALLY DETERMINED TRAIT, GLUCOSE-
     6-PHOSPHATE DEHYDROGENASE DEFICIENCY, WITH BEHAVIORAL
     MANIFESTATIONS IN SCHIZOPHRENIA. J LAB CLIN MED 62:319-329

531. BOWMAN,J.E., BREWER,G.J., FRISCHER,H., CARTER,J.L.,
     EISENSTEIN,R.B. AND BAYRAKCI,C., 1965, A RE-EVALUATION OF
     THE RELATIONSHIP BETWEEN GLUCOSE-6-PHOSPHATE DEHYDROGENASE
     DEFICIENCY AND THE BEHAVIORAL MANIFESTATIONS OF SCHIZOPHRENIA.
     J LAB CLIN MED 65:222-227

532. ZINKHAM,W.H., 1961, A DEFICIENCY OF GLUCOSE-6-PHOSPHATE
     DEHYDROGENASE ACTIVITY IN LENS FROM INDIVIDUALS WITH
     PRIMAQUINE-SENSITIVE ERYTHROCYTES. JOHNS HOPKINS MED J
     109:206-216

533. HELGE,H. AND BORNER,K., 1966, KONGENITALE NICHTSPHAEROZYTAERE
     HAEMOLYTISCHE ANAEMIE, KATARAKT UND GLUCOSE-6-PHOSPHAT-
     DEHYDROGENASE-MANGEL. DTSCH MED WOCHENSCHR 91:1584-1589

534. HARLEY,J.D., AGAR,N.S. AND GRUCA,M.A., 1975, CATARACTS WITH
     A GLUCOSE-6-PHOSPHATE DEHYDROGENASE VARIANT. BR MED J 2:86
     (CORRESPONDENCE)

535. ESCOBAR,M.A., HELLER,P. AND TROBAUGH JR,F.E., 1964, "COMPLETE"
     ERYTHROCYTE GLUCOSE-6-PHOSPHATE DEHYDROGENASE DEFICIENCY.
     ARCH INTERN MED 113:428-434

536. NAIK,S.N. AND ANDERSON,D.E., 1970, G-6-PD DEFICIENCY AND
     CANCER. LANCET 1:1060-1061

537. CASSIMOS,C., SKLAVUNU-TSURUKTOSGLU,S., CATRIU,D. AND
     PANAJIOTIDU,C., 1973, THE INCIDENCE OF G 6 PD DISTURBANCES
     IN CANCER PATIENTS. IRCS 73-3 27-2-2 (ABSTRACT)

538. BEACONSFIELD,P., RAINSBURY,R. AND KALTON,G., 1965, GLUCOSE-
     6-PHOSPHATE DEHYDROGENASE DEFICIENCY AND THE INCIDENCE OF
     CANCER. ONCOLOGY 19:11-19

539. NAIK,S.N. AND ANDERSON,D.E., 1971, THE ASSOCIATION BETWEEN
     GLUCOSE-6-PHOSPHATE DEHYDROGENASE DEFICIENCY AND CANCER IN
     AMERICAN NEGROES. ONCOLOGY 25:356-364

540. SULIS,E., 1972, G-6-PD DEFICIENCY AND CANCER. LANCET 1:1185

541. BOCK,H.E., WALLER,H.D., LOEHR,G.W. AND KARGES,O., 1958,
     BESONDERHEITEN IM FERMENTGEHALT VON MEGALOCYTEN. KLIN
     WOCHENSCHR 36:151-157

542. RAPPELLI,A., GLORIOSO,N., TEDDE,R., MADEDDU,P. AND CAMPUS,S.,
     1976, IMPAIRED RENIN RELEASE AFTER REPETITIVE UPRIGHT
     STIMULATION IN G-6-PD DEFICIENCY SUBJECTS. IRCS 4:423

543. BORKOWSKI,A.J., MARKS,P.A., KATZ,F.H. AND CHRISSTY,N.P.,
     1962, AN ABNORMAL PATHWAY OF STEROID METABOLISM IN PATIENTS
     WITH GLUCOSE- 6-PHOSPHATE DEHYDROGENASE DEFICIENCY. J CLIN
     INVEST 41:1346-1347 (ABSTRACT)

544. TARLOV,A.R., BREWER,G.J. AND SWANSON,S.H., 1961, THE EFFECT
     OF PRIMAQUINE ADMINISTRATION ON THE SERUM CHOLESTEROL OF
     DRUG-SENSITIVE AMER. NEGROES. CLINICAL RESEARCH 9:190

545. ADAMSON,J.E., TADDEO,R.J. AND GWYN,P.P., 1970, LOSS OF
     FLAPS DUE TO GLUCOSE-6-PHOSPHATE DEHYDROGENASE DEFICIENCY.
     PLAST RECONSTR SURG 46:301-304

546. MC INTIRE,M.S. AND ANGLE,C.R., 1972, AIR LEAD: RELATION TO
     LEAD IN BLOOD OF BLACK SCHOOL CHILDREN DEFICIENT IN GLUCOSE-
     6-PHOSPHATE DEHYDROGENASE. SCIENCE 177:520-522

547. DERN,R.J., BEUTLER,E. AND ALVING,A.S., 1954, THE HEMOLYTIC
     EFFECT OF PRIMAQUINE. II. THE NATURAL COURSE OF THE
     HEMOLYTIC ANEMIA AND THE MECHANISM OF ITS SELF-LIMITED
     CHARACTER. J LAB CLIN MED 44:171-175

548. GREENBERG,M.S. AND WONG,H., 1961, STUDIES ON THE DESTRUCTION OF GLUTATHIONE-UNSTABLE RED BLOOD CELLS. THE INFLUENCE OF FAVA BEANS AND PRIMAQUINE UPON SUCH CELLS IN VIVO. J LAB CLIN MED 57:733-747

549. BEUTLER,E., DERN,R.J. AND ALVING,A.S., 1954, THE HEMOLYTIC EFFECT OF PRIMAQUINE. IV. THE RELATIONSHIP OF CELL AGE TO HEMOLYSIS. J LAB CLIN MED 44:439-442

550. PANNACCIULLI,I., TIZIANELLO,A., AJMAR,F. AND SALVIDIO,E., 1965, THE COURSE OF EXPERIMENTALLY-INDUCED HEMOLYTIC ANEMIA IN A PRIMAQUINE- SENSITIVE CAUCASIAN. A CASE STUDY. BLOOD 25:92-95

551. SALVIDIO,E., PANNACCIULLI,I., TIZIANELLO,A. AND AJMAR,F., 1967, NATURE OF HEMOLYTIC CRISES AND THE FATE OF G-6-PD DEFICIENT, DRUG-DAMAGED ERYTHROCYTES IN SARDINIANS. N ENGL J MED 276:1339-1344

552. TIZIANELLO,A., PANNACCIULLI,I., AJMAR,F. AND SALVIDIO,E., 1968, SITES OF DESTRUCTION OF RED CELLS IN G-6-PD DEFICIENT CAUCASIANS AND IN PHENYLHYDRAZINE TREATED PATIENTS. SCAND. J HAEMATOL 5:116-128

553. SALVIDIO,E., PANNACCIULLI,I. AND TIZIANELLO,A., 1967, LA CAPACITA ERRITROPOIETICA DEI SOGGETTI CON DEFICIENZA DI G 6 PD ERITROCITARIA. ATTI ACCAD MED LOMB 22:16-18

554. MARSICANO JR,A.R., HUTTON,J.J. AND BRYANT,W.M., 1973, FATAL HEMOLYSIS FROM MAFENIDE TREATMENT OF BURNS IN A PATIENT WITH GLUCOSE-6-PHOSPHATE DEHYDROGENASE DEFICIENCY. PLAST RECONSTR SURG 52:197-199

555. KIMBRO JR,E.L., SACHS,M.V. AND TORBERT,J.V., 1957, MECHANISM OF THE HEMOLYTIC ANEMIA INDUCED BY NITROFURANTOIN (FURADANTIN). JOHNS HOPKINS MED J 101:245-257

556. DAWSON,J.P., THAYER,W.W. AND DESFORGES,J.F., 1958, ACUTE HEMOLYTIC ANEMIA IN THE NEWBORN INFANT DUE TO NAPHTHALENE POISONING. REPORT OF TWO CASES WITH INVESTIGATION INTO THE MECHANISM OF THE DISEASE. BLOOD 13:1113-1125

557. FLATZ,G., VOSS,B. AND VOSS,S., 1970, ZUR ANWENDUNG VON SULFAMETHOXYPYRAZIN BEI PERSONEN MIT MANGEL DER GLUCOSE-6-PHOSPHAT-DEHYDROGENASE DER ERYTHROCYTEN. KLIN WOCHENSCHR. 48:88-91

558. SZEINBERG,A., KELLERMANN,J., ADAM,A., SHEBA,C. AND RAMOT,B., 1960, HAEMOLYTIC JAUNDICE FOLLOWING ASPIRIN ADMINISTRATION TO A PATIENT WITH A DEFICIENCY OF GLUCOSE-6-PHOSPHATE DEHYDROGENASE IN ERYTHROCYTES. ACTA HAEMATOL 23:58-64

559. ZINKHAM,W.H. AND CHILDS,B., 1957, EFFECT OF NAPHTHALENE DERIVATIVES ON GLUTATHIONE METABOLISM OF ERYTHROCYTES FROM PATIENTS WITH NAPHTHALENE HEMOLYTIC ANEMIA. J CLIN INVEST 36:938-939

560. DOYEN,A., LEONARD,J., MBENDI,S. AND SONNET,J., 1967, INFLUENCE DES DOSES THERAPEUTIQUES DU CIBA 32644-BA SUR L'HEMATOPOIESE DES PATIENTS ATTEINTS DE BILHARZIOSE ET D'AMIBIASE. ACTA TROP (BASEL) 24:59-77

561. SZEINBERG,A., PRAS,M., SHEBA,C., ADAM,A. AND RAMOT,B.,
      1959, THE HEMOLYTIC EFFECT OF VARIOUS SULFONAMIDES ON
      SUBJECTS WITH A DEFICIENCY OF GLUCOSE-6-PHOSPHATE
      DEHYDROGENASE OF ERYTHROCYTES. ISR MED J 18:176

562. GAETANI,G.D., MARENI,C., RAVAZZOLO,R. AND SALVIDIO,E.,
      1976, HAEMOLYTIC EFFECT OF TWO SULPHONAMIDES EVALUATED BY
      A NEW METHOD. BR J HAEMATOL 32:183-191

563. WELT,S.I., JACKSON,E.H., KIRKMAN,H.N. AND PARKER,J.C.,
      1971, THE EFFECTS OF CERTAIN DRUGS ON THE HEXOSE MONOPHOSPHATE
      SHUNT OF HUMAN RED CELLS. ANN NY ACAD SCI 179:625-635

564. DERN,R.J., BEUTLER,E. AND ALVING,A.S., 1955, THE HEMOLYTIC
      EFFECT OF PRIMAQUINE. V. PRIMAQUINE SENSITIVITY AS A
      MANIFESTATION OF A MULTIPLE DRUG SENSITIVITY. J LAB CLIN
      MED 45:30-39

565. BEUTLER,E., 1959, THE HEMOLYTIC EFFECT OF PRIMAQUINE AND
      RELATED COMPOUNDS. A REVIEW. BLOOD 14:103-139

566. TADA,K., 1961, ENZYMATIC ANOMALY OF ERYTHROCYTES IN CONGENITAL
      NONSPHEROCYTIC HEMOLYTIC ANEMIA. TOHOKU J EXP MED 75:263-
      267

567. HOUSTON,I.B. AND BARLOW,A.M., 1959, ACUTE HAEMOLYTIC ANAEMIA
      AND METHAEMOGLOBINURIA PRODUCED BY PHENACETIN. LANCET
      2:1062-1065

568. BROWN,C.B., MC MILLAN,J.M., BATEMAN,C.J.T. AND CATTELL,W.R.,
      1972, ACUTE RENAL FAILURE FOLLOWING ANALGESIC OVERDOSE IN
      G6PD DEFICIENCY. BR J UROL 44:155-160

569. MILLAR,J., PELOQUIN,R. AND DE LEEUW,N.K.M., 1972, PHENACETIN-
      INDUCED HEMOLYTIC ANEMIA. CAN MED ASSOC J 106:770-775

570. GLADER,B., 1976, EVALUATION OF THE HEMOLYTIC ROLE OF ASPIRIN
      IN GLUCOSE-6-PHOSPHATE DEHYDROGENASE DEFICIENCY. J PEDIATR
      89:1027-1028

571. WORATHUMRONG,N. AND GRIMES,A.J., 1975, THE EFFECT OF O-
      SALICYLATE UPON PENTOSE PHOSPHATE PATHWAY ACTIVITY IN NORMAL
      AND G6PD-DEFICIENT RED CELLS. BR J HAEMATOL 30:225-231

572. KELLERMEYER,R.W., TARLOV,A.R., BREWER,G.J., CARSON,P.E.
      AND ALVING,A.S., 1962, HEMOLYTIC EFFECT OF THERAPEUTIC
      DRUGS. CLINICAL CONSIDERATIONS OF THE PRIMAQUINE-TYPE
      HEMOLYSIS. JAMA 180:388-394

573. HERMAN,J. AND BEN-MEIR,S., 1975, OVERT HEMOLYSIS IN PATIENTS
      WITH GLUCOSE-6-PHOSPHATE DEHYDROGENASE DEFICIENCY. ISR J
      MED SCI 2:340-344

574. SHAHIDI,N.T. AND WESTRING,D.W., 1970, ACETYLSALICYLIC ACID-
      INDUCED HEMOLYSIS AND ITS MECHANISM. J CLIN INVEST 49:1334-
      1340

575. SARTORI,E. AND PANIZON,E., 1957, NUOVE PROSPETTIVE NELLO
      STUDIO DEL FAVISMO. STUDI SASSARESI 35:363

576. BEUTLER,E., 1960, DRUG-INDUCED HEMOLYTIC ANEMIA (PRIMAQUINE SENSITIVITY). THE METABOLIC BASIS OF INHERITED DISEASE STANBURY,J.B., WYNGAARDEN,J.B. AND FREDRICKSON,D.S. ED. 1031-1067, MC GRAW-HILL, NEW YORK

577. BERNASCONI,C., BEDARIDA,G., POLLINI,G. AND SARTORI,S., 1961, STUDIO DEL MECCANISMO DI EMOLISI IN UN CASO DI ANEMIA EMOLITICA ACQUISITA DA PIRAMIDONE. HAEMATOL ARCH 46:697-720

578. DIMOPOULOS,C., MORAKIS,A., DIMOPOULOS,B., ZERVAS,A., PANAYIOTIDES,N. AND DOUTSIAS,A., 1973, ANEMIE HEMOLYTIQUE AIGUE CONSECUTIVE A L'ADMINISTRATION DE NITROFURANE ET DE NOVALGINE CHEZ DEUX MALADES PRESENTANT UN DEFICIT EN GLUCOSE 6-PHOSPHATE-DEHYDROGENASE ERYTHROCYTAIRE. J UROL NEPHROL (PARIS) 79:524-528

579. SZEINBERG,A., SHEBA,C., HIRSCHORN,N. AND BODONYI,E., 1957, CHEMICAL STUDIES ON ERYTHROCYTES IN CASES OF HAEMOLYTIC ANAEMIA DUE TO VICIA FABA, SULPHONAMIDES AND P-AMINOSALICYLIC ACID. BULL RES COUNC OF ISRAEL 6E:115-118

580. SZEINBERG,A., SHEBA,C. AND ADAM,A., 1958, SELECTIVE OCCURRENCE OF GLUTATHIONE INSTABILITY IN RED BLOOD CORPUSCLES OF THE VARIOUS JEWISH TRIBES. BLOOD 13:1043-1053

581. LESOBRE,B., HOMBERG,J.C., SEGER,J., KOURILSKY,R. AND PIERON,R., 1970, G-6-PD DEFICIENCY REVEALED DURING PAS THERAPY. SEM HOP PARIS 46:1361-1368

582. MESSERSCHMITT,J., SUAUDEAU,C., BENALLEGUE,V.R., FABRE,S., BON,J., ANDRE,L., KHATI,B., DUBOIS,M., BENABDALLAH,S. AND KOTCHOYAN,P., 1967, DEFAUT EN G-6-PD ET ANEMIES HEMOLYTIQUES EN ALGERIE. NOUV REV FR HEMATOL 7:827-840

583. MUNROE,W.D., LAWSON,W.J. AND HOLCOMB,T.M., 1964, HEMOLYTIC ANEMIA DUE TO AMINOSALICYLIC ACID. AM J DIS CHILD 108:425-429

584. SANSONE,G. AND SEGNI,G., 1958, L'ANEMIA EMOLITICA ACUTA DA SULFAMIDE E QUELLA DA PAS: DIFFERENZE PATOGENETICHE. BULL SOC ITAL BIOL SPER 34:1556-1558

585. MC CURDY,P.R. AND DONOHOE,R.F., 1966, PYRIDOXINE-RESPONSIVE ANEMIA CONDITIONED BY ISONICOTINIC ACID HYDRAZIDE. BLOOD 27:352-362

586. RYAN,B.P.K. AND PARSONS,J.C., 1961, GLUCOSE-6-PHOSPHATE DEHYDROGENASE ACTIVITY IN ANAEMIC PAPUANS. MED J AUST 2:502-506

587. RAKITZIS,E.T., 1964, TEST FOR GLUCOSE-6-PHOSPHATE DEHYDROGENASE DEFICIENCY. LANCET 2:1182-1183

588. JACOB,H. AND JANDL,J.H., 1966, A SIMPLE VISUAL SCREENING TEST FOR G-6-PD DEFICIENCY EMPLOYING ASCORBATE AND CYANIDE. N ENGL J MED 274:1162-1167

589. SZEINBERG,A., ADAM,A., MYERS,F., SHEBA,C. AND RAMOT,B., 1959, A HEMATOLOGICAL SURVEY OF INDUSTRIAL WORKERS WITH ENZYME-DEFICIENT ERYTHROCYTES. AMA ARCHIVES OF INDUSTRIAL HEALTH 20:510-516

590. UDOMRATN,T., STEINBERG,M.H., CAMPBELL JR,G.D. AND OELSHLEGEL
      JR,F.J., 1977, EFFECTS OF ASCORBIC ACID ON GLUCOSE-6-
      PHOSPHATE DEHYDROGENASE-DEFICIENT ERYTHROCYTES: STUDIES IN
      AN ANIMAL MODEL. BLOOD 49:471-475

591. CAMPBELL JR,G.D., STEINBERG,M.H. AND BOWER,J.D., 1975,
      ASCORBIC ACID-INDUCED HEMOLYSIS IN G-6-PD DEFICIENCY. ANN
      INTERN MED 82:810 (LETTER)

592. LARIZZA,P., BRUNETTI,P. AND GRIGNANI,F., 1960, ANEMIE
      EMOLITICHE ENZIMOPENICHE. HAEMATOLOGICA (PAVIA) 45:1-90,
      129-212

593. CHATTERJI,S.C. AND DAS,P.K., 1963, CHLORAMPHENICOL INDUCED
      HAEMOLYTIC ANAEMIA DUE TO ENZYMATIC DEFICIENCY OF
      ERYTHROCYTES. J INDIAN MED ASSOC 40:172-174

594. BAKSHI,S. AND SINGH,J., 1972, ACUTE HAEMOLYTIC ANAEMIA IN
      TYPHOID FEVER. INDIAN J PEDIATR 39:270-273

595. CHAN,T.K., CHESTERMAN,C.N., MC FADZEAN,A.J.S. AND TODD,D.,
      1971, THE SURVIVAL OF GLUCOSE-6-PHOSPHATE DEHYDROGENASE-
      DEFICIENT ERYTHROCYTES IN PATIENTS WITH TYPHOID FEVER ON
      CHLORAMPHENICOL THERAPY. J LAB CLIN MED 77:177-184

596. KOSOWER,N.S. AND KOSOWER,E.M., 1967, DOES 3,4-
      DIHYDROXYPHENYLALANINE PLAY A PART IN FAVISM?. NATURE
      215:285-286

597. BEUTLER,E., 1970, L-DOPA AND FAVISM. BLOOD 36:523-525
      (EDITORIAL)

598. GAETANI,G., SALVIDIO,E., PANNACCIULLI,I., AJMAR,F. AND
      PARAVIDINO,G., 1970, ABSENCE OF HAEMOLYTIC EFFECTS OF L-
      DOPA ON TRANSFUSED G6PD-DEFICIENT ERYTHROCYTES. EXPERIENTIA
      26:785-786

599. SNYDER,L.M., EDELSTEIN,L., FORTIER,N., CARIGLIA,N., JACOBS,J.
      AND CIPRO,D., 1974, THE PROTECTIVE EFFECT OF L-DOPA ON
      HEINZ BODY FORMATION IN G6PD DEFICIENT RED CELLS. EXPERIENTIA
      30:85-86

600. AWASTHI,Y.C., SRIVASTAVA,S.K., SNYDER,L.M., EDELSTEIN,L.
      AND FORTIER,N.L., 1977, L-DOPA PEROXIDASE ACTIVITY OF HUMAN
      ERYTHROCYTE CATALASE. J LAB CLIN MED 89:763-769

601. GANZONI,A. AND RHOMBERG,F., 1965, HEMOLYTIC CRISIS IN
      GLUCOSE-6-PHOSPHATE DEHYDROGENASE DEFICIENCY AND LEAD
      POISONING. ACTA HAEMATOL 34:338-346

602. WESTRING,D.W. AND CALAS,C., 1968, HEMOLYTIC EFFECT OF
      ESTROGEN ON G-6-PD DEFICIENT ERYTHROCYTES. CLINICAL RESEARCH
      16:544 (ABSTRACT)

603. BREWER,G.J. AND TARLOV,A.R., 1961, STUDIES ON THE MECHANISM
      OF PRIMAQUINE-TYPE HEMOLYSIS: THE EFFECT OF METHYLENE
      BLUE. CLINICAL RESEARCH 9:65 (ABSTRACT)

604. ROSEN,P.J., JOHNSON,C., MC GEHEE,W.G. AND BEUTLER,E., 1971,
      FAILURE OF METHYLENE BLUE TREATMENT IN TOXIC
      METHEMOGLOBINEMIA. ASSOCIATION WITH GLUCOSE-6-PHOSPHATE
      DEHYDROGENASE DEFICIENCY. ANN INTERN MED 75:83-86

605. BELTON,E.M. AND JONES,R.V.,.1965, HAEMOLYTIC ANAEMIA DUE
TO NALIDIXIC ACID. LANCET 2:691

606. MANDAL,B.K. AND STEVENSON,J., 1970, HAEMOLYTIC CRISIS
PRODUCED BY NALIDIXIC ACID. LANCET 1:614 (LETTER)

607. ALLESIO,L. AND MORSELLI,G., 1972, OCCUPATIONAL EXPOSURE TO
NALIDIXIC ACID. BR MED J 4:110-111 (LETTER)

608. VARGAS,L.P. AND GONZALES,C.S., 1967, HAEMOLYTIC ANAEMIA
AFTER NALIDIXIC ACID. LANCET 2:97-98 (LETTER)

609. VALAES,T., DOXIADIS,S. AND FESSAS,P., 1963, ACUTE HEMOLYSIS
DUE TO NAPHTHALENE INHALATION. J PEDIATR 63:904-915

610. SANSONE,G., 1958, L'ANEMIA EMOLITICA ACUTA DE INGESTIONE
ACCIDENTALE DI NAFTALINA NEL BAMBINO. HAEMATOLOGICA (LATINA)
1:45-60

611. GILLES,H.M. AND TAYLOR,B.G., 1961, THE EXISTENCE OF THE
GLUCOSE-6-PHOSPHATE DEHYDROGENASE DEFICIENCY TRAIT IN
NIGERIA AND ITS CLINICAL IMPLICATIONS. ANN TROP MED PARASITOL
55:64-70

612. GILLES,H.M. AND IKEME,A.C., 1960, HEMOGLOBINURIA AMONG
ADULT NIGERIANS DUE TO GLUCOSE-6-PHOSPHATE DEHYDROGENASE
DEFICIENCY WITH DRUG SENSITIVITY. LANCET 2:889-891

613. SANSONE,G. AND SEGNI,G., 1958, DIFETTO BIOCHIMICO
ERITROCITARIO, A CARATTERE GENETICO, IN UN BAMBINO CON
ANEMIA EMOLITICA ACUTA DA NAFTALINA. BULL SOC ITAL BIOL
SPER 34:615-617

614. MICHOT,F., RASTETTER,J. AND GRONAUER,H., 1966, DURCH NEO-
SALVARSAN AUSGELOESTE HAEMOLYSE BEI GLUKOSE-6-PHOSPHAT-
DEHYDROGENASE-MANGEL, KOMBINIERT MIT HEPATISCHEM ICTERUS.
SCHWEIZ MED WOCHENSCHR 96:985-987

615. LAPIERRE,J., HOLLER,C., TOURTE-SCHAEFER,C., LEBAS-SAISON,E.,
LAUNOIS,J.P. AND CACHIN,M., 1976, HAEMOLYTIC ANAEMIA
FOLLOWING ANTI-BILHARZIA TREATMENT USING NIRIDAZOLE IN A
WOMAN OF CARIBBEAN ORIGIN WITH G PD DEFICIENCY. NOUV PRESSE
MED 5:147

616. MC CAFFREY,R.P., FARID,Z. AND KENT,D.C., 1972, ACUTE
HAEMOLYSIS WITH AMBILHAR TREATMENT IN GLUCOSE-6-PHOSPHATE
DEHYDROGENASE DEFICIENCY. TRANS R SOC TROP MED HYG 66:795-
797

617. THOMAS,M., AGNUS,D., POIROT,J.-.L. AND GOLVAN,Y.-.J., 1976,
HEMOLYSIS INDUCED BY NIRIDAZOLE IN TWO PATIENTS WITH
DEFICIENCY OF G-6-PD. NOUV PRESSE MED 5:1537-1538

618. SONNET,J., VANDEPITTE,J. AND HAUMONT,A., 1959, ANEMIE
HEMOLYTIQUE PAR LA NITROFURAZONE REVELATRICE D'UNE DEFICIENCE
GLOBULAIR EN GLUCOSE-6-PHOSPHATE DEHYDROGENASE. ANN SOC
BELG MED TROP 39:691-702

619. JEANNET,M., PERRIER,C.V. AND TOENZ,O., 1964, ANEMIE
HEMOLYTIQUE AIGUE PAR LA NITROFURANTOINE CHEZ UNE IRANIENNE
PRESENTANT UN DEFICIT EN GLUCOSE-6-PHOSPHATE DEHYDROGENASE
ERYTHROCYTAIRE. SCHWEIZ MED WOCHENSCHR 94:939-943

620. ZAIL,S.S., CHARLTON,R.W. AND BOTHWELL,T.H., 1962, THE
     HAEMOLYTIC EFFECT OF CERTAIN DRUGS IN BANTU SUBJECTS WITH
     A DEFICIENCY OF GLUCOSE-6-PHOSPHATE DEHYDROGENASE. S AFR
     J MED SCI 27:95-99

621. SZEINBERG,A., ADAM,A. AND SHEBA,C., 1962, THE EFFECT OF IN
     VITRO INCUBATION WITH NITROFURANTOIN ON VIABILITY OF NORMAL
     AND ENZYME DEFICIENT RED CELLS. PROC TEL-HASHOMER HOSPITAL
     1:49-52

622. ROBERTSON,D.H.H., 1961, NITROFURAZONE-INDUCED HAEMOLYTIC
     ANAEMIA IN A REFRACTORY CASE OF TRYPANOSOMA RHODESIENSE
     SLEEPING SICKNESS: THE HAEMOLYTIC TRAIT & SELF-LIMITING
     HAEMOLYTIC ANAEMIA. ANN TROP MED PARASITOL 55:49-64

623. BUCKLEY,R.D., HACKNEY,J.D., CLARK,K. AND POSIN,C., 1975,
     OZONE AND HUMAN BLOOD. ARCH ENVIRON HEALTH 30:40-43

624. CALABRESE,E.J., KOJOLA,W.H. AND CARNOW,B.W., 1977, OZONE:
     A POSSIBLE CAUSE OF HEMOLYTIC ANEMIA IN GLUCOSE-6-PHOSPHATE
     DEHYDROGENASE DEFICIENT INDIVIDUALS. JOURNAL OF TOXICOLOGY
     AND ENVIRONMENTAL HEALTH 2:709-712

625. HOCKWALD,R.S., ARNOLD,J., CLAYMAN,C.B. AND ALVING,A.S.,
     1952, STATUS OF PRIMAQUINE. IV. TOXICITY OF PRIMAQUINE IN
     NEGROES. JAMA 149:1568-1570

626. GEORGE,J.N., SEARS,D.A., MC CURDY,P. AND CONRAD,M.E., 1967,
     PRIMAQUINE SENSITIVITY IN CAUCASIANS: HEMOLYTIC REACTIONS
     INDUCED BY PRIMAQUINE IN G-6-PD DEFICIENT SUBJECTS. J LAB
     CLIN MED 70:80-93

627. CHAN,T.K., TODD,D. AND TSO,S.C., 1976, DRUG-INDUCED HAEMOLYSIS
     IN GLUCOSE-6-PHOSPHATE DEHYDROGENASE DEFICIENCY. BR MED J
     2:1227-1229

628. BREWER,G.J. AND ZARAFONETIS,J.D., 1976, THE HAEMOLYTIC
     EFFECT OF VARIOUS REGIMENS OF PRIMAQUINE WITH CHLOROQUINE
     IN AMERICAN NEGROES WITH G6PD DEFICIENCY AND THE LACK OF
     AN EFFECT OF VARIOUS ANTIMALARIAL SUPPRESSIVE AGENTS ON
     ERYTHROCYTE METABOLISM. BULL WHO 36:303-308

629. ZIAI,M., AMIRHAKIMI,G.H., REINHOLD,J.G., TABATABEE,M.,
     GETTNER,M.E., BOWMAN,J.E. AND KAMAL,D., 1967, MALARIA
     PROPHYLAXIS AND TREATMENT IN G-6-PD DEFICIENCY. CLIN PEDIATR
     6:242-243

630. GLASS,L., RAJEGOWDA,B.K., BOWEN,E. AND EVANS,H.E., 1973,
     EXPOSURE TO QUININE AND JAUNDICE IN A GLUCOSE-6-PHOSPHATE
     DEHYDROGENASE- DEFICIENT NEWBORN INFANT. J PEDIATR 82:734-
     735

631. HEINRICH,R.A., SMITH,T.C. AND BUCHANAN,R.A., 1971, A
     PHARMACOLOGICAL STUDY OF A NEW SULFONAMIDE IN GLUCOSE-6-
     PHOSPHATE DEHYDROGENASE DEFICIENT SUBJECTS. J CLIN PHARMACOL
     428-432

632. KELLERMEYER,R.W., TARLOV,A.R., SCHRIER,S.L. AND ALVING,A.S.,
     1958, HEMOLYTIC EFFECT OF COMMONLY USED DRUGS ON ERYTHROCYTES
     DEFICIENT IN GLUCOSE-6-PHOSPHATE DEHYDROGENASE. J LAB CLIN
     MED 52:827-828 (ABSTRACT)

633. BROWN,A. AND CEVIK,N., 1965, HEMOLYSIS AND JAUNDICE IN THE NEWBORN FOLLOWING MATERNAL TREATMENT WITH SULFAMETHOXYPYRIDAZINE (KYNEX). PEDIATRICS 36:742-744

634. BANNERT,N., THAL,W. AND LUBAS,E., 1969, GLUCOSE-6-PHOSPHATDEHYDROGENASE-MANGEL ALS URSACHE DES HAEMOLYTISCHEN IKTERUS BEI EINER DEUTSCHEN FAMILIE. MONATSSCHR KINDERHEILKD 117:675-679

635. NORDEN,C.W., DESFORGES,J.F. AND KASS,E.H., 1968, HEMOLYTIC EFFECT OF SULFONAMIDES IN PATIENTS WITH ERYTHROCYTES DEFICIENT IN GLUCOSE-6-PHOSPHATE DEHYDROGENASE. N ENGL J MED 279:30-31

636. ALLEN JR,S.D. AND WILKERSON,J.L., 1972, THE IMPORTANCE OF GLUCOSE-6-PHOSPHATE DEHYDROGENASE SCREENING IN A UROLOGIC PRACTICE. J UROL 107:304-305

637. CHAN,T.K. AND MC FADZEAN,A.J.S., 1974, HAEMOLYTIC EFFECT OF TRIMETHOPRIM:SULPHAMETHOXAZOLE IN G-6-PD DEFICIENCY. TRANS R SOC TROP MED HYG 68:61-62

638. OWUSU,S.K., 1972, ACUTE HAEMOLYSIS COMPLICATING CO-TRIMOXAZOLE THERAPY FOR TYPHOID FEVER IN A PATIENT WITH G.-6-P.D. DEFICIENCY. LANCET 2:819 (LETTER TO THE EDITOR)

639. DESFORGES,J.F., THAYER,W.W. AND DAWSON,J.P., 1959, HEMOLYTIC ANEMIA INDUCED BY SULFOXONE THERAPY, WITH INVESTIGATIONS INTO THE MECHANISMS OF ITS PRODUCTION. AM J MED 27:132-136

640. DEGOWIN,R.L., EPPES,R.B., POWELL,R.D. AND CARSON,P.E., 1966, THE HAEMOLYTIC EFFECTS OF DIAPHENYLSULFONE (DDS) IN NORMAL SUBJECTS AND IN THOSE WITH GLUCOSE-6-PHOSPHATE-DEHYDROGENASE DEFICIENCY. BULL WHO 35:165-179

641. CHERNOF,D., 1967, DAPSONE-INDUCED HEMOLYSIS AND G 6 PD DEFICIENCY. JAMA 201:554-556

642. GLADER,B.E. AND CONRAD,M.E., 1973, HEMOLYSIS BY DIPHENYLSULFONES: COMPARATIVE EFFECTS OF DDS AND HYDROXYLAMINE-DDS. J LAB CLIN MED 81:267-272

643. CUCINELL,S.A., REBERT,C. AND CLYDE,D., 1974, CLINICAL PHARMACOLOGY OF DIFORMYLDAPSONE. J CLIN PHARMACOL 14:51-57

644. SALVIDIO,E., PANNACCIULLI,I., AJMAR,F., GAETANI,G., GHIO,R., MOLININO,M. AND GARRE,C., 1972, HEMOLYTIC SIDE EFFECTS OF SOME ANTIMALARIAL DRUGS. BASIC RES MALARIA 39:83-100

645. TEUNIS,B.S., LEFTWICH,E.I. AND PIERCE,L.E., 1970, ACUTE METHEMOGLOBINEMIA AND HEMOLYTIC ANEMIA DUE TO TOLUIDINE BLUE. ARCH SURG 101:527-531

646. DJERASSI,L.S. AND VITANY,L., 1975, HAEMOLYTIC EPISODE IN G6 PD DEFICIENT WORKERS EXPOSED TO TNT. BR J IND MED 32:54-58

647. ALLISON,A.C., 1955, DANGER OF VITAMIN K TO NEWBORN. LANCET 1:669 (LETTER)

648. CROSSE,V.M., MEYER,T.C. AND GERRARD,J.W., 1955, KERNICTERUS
     AND PREMATURITY. ARCH DIS CHILD 30:501-508

649. HARLEY,J.D., 1961, ACUTE HAEMOLYTIC ANAEMIA IN MEDITERRANEAN
     CHILDREN WITH GLUCOSE-6-PHOSPHATE DEHYDROGENASE-DEFICIENT
     ERYTHROCTES. AUST ANN MED 10:192-200

650. ZINKHAM,W.H., 1963, PERIPHERAL BLOOD AND BILIRUBIN VALUES
     IN NORMAL FULL-TERM PRIMAQUINE- SENSITIVE NEGRO INFANTS:
     EFFECT OF VITAMIN K. PEDIATRICS 31:983-995

651. STOCKS,J., KEMP,M. AND DORMANDY,T.L., 1971, INCREASED
     SUSCEPTIBILITY OF RED-BLOOD-CELL LIPIDS TO AUTOOXIDATION
     IN HAEMOLYTIC STATES. LANCET 1:266-269

652. PINKHAS,J., DJALDETTI,M., JOSHUA,H., RESNICK,C. AND DE
     VRIES,A., 1963, SULFHEMOGLOBINEMIA AND ACUTE HEMOLYTIC
     ANEMIA WITH HEINZ BODIES FOLLOWING CONTACT WITH A FUNGICIDE-
     ZINC ETHYLENE BISIDITHIOCARBAMATE IN SUBJECT WITH GLUCOSE-
     6-PHOSPHATE DEHYDROGENASE DEFICIENCY AND HYPO- CATALASEMIA.
     BLOOD 21:484-494

653. COTTON,D.W.K. AND SUTORIUS,A.H.M., 1971, INHIBITING EFFECT
     OF SOME ANTIMALARIAL SUBSTANCES ON GLUCOSE-6-PHOSPHATE
     DEHYDROGENASE. NATURE 233:197

654. DESFORGES,J.F., KALAW,E. AND GILCHRIST,P., 1960, INHIBITION
     OF GLUCOSE-6-PHOSPHATE DEHYDROGENASE BY HEMOLYSIS INDUCING
     DRUGS. J LAB CLIN MED 55:757-766

655. LIEBOWITZ,J. AND COHEN,G., 1968, INCREASED HYDROGEN PEROXIDE
     LEVELS IN GLUCOSE 6-PHOSPHATE DEHYDROGENASE DEFICIENT
     ERYTHROCYTES EXPOSED TO ACETYLPHENYLHYDRAZINE. BIOCHEM
     PHARMACOL 17:983-988

656. COHEN,G. AND HOCHSTEIN,P., 1964, GENERATION OF HYDROGEN
     PEROXIDE IN ERYTHROCYTES BY HEMOLYTIC AGENTS. BIOCHEMISTRY
     3:895-900

657. CARRELL,R.W., WINTERBOURN,C.C. AND RACHMILEWITZ,E.A., 1975,
     ACTIVATED OXYGEN AND HAEMOLYSIS. BR J HAEMATOL 30:259-264

658. BEUTLER,E. AND TEEPLE,L., 1969, THE EFFECT OF OXIDIZED
     GLUTATHIONE (GSSG) ON HUMAN ERYTHROCYTE HEXOKINASE ACTIVITY.
     ACTA BIOL MED GER 22:707-711

659. GOLDSTEIN,B.D. AND MC DONAGH,E.M., 1976, SPECTROFLUORESCENT
     DETECTION OF IN VIVO RED CELL LIPID PEROXIDATION IN PATIENTS
     TREATED WITH DIAMINODIPHENYLSULFONE. J CLIN INVEST 57:1302-
     1307

660. BUNN,H.E.F. AND JANDL,J.H., 1966, EXCHANGE OF HEME AMONG
     HEMOGLOBIN MOLECULES. PROC NATL ACAD SCI USA 56:974-978

661. BEUTLER,E., BALUDA,M.C. AND KELLY,B.M., 1962, THE ROLE OF
     METHEMOGLOBIN IN THE MECHANISM OF DRUG-INDUCED HEMOLYTIC
     ANEMIA. PROC. IX CONG. INTNATL. SOC. OF HEMAT. MEXICO CITY
     233-244

662. RENTSCH,G., 1967, GENESIS OF HEINZ BODIES AND METHEMOGLOBIN FORMATION. BIOCHEM PHARMACOL 17:423-427

663. FINCH,C.A., 1948, METHEMOGLOBINEMIA AND SULFHEMOGLOBINEMIA. N ENGL J MED 239:470-478

664. WARBURG,C., KUBOWITZ,F. AND CHRISTIAN,W., 1931, UEBER DIE WIRKUNG VON PHENYLHYDRAZINE UND PHENYLHYDROXLAMIN AUF DEN STOFFWECHSEL DER ROTEN BLUTZELLEN (METHODE ZUR MESSUNG DES STOFFWECHSELS ROTER BLUTZELLEN). BIOCHEM Z 242:170-205

665. PEISACH,J., BLUMBERG,W.E. AND RACHMILEWITZ,E.A., 1975, THE DEMONSTRATION OF FERRIHEMOCHROME INTERMEDIATES IN HEINZ BODY FORMATION FOLLOWING THE REDUCTION OF OXYHEMOGLOBIN A BY ACETYLPHENYLHYDRAZINE. BIOCHIM BIOPHYS ACTA 393:404-418

666. RACHMILEWITZ,E.A., HARARI,E. AND WINTERHALTER,K.H., 1974, SEPARATION OF ALPHA- AND BETA-CHAINS OF HEMOGLOBIN A BY ACETYLPHENYLHYDRAZINE. BIOCHIM BIOPHYS ACTA 371:402-407

667. ITANO,H.A., HOLLISTER,D.W., FOGARTY JR,W.M. AND MANNEN,S., 1974, EFFECT OF RING SUBSTITUTION ON THE HEMOLYTIC ACTION OF ARYLHYDRAZINES. PROC SOC EXP BIOL MED 147:656-658

668. ITANO,H.A. AND MANNEN,S., 1976, REACTIONS OF PHENYLDIAZENE AND RING-SUBSTITUTED PHENYLDIAZENES WITH FERRIHEMOGLOBIN. BIOCHIM BIOPHYS ACTA 421:87-96

669. ITANO,H.A., HOSOKAWA,K. AND HIROTA,K., 1976, INDUCTION OF HAEMOLYTIC ANAEMIA BY SUBSTITUTED PHENYLHYDRAZINES. BR J HAEMATOL 256:665-667

670. ITANO,H.A., HIROTA,K. AND HOSOKAWA,K., 1975, MECHANISM OF INDUCTION OF HAEMOLYTIC ANAEMIA BY PHENYLHYDRAZINE. NATURE 256:665-667

671. ITANO,H.A., HIROTA,K. AND VEDVICK,T.S., 1977, LIGANDS AND OXIDANTS IN FERRIHEMOCHROME FORMATION AND OXIDATIVE HEMOLYSIS. PROC NATL ACAD SCI USA 74:2556-2560

672. LARCAN,A., KAIFFER,M., MAITREHANCHE,M., GENETET,B. AND VIGNERON,C., 1972, INSUFFISANCE RENALE AIGUE. REVELATRICE D'UN DEFICIT EN GLUCOSE- 6-PHOSPHATE DESHYDROGENASE: GRAVITE DE L'HEMOLYSE ISTROGENE. NOUV PRESSE MED 35:2299-2304

673. OWUSU,S.K., FOLI,A.K., KONOTEY HULU,F.I.D., ADDY,J.H., JANOSI,M. AND LARBI,E.B., 1972, ACUTE REVERSIBLE RENAL FAILURE ASSOCIATED WITH GLUCOSE-6-PHOSPHATE DEHYDROGENASE DEFICIENCY. LANCET 2:1255-1257

674. WHELTON,A., DONADIO JR,J.V. AND ELISBERG,B.L., 1968, ACUTE RENAL FAILURE COMPLICATING RICKETTSIAL INFECTIONS IN GLUCOSE-6-PHOSPHATE DEHYDROGENASE-DEFICIENT INDIVIDUALS. ANN INTERN MED 69:323-328

675. GULATI,P.D. AND RIZVI,S.N.A., 1976, ACUTE REVERSIBLE RENAL FAILURE IN G-6 PD-DEFICIENT SIBLINGS. POSTGRAD MED J 52:83-85

676. ANGLE,C.R., 1972, GLUCOSE-6-PHOSPHATE DEHYDROGENASE DEFICIENCY
     AND ACUTE RENAL FAILURE. LANCET 2:134

677. PHILLIPS,S.M. AND SILVERS,N.P., 1969, GLUCOSE-6-PHOSPHATE
     DEHYDROGENASE DEFICIENCY, INFECTIOUS HEPATITIS, ACUTE
     HEMOLYSIS, AND RENAL FAILURE. ANN INTERN MED 70:99-104

678. LWANGA,D. AND WING,A.J., 1970, RENAL COMPLICATIONS ASSOCIATED
     WITH TYPHOID FEVER. EAST AFR MED J 47:146-152

679. CONTE,J., DURAND,D., TON THAT,H. AND SUC,J.M., 1973, ACUTE
     RENAL FAILURE AND HEMOLYTIC ANEMIA DUE TO RED CELL G6PD
     DEFICIENCY FIRST MANIFESTED AFTER CHLOROQUINE ADMINISTRATION.
     J UROL NEPHROL 79:756-763 (EXCERPTA MEDICA VOL. II.I NO.
     71)

680. BURKA,E.R., WEAVER III,Z. AND MARKS,P.A., 1966, CLINICAL
     SPECTRUM OF HEMOLYTIC ANEMIA ASSOCIATED WITH G 6 PD
     DEFICIENCY. ANN INTERN MED 64:817-825

681. MENGEL,C.E., METZ,E. AND YANCEY,W.S., 1967, ANEMIA DURING
     ACUTE INFECTIONS. ROLE OF GLUCOSE-6-PHOSPHATE DEHYDROGENASE
     DEFICIENCY IN NEGROES. ARCH INTERN MED 119:287-290

682. WILLIAMS,A.O., TUGWELL,P. AND EDINGTON,G.M., 1976, GLUCOSE-
     6-PHOSPHATE DEHYDROGENASE DEFICIENCY AND LOBAR PNEUMONIA.
     ARCH PATHOL LAB MED 100:25-31

683. BERRY,D.H. AND VIETTI,T.J., 1965, CLINICAL MANIFESTATIONS
     OF PRIMAQUINE-SENSITIVE ANEMIA. AM J DIS CHILD 110:166-171

684. TUGWELL,P., 1973, GLUCOSE-6-PHOSPHATE-DEHYDROGENASE DEFICIENCY
     IN NIGERIANS WITH JAUNDICE ASSOCIATED WITH LOBAR PNEUMONIA.
     LANCET 1:968-969

685. LAMPE,R.M., KIRDPON,S., MANSUWAN,P. AND BENENSON,M.W.,
     1975, GLUCOSE-6-PHOSPHATE DEHYDROGENASE DEFICIENCY IN THAI
     CHILDREN WITH TYPHOID FEVER. J PEDIATR 87:576-578

686. HERSKO,C. AND VARDY,P.A., 1967, HAEMOLYSIS IN TYPHOID FEVER
     IN CHILDREN WITH G-6-PD DEFICIENCY. BR MED J 1:214-215

687. CHAN,T.K., 1972, G-6-PD DEFICIENCY, TYPHOID, AND CO-
     TRIMOXAZOLE. LANCET 2:1258

688. HARLEY,J.D., 1962, ACUTE HAEMOLYTIC ANAEMIA IN MEDITERRANEAN
     CHILDREN WITH GLUCOSE-6-PHOSPHATE DEHYDROGENASE-DEFICIENT
     ERYTHROCYTES. BLOOD 19:257-258 (ABSTRACT)

689. CONSTANTOPOULOS,A., ECONOMOPOULOS,P. AND KANDYLAS,J., 1973,
     FULMINANT DIARRHEA AND ACUTE HEMOLYSIS DUE TO G.-6-P.D.
     DEFICIENCY IN SALMONELLOSIS. LANCET 1:1522

690. ARCURI,F. AND ROBERT,L., 1969, ANEMIA EMOLITICA ACUTA IN
     CORSO DI SEPSI DA PROTEUS MORGANII IN SOGGETTO CARENTE DI
     GLUCOSIO-6-FOSFATO DEIDROGENASI ERITOCITARIA. GIORNALE DI
     MALATTIE INFETTIVE E PARASSITARIE 21:257

691. CONRAD,M.E., SCHWARTZ,F.D. AND YOUNG,A.A., 1964, INFECTIOUS
     HEPATITIS - A GENERALIZED DISEASE. A STUDY OF RENAL, GASTRO-
     INTESTINAL AND HEMATOLOGIC ABNORMALITIES. AM J MED 37:789-
     801

692. KATTAMIS,C.A. AND TJORTJATOU,F., 1970, THE HEMOLYTIC PROCESS OF VIRAL HEPATITIS IN CHILDREN WITH NORMAL OR DEFICIENT GLUCOSE-6-PHOSPHATE DEHYDROGENASE ACTIVITY. J PEDIATR 77:422-430

693. SALEN,G., GOLDSTEIN,F., HAURANI,F. AND WIRTS,C.W., 1966, ACUTE HEMOLYTIC ANEMIA COMPLICATING VIRAL HEPATITIS IN PATIENTS WITH GLUCOSE-6-PHOSPHATE DEHYDROGENASE DEFICIENCY. ANN INTERN MED 65:1210-1220

694. BOON,W.H., 1966, VIRAL HEPATITIS IN G-6-PD DEFICIENCY. LANCET 1:882-883

695. FRIED,D., GOTLIEB,A. AND ROITMAN,A., 1977, INFECTIOUS HEPATITIS WITH EXCESSIVE HYPERBILIRUBINEMIA AND A HEMOLYTIC CRISIS IN AN 8-YEAR-OLD BOY. CLIN PEDIATR 16:482-483

696. HENNEMAN,D.H., ALTSCHULE,M.D. AND GONCZ,R.M., 1954, GLUTATHIONE IN HUMAN DISEASE. GLUTATHIONE. A SYMPOSIUM COLOWICK,S., LAZAROW,A., RACKER,E., SCHWARZ,D.R., STADTMAN,E. AND WAELSCH,H. ED. 299-310, ACADEMIC PRESS, NEW YORK

697. GANT,F.L. AND WINKS JR,G.F., 1961, PRIMAQUINE SENSITIVE HEMOLYTIC ANEMIA COMPLICATING DIABETIC ACIDOSIS. CLINICAL RESEARCH 9:27

698. GELLADY,A. AND GREENWOOD,R.D., 1972, G-6-PD HEMOLYTIC ANEMIA COMPLICATING DIABETIC KETOACIDOSIS. J PEDIATR 80:1037-1038

699. OCKEL,E., RAPOPORT,S., HINTERBERGER,U. AND GERISCHERMOTHES,W., 1962, DIE PH-ABHAENGIGKEIT DER ANAEROBEN GLYKOLYSE UND DER HEXOKINASE. FOLIA HAEMATOL (LEIPZ) 78:477-480

700. BEUTLER,E. AND GUINTO,E., 1974, THE REDUCTION OF GLYCERALDEHYDE BY HUMAN ERYTHROCYTES. L-HEXONATE DEHYDROGENASE ACTIVITY. J CLIN INVEST 53:1258-1264

701. GLADER,B., 1975, ROLE OF ELEVATED GLUCOSE CONCENTRATIONS IN THE HEMOLYSIS OF GLUCOSE-6- PHOSPHATE DEHYDROGENASE DEFICIENT ERYTHROCYTES. PROC SOC EXP BIOL MED 148:50-53

702. BEUTLER,E. AND GUINTO,E., 1974, MECHANISM OF STIMULATION OF THE HEXOSE MONOPHOSPHATE SHUNT OF ERYTHROCYTES BY PYRUVATE. ENZYME 18:7-18

703. SCHAERER,K., HERZKA,H. AND MARTI,H.R., 1963, KERNICTERUS BEI MANGEL AN GLUKOSE-6-PHOSPHAT-DEHYDROGENASE DER ERYTHROCYTEN. HELV PAEDIATR ACTA 2:148-162

704. LU,T.C., WEI,H. AND BLACKWELL,R.Q., 1966, INCREASED INCIDENCE OF SEVERE HYPERBILIRUBINEMIA AMONG NEWBORN CHINESE INFANTS WITH G-6-PD DEFICIENCY. PEDIATRICS 37:994-999

705. PANIZON,F., 1960, L'ICTERE GRAVE DU NOUVEAU-NE ASSOCIE A UNE DEFICIENCE EN GLUCOSE-6-PHOSPHATE DEHYDROGENASE. BIOL NEONATE 2:167-177

706. DOXIADIS,S.A., FESSAS,P. AND VALAES,T., 1960, ERYTHROCYTE ENZYME DEFICIENCY IN UNEXPLAINED KERNICTERUS. LANCET 2:44

707. PANIZON,F., 1960, ERYTHROCYTE ENZYME DEFICIENCY IN UNEXPLAINED
     KERNICTERUS. LANCET 2:1093

708. WOODFIELD,D.G. AND BIDDULPH,J., 1975, NEONATAL JAUNDICE
     AND GLUCOSE-6-PHOSPHATE DEHYDROGENASE DEFICIENCY IN PAPUA
     NEW GUINEA. MED J AUST 1:443-446

709. MELONI,T., COSTA,S. AND CUTILLO,S., 1975, HAPTOGLOBIN,
     HEMOPEXIN, HEMOGLOBIN AND HEMATOCRIT IN NEWBORNS WITH
     ERYTHROCYTE GLUCOSE-6-PHOSPHATE DEHYDROGENASE DEFICIENCY.
     ACTA HAEMATOL 54:284-288

710. IFEKWUNIGWE,A.E. AND LUZZATTO,L., 1966, KERNICTERUS IN G.-
     6-P.D.-DEFICIENCY. LANCET 1:667

711. BROWN,W.R. AND BOON,W.H., 1968, HYPERBILIRUBINEMIA AND
     KERNICTERUS IN GLUCOSE-6-PHOSPHATE DEHYDROGENASE-DEFICIENT
     INFANTS IN SINGAPORE. PEDIATRICS 41:1055-1062

712. STERN,L., CAMERON,D. AND DALLAIRE,L., 1968, NEONATAL JAUNDICE
     ASSOCIATED WITH ERYTHROCYTE GLUCOSE-6-PHOSPHATE DEHYDROGENASE
     DEFICIENCY IN A NON-MEDITERRANEAN CAUCASIAN INFANT WITH
     TRISOMIC DOWN*S SYNDROME. CAN MED ASSOC J 98:1196-1197

713. WEATHERALL,D.J., 1960, ENZYME DEFICIENCY IN HAEMOLYTIC
     DISEASE OF THE NEWBORN. LANCET 2:835-837

714. SZEINBERG,A., OLIVER,M., SCHMIDT,R., ADAM,A. AND SHEBA,C.,
     1963, GLUCOSE-6-PHOSPHATE DEHYDROGENASE DEFICIENCY AND
     HAEMOLYTIC DISEASE. ARCH DIS CHILD 38:23-28

715. FREIER,S., MAYER,K., ABRAHAMOV,A. AND LEVENE,C., 1965,
     NEONATAL JAUNDICE IN INFANTS WITH ENZYMATIC DEFECT OF THE
     RED BLOOD CELL. ISR J MED SCI 1:844-847

716. DREW,J.H., SMITH,M.B. AND KITCHEN,W.H., 1977, GLUCOSE-6-
     PHOSPHATE DEHYDROGENASE DEFICIENCY IN IMMIGRANT GREEK
     INFANTS. J PEDIATR 90:659-660

717. PERKINS,R.P., 1976, THE SIGNIFICANCE OF GLUCOSE-6-PHOSPHATE
     DEHYDROGENASE DEFICIENCY IN PREGNANCY. AM J OBSTET GYNECOL
     125:215-223

718. KARAYALCIN,G., KIM,K.Y., ABALLI,A.J. AND LANZKOWSKY,P.,
     1973, GLUCOSE-6-PHOSPHATE DEHYDROGENASE (G-6-PD) DEFICIENCY
     AND HYPERBILIRUBINEMIA IN BLACK AMERICAN TERM INFANTS.
     AMERICAN SOCIETY OF HEMATOLOGY (ABSTRACT 165) P92

719. LOPEZ,R. AND COOPERMAN,J.M., 1971, GLUCOSE-6-PHOSPHATE
     DEHYDROGENASE DEFICIENCY AND HYPERBILIRUBINEMIA IN THE
     NEWBORN. AM J DIS CHILD 122:66-70

720. ESHAGHPOUR,E., OSKI,F.A. AND WILLIAMS,M., 1967, THE
     RELATIONSHIP OF ERYTHROCYTE GLUCOSE-6-PHOSPHATE DEHYDROGENASE
     DEFICIENCY TO HYPERBILIRUBINEMIA IN NEGRO PREMATURE INFANTS.
     J PEDIATR 70:595-601

721. LEVIN,S.E., CHARLTON,R.W. AND FREIMAN,I., 1964, GLUCOSE-6-
     PHOSPHATE DEHYDROGENASE DEFICIENCY AND NEONATAL JAUNDICE
     IN SOUTH AFRICAN BANTU INFANTS. J PEDIATR 65:757-764

722. BIENZLE,U., EFFIONG,C. AND LUZZATTO,L., 1976, ERYTHROCYTE
     GLUCOSE 6-PHOSPHATE DEHYDROGENASE DEFICIENCY (G6PD TYPE A-
) AND NEONATAL JAUNDICE. ACTA PAEDIATR SCAND 65:701-703

723. ZINKHAM,W.H. AND CHILDS,B., 1958, A DEFECT IN GSH METABOLISM
     IN ERYTHROCYTES FROM PATIENTS WITH A NAPHTHALENE-INDUCED
     HEMOLYTIC ANEMIA. PEDIATRICS 22:461-471

724. MALAKA-ZAFIRIU,K., TSIURES,J. AND CASSIMOS,C., 1975, D-
     GLUCARIC ACID EXCRETION IN NEWBORNS WITH SEVERE JAUNDICE
     OF UNKNOWN ETIOLOGY AND DUE TO GLUCOSE-6-PHOSPHATE
     DEHYDROGENASE DEFICIENCY IN GREECE. HELV PAEDIATR ACTA
     30:201-207

725. MALAKA-ZAFIRIU,K., TSIURES,I., DANIELIDES,B. AND CASSIMOS,C.,
     1973, SALICYLAMIDE GLUCURONIDE FORMATION IN NEWBORNS WITH
     SEVERE JAUNDICE OF UNKNOWN ETIOLOGY AND DUE TO GLUCOSE 6
     PHOSPHATE DEHYDROGENASE DEFICIENCY IN GREECE. HELV PAEDIATR
     ACTA 28:323-329

726. KATTAMIS,C.A., KYRIAZAKOU,M. AND CHAIDAS,S., 1969, FAVISM.
     CLINICAL AND BIOCHEMICAL DATA. J MED GENET 6:34-41

727. SARTORI,E., 1971, ON THE PATHOGENESIS OF FAVISM. J MED
     GENET 8:462-467

728. KATTAMIS,C., 1971, FAVISM IN BREAST-FED INFANTS. ARCH DIS
     CHILD 46:741

729. EMANUEL,B. AND SCHOENFELD,A., 1961, FAVISM IN A NURSING
     INFANT. J PEDIATR 58:263-266

730. LUISADA,L., 1941, FAVISM: SINGULAR DISEASE AFFECTING CHIEFLY
     RED BLOOD CELLS. MEDICINE (BALTIMORE) 20:229-250

731. SANSONE,G., PIGA,A.M. AND SEGNI,G., 1958, IL FAVISMO MINERVA
     MEDICA, TORINO

732. DACIE,J.V., 1967, THE HAEMOLYTIC ANAEMIAS, PART IV P. 1057,
     2ND EDITION, GRUNE & STRATTON, NEW YORK

733. SYMVOULIDIS,A., VOUDICLARIS,S., MOUNTOKALAKIS,T. AND
     POUGOUNIAS,H., 1972, ACUTE RENAL FAILURE IN G.-6-P.D.
     DEFICIENCY. LANCET 2:819-820 (LETTER TO THE EDITOR)

734. DAVIES,P., 1962, FAVISM: A FAMILY STUDY. Q J MED 31:157-
     177

735. HOLT,J.M. AND SLADDEN,R.A., 1965, FAVISM IN ENGLAND--TWO
     MORE CASES. ARCH DIS CHILD 40:271-273

736. SROCZYNSKA,M. AND SYCHLOWY,A., 1973, FAWIZM-PRZELOM
     HEMOLITYCZNY W PRZEBIEGU NIEDOBORU DEHYDROGENAZY GLUKOZO-
     6-FOSFORANOWEJ W KRWINKACH CZERWONYCH. POL TYG LEK 28:744-
     745

737. KAHN,A., MARIE,J., DESBOIS,J.-.C. AND BOIVIN,P., 1976,
     FAVISM IN A PORTUGUESE FAMILY DUE TO A DEFICIENT GLUCOSE-
     6-PHOSPHATE DEHYDROGENASE VARIANT OF 'CANTON' OR 'CANTON-
     LIKE' TYPE 1. ACTA HAEMATOL 56:58-64

738. PANICH,V. AND NA NAKORN,S., 1973, ACUTE HEMOLYSIS IN G-6-
      PD UNION (THAI) REPORT ON FOUR CASES. J MED ASSOC THAI
      56:241-249

739. SZEINBERG,A. AND CHARI BITRON,A., 1957, BLOOD GLUTATHIONE
      CONCENTRATION AFTER HAEMOLYTIC ANEMIA DUE TO VICIA FABA OR
      SULPHONAMIDES. ACTA HAEMATOL 18:229-233

740. DU,S.-.D., 1952, FAVISM IN WEST CHINA. CHIN MED J 70:17-26

741. CROSBY,W.H., 1956, FAVISM IN SARDINIA (NEWSLETTER). BLOOD
      11:91-92

742. SANSONE,G. AND SEGNI,G., 1956, PRIME DETERMINAZIONI DEL
      GLUTATIONE (GSH) EMATICO NEL FAVISMO. BOLL SOC ITAL BIOL
      SPER 32:456-458

743. ZINKHAM,W.H., LENHARD JR,R.E. AND CHILDS,B., 1958, A
      DEFICIENCY OF GLUCOSE-6-PHOSPHATE DEHYDROGENASE ACTIVITY
      IN ERYTHROCYTES FROM PATIENTS WITH FAVISM. JOHNS HOPKINS
      MED J 102:169-175

744. PANIZON,F. AND VULLO,C., 1961, THE MECHANISM OF HAEMOLYSIS
      IN FAVISM. ACTA HAEMATOL 26:337-343

745. STAMATOYANNOPOULOS,G., FRASER,G.R., MOTULSKY,A.G., FESSAS,P.,
      AKRIVAKIS,A. AND PAPAYANNOPOULOU,T.H., 1966, ON THE FAMILIAL
      PREDISPOSITION TO FAVISM. AM J HUM GENET 18:253-263

746. CASSIMOS,C.H.R., MALAKA ZAFIRIU,K. AND TSIURES,J., 1974,
      URINARY D-GLUCARIC ACID EXCRETION IN NORMAL AND G-6-PD
      DEFICIENT CHILDREN WITH FAVISM. J PEDIATR 84:871-872

747. CASSIMOS,C.H.R., TSIURES,I. AND DANIELIDES,B., 1973,
      DISTURBANCES OF SALICYLAMIDE GLUCURONIDE FORMATION IN NORMAL
      AND G-6-PD DEFICIENT CHILDREN. IRCS HEMATOLOGY (73-3) 17-
      3-1

748. CUTILLO,S., COSTA,S., VINTULEDDU,M.C. AND MELONI,T., 1976,
      SALICYLAMIDE-GLUCURONIDE FORMATION IN CHILDREN WITH FAVISM
      AND IN THEIR PARENTS. ACTA HAEMATOL 55:296-299

749. ROTH,K.L. AND FRUMIN,A.M., 1960, STUDIES ON THE HEMOLYTIC
      PRINCIPLE OF THE FAVA BEAN. J LAB CLIN MED 56:695-700

750. FIORELLI,G., PODDA,M., CORRIAS,A. AND FARGION,S., 1974,
      THE RELEVANCE OF IMMUNE REACTIONS IN ACUTE FAVISM. ACTA
      HAEMATOL 51:211-218

751. MAGER,J., GLASER,G., RAZIN,A., IZAK,G., BIEN,S. AND NOAM,M.,
      1965, METABOLIC EFFECTS OF PYRIMIDINES DERIVED FROM FAVA
      BEAN GLYCOSIDES ON HUMAN ERYTHROCYTES DEFICIENT IN GLUCOSE-
      6-PHOSPHATE DEHYDROGENASE. BIOCHEM BIOPHYS RES COMMUN
      20:235-240

752. RAZIN,A., HERSHKO,A., GLASER,G. AND MAGER,J., 1968, THE
      OXIDANT EFFECT OF ISOURAMIL ON RED CELL GLUTATHIONE AND
      ITS SYNERGISTIC ENCHANCEMENT BY ASCORBIC ACID OR 3,4-
      DIHYDROXYPHENYLALANINE. POSSIBLE RELATION TO THE PATHOGENESIS
      OF FAVISM. ISR J MED SCI 4:852-857

753. FLOHE,L., NIEBCH,G. AND REIBER,H., 1971, ZUR WIRKUNG VON DIVICIN IN MENSCHLICHEN ERYTHROCYTEN. Z KLIN CHEM KLIN BIOCHEM 9:431-437

754. BOTTINI,E., 1973, FAVISM: CURRENT PROBLEMS AND INVESTIGATIONS. J MED GENET 10:154-157

755. PODDA,M., FIORELLI,G., IDEO,G., SPANO,G. AND DIOGUARDI,N., 1969, IN VITRO EFFECT OF A FAVA BEAN EXTRACT AND OF ITS FRACTIONS ON REDUCED GLUTATHIONE IN GLUCOSE-6-PHOSPHATE DEHYDROGENASE DEFICIENT RED CELLS. FOLIA HAEMATOL (LEIPZ) 91:51-55

756. BOTTINI,E., LUCARELLI,P., SPENNATI,G.F., BUSINCO,L. AND PALMARINO,R., 1970, PRESENCE IN VICIA FABA OF DIFFERENT SUBSTANCES WITH ACTIVITY IN VITRO ON GD (-) MED RED BLOOD CELL REDUCED GLUTATHIONE. CLIN CHIM ACTA 30:831-834

757. VUOPIO,P., HARKONEN,M., HELSKE,T. AND NAEVERI,H., 1975, RED CELL GLUCOSE-6-PHOSPHATE DEHYDROGENASE DEFICIENCY IN FINLAND. CHARACTERIZATION OF A NEW VARIANT WITH SEVERE ENZYME DEFICIENCY. SCAND J HAEMATOL 15:145-152

758. SONNET,J., LIEVENS,M., VERPOORTEN,C., KRIEKEMANS,J. AND EECKELS,R., 1974, SPORADIC G6PD DEFICIENCY WITH HAEMOLYTIC ANAEMIA IN TWO CHILDREN OF WEST EUROPEAN ANCESTRY. BR J HAEMATOL 28:299-310

759. ZINKHAM,W.H. AND LENHARD,R.E., 1959, METABOLIC ABNORMALITIES OF ERYTHROCYTES FROM PATIENTS WITH CONGENITAL NONSPHEROCYTIC HEMOLYTIC ANEMIA. J PEDIATR 55:319-336

760. HUSKISSON,E.C., MURPHY,B. AND WEST,C., 1970, GLUCOSE-6-PHOSPHATE DEHYDROGENASE DEFICIENCY AND CHRONIC HAEMOLYSIS IN AN ENGLISH FAMILY. J CLIN PATHOL 23:135-139

761. SCHROETER,W., DRESCHER,J. AND FISCHER,K., 1967, UEBER EINE SELTENE FORM DES GLUCOSE-6-PHOSPHATDEHYDROGENASE-MANGELS MIT KONGENITALER NICHTSPHAEROCYTAERER HAEMOLYTISCHER ANAEMIE. KLIN WOCHENSCHR 45:355-362

762. PUXEDDU,A., SANTEUSANIO,F., MIGLIORINI,E., SIRACUSA,A. AND MERLITTI,A., 1968, STUDIO DI UN GRUPPO FAMILIARE UMBRO-MARCHIGIANO CON ANEMIA EMOLITICA CONGENITA NON SFEROCITICA DA CARENZA DI GLUCOSIO-6-FOSFATO-DEIDROGENASI (G6-PD). HAEMATOLOGICA ARCHIVIO 53:30-52

763. ABE,T., TAKAFUJI,H., YAMAMOTO,M., DAIMON,S., NAKAJIMA,K., AGASAWARA,K., TAKINO,T., FUJIKI,N., NISHINA,T. AND MIWA,S., 1968, KONGENITALE NICHTSPHAEROZYTARE HAEMOLYTISCHE ANAMIEN DURCH MANGEL AN GLUCOSE-6-PHOSPHAT-DEHYDROGENASE DER ERYTHROZYTEN IN EINER JAPANISCHEN. BLUT 17:143-151

764. ENGSTROM,P.F. AND BEUTLER,E., 1970, G-6-PD TRIPLER: A UNIQUE VARIANT ASSOCIATED WITH CHRONIC HEMOLYTIC DISEASE. BLOOD 36:10-13

765. KOJIMA,H., 1972, CONGENITAL NONSPHEROCYTIC HEMOLYTIC DISEASE (CNHD) DUE TO A G-6-PD VARIANT: G-6-PD KYOTO. ACTA HAEMATOL JAP 35:32-38

766. STREIFF,F. AND VIGNERON,C., 1971, CHRONIC HAEMOLYTIC ANEMIA
      DUE TO A DEFECT OF GLUCOSE-6-PHOSPHATE DEHYDROGENASE (G6PD)
      IN A LORRAINE FAMILY. DEMONSTRATION OF A NEW TYPE OF THE
      ENZYME: GD(-) NANCY. NOUV REV FR HEMATOL 11:279-290

767. SHAHIDI,N.T. AND DIAMOND,L.K., 1959, ENZYME DEFICIENCY IN
      ERYTHROCYTES IN CONGENITAL NONSPHEROCYTIC HEMOLYTIC ANEMIA.
      PEDIATRICS 24:245-253

768. MILLS,G.C., ALPERIN,J.B. AND TRIMMER,K.B., 1975, STUDIES
      ON VARIANT GLUCOSE-6-PHOSPHATE DEHYDROGENASES: G6PD FORT
      WORTH. BIOCHEM MED 13:264-275

769. KUEHBOECK,V.J., PIETSCHMANN,H. AND ROTHENBUCHNER,G., 1969,
      ENZYMOPENISCHE HAEMOLYTISCHE ANAEMIE BEI EINER
      OESTERREICHISCHEN FAMILIE. WIEN KLIN WOCHENSCHR 81:135-137

770. BEUTLER,E. AND FAIRBANKS,V.F., 1962, THE NORMAL HUMAN FEMALE
      AS A MOSAIC OF X-CHROMOSOME ACTIVITY: STUDIES USING GLUCOSE-
      6-PHOSPHATE DEHYDROGENASE AS A GENETIC MARKER. PROC IX CONG
      INTNATL SOC HEMAT, MEXICO CITY 43-53

771. BEUTLER,E., ROBSON,M. AND BUTTENWIESER,E., 1957, THE
      MECHANISM OF GLUTATHIONE DESTRUCTION AND PROTECTION IN
      DRUG-SENSITIVE AND NON-SENSITIVE ERYTHROCYTES. IN VITRO
      STUDIES. J CLIN INVEST 36:617-628

772. ZINKHAM,W.H., 1959, AN IN VITRO ABNORMALITY OF GLUTATHIONE
      METABOLISM IN ERYTHROCYTES FROM NORMAL NEWBORNS: MECHANISM
      AND CLINICAL SIGNIFICANCE. PEDIATRICS 23:18-23

773. SWARUP,S., GHOSH,S.K. AND CHATTERJEA,J.B., 1960, GLUTATHIONE
      STABILITY TEST IN HAEMOGLOBIN E-THALASSEMIA DISEASE. NATURE
      188:153

774. DESFORGES,J.F., 1962, GLUTATHIONE INSTABILITY IN NORMAL
      BLOOD. BLOOD 20:186-195

775. MOELLER,N.P.H. AND STEENSGAARD,J., 1971, STUDIES ON THE
      GLUTATHIONE STABILITY OF NORMAL AND GLUCOSE-6-PHOSPHATE-
      DEFICIENT HUMAN ERYTHROCYTES. SCAND J CLIN LAB INVEST
      28:277-282

776. GLOCK,G.E. AND MC LEAN,P., 1953, FURTHER STUDIES ON THE
      PROPERTIES AND ASSAY OF GLUCOSE-6-PHOSPHATE DEHYDROGENASE,
      AND 6-PHOSPHOGLUCONATE DEHYDROGENASE OF RAT LIVER. BIOCHEM
      J 55:400-408

777. BREWSTER,M.A., BERRY,D.H. AND MURPHEY,M.N., 1974, AUTOMATED
      REACTION RATE ANALYSIS OF ERYTHROCYTE GLUCOSE-6-PHOSPHATE
      DEHYDROGENASE AND GLUTATHIONE REDUCTASE ACTIVITIES. BIOCHEM
      MED 10:229-235

778. MARKS,P.A., 1958, RED CELL GLUCOSE-6-PHOSPHATE AND 6-
      PHOSPHOGLUCONIC DEHYDROGENASES AND NUCLEOSIDE PHOSPHORYLASE.
      SCIENCE 127:1338-1339

779. CATALANO,E.W., JOHNSON,G.F. AND SOLOMON,H.M., 1975,
      MEASUREMENT OF ERYTHROCYTE GLUCOSE-6-PHOSPHATE DEHYDROGENASE
      ACTIVITY WITH A CENTRIFUGAL ANALYZER. CLIN CHEM 21:134-138

780. BISHOP,C., 1966, ASSAY OF GLUCOSE-6-PHOSPHATE DEHYDROGENASE
      (E.C. 1.1.1.49) AND 6-PHOSPHOGLUCONATE DEHYDROGENASE (E.C.
      1.1.1.43) IN RED CELLS. J LAB CLIN MED 68:149-155

781. ELLS,H.A. AND KIRKMAN,H.N., 1961, A COLORIMETRIC METHOD
      FOR ASSAY OF ERYTHROCYTIC GLUCOSE-6-PHOSPHATE DEHYDROGENASE.
      PROC SOC EXP BIOL MED 106:607-609

782. LOWE,M.L., STELLA,A.F., MOSHER,B.S., GIN,J.B. AND
      DEMETRIOU,J.A., 1972, MICROFLUOROMETRY OF GLUCOSE-6-PHOSPHATE
      DEHYDROGENASE AND 6-PHOSPHOGLUCONATE DEHYDROGENASE IN RED
      CELLS. CLIN CHEM 18:440-445

783. BENI,A., FIORITONI,G., SALVATI,A.M., TENTORI,L. AND
      TORLONTANO,G., 1973, QUANTITATION OF THE ULTRAVIOLET LIGHT
      TEST FOR ERYTHROCYTE GLUCOSE 6- PHOSPHATE DEHYDROGENASE,
      PYRUVATE KINASE AND GLUTATHIONE REDUCTASE. CLIN CHIM ACTA
      49:41-48

784. TAN,I.K. AND WHITEHEAD,T.P., 1969, AUTOMATED FLUOROMETRIC
      DETERMINATION OF GLUCOSE-6-PHOSPHATE DEHYDROGENASE (G 6
      PD) AND 6-PHOSPHOGLUCONATE DEHYDROGENASE (6PGD) ACTIVITIES
      IN RED BLOOD CELLS. CLIN CHEM 15:467-478

785. MOTULSKY,A.G. AND CAMPBELL-KRAUT,J.M., 1961, POPULATION
      GENETICS OF GLUCOSE-6-PHOSPHATE DEHYDROGENASE DEFICIENCY
      OF THE RED CELL. PROC.CONF.ON GENETIC POLYMORPHISMS AND
      GEOGRAPHIC VARIATIONS IN DISEASE BLUMBERG,B.S. ED. 159-180,
      GRUNE & STRATTON, NEW YORK

786. BERNSTEIN,R.E., 1963, BRILLIANT CRESYL BLUE SCREENING TEST
      FOR DEMONSTRATING GLUCOSE-6-PHOSPHATE DEHYDROGENASE DEFICIENCY
      IN RED CELLS. CLIN CHIM ACTA 8:158-160

787. TOENZ,O. AND BETKE,K., 1962, EINFACHER FARBTEST ZUR BESTIMMUNG
      DER GLUCOSE-6-PHOSPHATDEHYDROGENASE IN MENSCHLICHEN
      ERYTHROCYTEN. KLIN WOCHENSCHR 40:649-653

788. MARTI,H.R., 1968, SEMIQUANTITATIVE ASSAY OF ERYTHROCYTE
      GLUCOSE-6-PHOSPHATE DEHYDROGENASE ACTIVITY BY A NEW
      MODIFICATION OF THE MOTULSKY TEST. EXPERIENTIA 24:416

789. BERNSTEIN,R.E., 1962, A RAPID SCREENING DYE TEST FOR THE
      DETECTION OF GLUCOSE-6-PHOSPHATE DEHYDROGENASE DEFICIENCY
      IN RED CELLS. NATURE 194:192-193

790. FRISCHER,H., CARSON,P.E., BOWMAN,J.E. AND RIECKMANN,K.H.,
      1973, VISUAL TEST FOR ERYTHROCYTIC GLUCOSE-6-PHOSPHATE
      DEHYDROGENASE, 6-PHOSPHOGLUCONIC DEHYDROGENASE, AND
      GLUTATHIONE REDUCTASE DEFICIENCIES. J LAB CLIN MED 81:613-
      624

791. FAIRBANKS,V.F. AND BEUTLER,E., 1962, A SIMPLE METHOD FOR
      DETECTION OF ERYTHROCYTE GLUCOSE-6-PHOSPHATE DEHYDROGENASE
      DEFICIENCY (G-6-PD SPOT TEST). BLOOD 20:591-601

792. SASS,M.D., CARUSO,C.J. AND AXELROD,D.R., 1966, RAPID
      SCREENING FOR D-GLUCOSE-6-PHOSPHATE: NADP OXIDOREDUCTASE
      DEFICIENCY WITH METHYLENE BLUE. J LAB CLIN MED 68:156-162

793. GIBBS,W.N., 1974, THE METHYLENE BLUE REDUCTION TEST: EVALUATION OF A SCREENING METHOD FOR GLUCOSE-6-PHOSPHATE DEHYDROGENASE DEFICIENCY. AM J TROP MED HYG 23:1197-1202

794. OSKI,F.A. AND GROWNEY,P.M., 1965, A SIMPLE MICROMETHOD FOR THE DETECTION OF ERYTHROCYTE GLUCOSE-6-PHOSPHATE DEHYDROGENASE DEFICIENCY. J PEDIATR 66:90-93

795. BREWER,G.J., TARLOV,A.R. AND ALVING,A.S., 1962, THE METHEMOGLOBIN REDUCTION TEST FOR PRIMAQUINE-TYPE SENSITIVITY OF ERYTHROCYTES. JAMA 180:386-388

796. BAPAT,J.P., BAXI,A.J. AND BHATIA,H.M., 1976, IS METHEMOGLOBIN REDUCTION TEST A TRUE INDEX OF G-6-PD DEFICIENCY. INDIAN J MED RES 64:1687-1690

797. FAIRBANKS,V.F. AND FERNANDEZ,M.N., 1969, THE IDENTIFICATION OF METABOLIC ERRORS ASSOCIATED WITH HEMOLYTIC ANEMIA. JAMA 208:316-320

798. ZURCHER,C., KUIJLMAN,F.F., SASS,F., ZURCHER,T., LOOS,J.A. AND PRINS,H.K., 1969, GLUCOSE-6-PHOSPHATE DEHYDROGENASE DEFICIENCY IN FEMALES, DIAGNOSED BY PARTIAL INHIBITION OF GLUTATHIONE REDUCTASE ACTIVITY IN THE ERYTHROCYTES AFTER INCUBATION WITH CHROMATE. CLIN CHIM ACTA 25:139-146

799. KOUTRAS,G.A., SCHNEIDER,A.S., HATTORI,M. AND VALENTINE,W.N., 1965, STUDIES ON CHROMATED ERYTHROCYTES. MECHANISMS OF CHROMATE INHIBITION OF GLUTATHIONE REDUCTASE. BR J HAEMATOL 11:360-369

800. BEUTLER,E., 1966, A SERIES OF NEW SCREENING PROCEDURES FOR PYRUVATE KINASE DEFICIENCY, GLUCOSE-6-PHOSPHATE DEHYDROGENASE DEFICIENCY, AND GLUTATHIONE REDUCTASE DEFICIENCY. BLOOD 28:553-562

801. BEUTLER,E. AND MITCHELL,M., 1968, SPECIAL MODIFICATIONS OF THE FLUORESCENT SCREENING METHOD FOR GLUCOSE-6-PHOSPHATE DEHYDROGENASE DEFICIENCY. BLOOD 32:816-818

802. WHITE,P.A., 1972, SPECIAL MODIFICATIONS OF THE FLUORESCENT SCREENING TEST FOR GLUCOSE 6 PHOSPHATE DEHYDROGENASE DEFICIENCY. AUST J MED TECHNOL 3:133-136 (CITED IN EXCERPTA MEDICA VOL. 10.2, NO. 502)

803. HERZ,F., KAPLAN,E. AND SCHEYE,E.S., 1970, DIAGNOSIS OF ERYTHROCYTE GLUCOSE-6-PHOSPHATE DEHYDROGENASE DEFICIENCY IN THE NEGRO MALE DESPITE HEMOLYTIC CRISIS. BLOOD 35:90-93

804. SZEINBERG,A. AND PELED,N., 1973, DETECTION OF GLUCOSE-6-PHOSPHATE DEHYDROGENASE DEFICIENCY IN THE NEWBORN USING BLOOD SPECIMENS DRIED ON FILTER PAPER. ISR J MED SCI 9:1353-1354

805. DOW,P.A., PETTEWAY,M.B. AND ALPERIN,J.B., 1974, SIMPLIFIED METHOD FOR G6PD SCREENING USING BLOOD COLLECTED ON FILTER PAPER. AM J PATHOL 61:333-336

806. GUIDI,G., SOLERO,P. AND SCHIAVON,R., 1976, DEFICIT ERITROCITARIO DI GLUCOSIO-6-FOSFATO DEIDROGENASI: UN SEMPLICE E RAPIDO PROCEDIMENTO DI SCREENING. LAB 3:495-498

807. RINGELHAHN,B., 1972, A SIMPLE LABORATORY PROCEDURE FOR THE
      RECOGNITION OF A- (AFRICAN TYPE) G6PD DEFICIENCY IN ACUTE
      HAEMOLYTIC CRISIS. CLIN CHIM ACTA 36:272-274

808. SMITH,J.E., 1971, A MODIFIED SCREENING METHOD FOR ESTIMATING
      ERYTHROCYTE GLUCOSE-6-PHOSPHATE DEHYDROGENASE. RES VET SCI
      12:198-199

809. YEUNG,C.Y., LAI,H.C. AND LEUNG,N.K., 1970, FLUORESCENT SPOT
      TEST FOR SCREENING ERYTHROCYTE GLUCOSE-6-PHOSPHATE
      DEHYDROGENASE DEFICIENCY IN NEWBORN BABIES. J PEDIATR
      76:931-934

810. DICKSON,L.G., JOHNSON,C.B. AND JOHNSON,D.P., 1973, AUTOMATED
      FLUOROMETRIC METHOD FOR SCREENING FOR ERYTHROCYTE GLUCOSE-
      6- PHOSPHATE DEHYDROGENASE DEFICIENCY. CLIN CHEM 19:301-
      303

811. MAPLES,J.S., DICKSON,L.G. AND UDDIN,D.E., 1973, COUPLING
      OF GLUCOSE-6-PHOSPHATE DEHYDROGENASE AND HEMOGLOBIN S
      SCREENING TO AUTOMATED DETERMINATIONS OF BLOOD GROUP AND
      TYPE. CLIN CHEM 19:1389-1391

812. BEUTLER,E., 1975, RED CELL METABOLISM. A MANUAL OF
      BIOCHEMICAL METHODS 2ND EDITON , GRUNE & STRATTON, NEW YORK

813. PENTON,E., PASCUAL,C., LLANES,A. AND THIELMANN,K., 1972,
      THE ACTIVITY OF GLUCOSE-6-PHOSPHATE DEHYDROGENASE IN WHOLE
      BLOOD SAMPLES DRIED AND STORED ON FILTER PAPER. ACTA BIOL
      MED GER 28:177-180

814. SCHOOS-BARBETTE,S., DODINVAL-VERSIE,J. AND LAMBOTTE,C.,
      1976, MODIFICATION OF NEONATAL SCREENING TEST FOR ERYTHROCYTE
      GLUCOSE-6-PHOSPHATE DEHYDROGENASE DEFICIENCY. CLIN CHIM
      ACTA 71:239-244

815. BEUTLER,E., 1969, G-6-PD ACTIVITY OF INDIVIDUAL ERYTHROCYTES
      AND X-CHROMOSOMAL INACTIVATION. BIOCHEMICAL METHODS IN RED
      CELL GENETICS YUNIS,J.J. ED. 95-113, ACADEMIC PRESS, NEW
      YORK

816. BEUTLER,E., DERN,R.J. AND BALUDA,M.C., 1963, A NEW TECHNIQUE
      FOR THE ASCERTAINMENT OF HETEROZYGOTES FOR G-6-PD DEFICIENCY.
      PROC 9TH CONGR EUROP SOC HAEMAT 675-684, S. KARGER, BASEL

817. KLEIHAUER,E. AND BETKE,K., 1963, ELUTION PROCEDURE FOR THE
      DEMONSTRATION OF METHAEMOGLOBIN IN RED CELLS OF HUMAN BLOOD
      SMEARS. NATURE 199:1196-1197

818. GALL JR,J.C., BREWER,G.J. AND DERN,R.J., 1965, STUDIES OF
      GLUCOSE-6-PHOSPHATE DEHYDROGENASE ACTIVITY OF INDIVIDUAL
      ERYTHROCYTES: THE METHEMOGLOBIN-ELUTION TEST FOR
      IDENTIFICATION OF FEMALES HETEROZYGOUS FOR G6PD DEFICIENCY.
      AM J HUM GENET 17:359-368

819. FAIRBANKS,V.F. AND LAMPE,L.T., 1968, A TETRAZOLIUM-LINKED
      CYTOCHEMICAL METHOD FOR ESTIMATION OF GLUCOSE-6-PHOSPHATE
      DEHYDROGENASE ACTIVITY IN INDIVIDUAL ERYTHROCYTES:
      APPLICATIONS IN THE STUDY OF HETEROZYGOTES FOR GLUCOSE-6-
      PHOSPHATE DEHYDROGENASE DEFICIENCY. BLOOD 31:589-603

820. GORDON,P.A. AND STUART,J., 1974, RED CELL CYTOCHEMISTRY IN GLUCOSE-6-PHOSPHATE DEHYDROGENASE DEFICIENCY. BR J HAEMATOL 27:358

821. ROZENSZAJN,L.A., SHOHAM,D. AND MENASHI,T., 1972, EVALUATION OF GLUCOSE-6-PHOSPHATE DEHYDROGENASE IN SINGLE ERYTHROCYTES IN HUMAN BLOOD SMEARS. ACTA HAEMATOL 47:303-310

822. SMITH,M.B. AND WHITESIDE,M.G., 1974, THE DETECTION OF HETEROZYGOUS GLUCOSE-6-PHOSPHATE DEHYDROGENASE DEFICIENCY IN MEDITERRANEANS BY COMPARATIVE ENZYME ASSAY. MED J AUST 1:133-135

823. MELONI,T., DORF,A. AND CUTILLO,S., 1972, EFFECT OF BARBITURIC ACID ON HYPERBILIRUBINEMIA IN NEWBORN INFANTS WITH GLUCOSEPHOSPHATE DEHYDROGENASE DEFICIENCY IN THE ERYTHROCYTES. HELV PAEDIATR ACTA 27:197-202

824. MELONI,T., CAGNAZZO,G., DORE,A. AND CUTILLO,S., 1973, PHENOBARBITAL FOR PREVENTION OF HYPERBILIRUBINEMIA IN GLUCOSE-6-PHOSPHATE DEHYDROGENASE DEFICIENT NEWBORN INFANTS. J PEDIATR 82:1048-1051

825. MELONI,T., COSTA,S., DORE,A. AND CUTILLO,S., 1974, PHOTOTHERAPY FOR NEONATAL HYPERBILIRUBINEMIA IN MATURE NEWBORN INFANTS WITH ERYTHROCYTE G-6-PD DEFICIENCY. J PEDIATR 85:560-562

826. BENOEHR,H.C., KLUMPP,F. AND WALLER,H.D., 1971, GLUCOSE-6-PHOSPHATE DEHYDROGENASE TYP SCHWABEN. DTSCH MED WOCHENSCHR 96:1029-1032

827. WANG,Y.M., PATTERSON,H.J. AND VAN EYS,J., 1971, THE POTENTIAL USE OF XYLITOL IN GLUCOSE-6-PHOSPHATE DEHYDROGENASE DEFICIENCY ANEMIA. J CLIN INVEST 50:1421-1428

828. WANG,Y.M., KING,S.M. AND VAN EYS,J., 1974, ISOCITRATE METABOLISM IN NORMAL AND GLUCOSE-6-PHOSPHATE DEHYDROGENASE DEFICIENT RED CELLS. BIOCHEM MED 11:327-337

829. SALVIDIO,E., PANNACCIULLI,I., AJMAR,F., GARRE,C., GAETANI,G., GHIO,R., MOLININO,M. AND RAVAZZOLO,R., 1972, GLUCOSE-6-PHOSPHATDEHYDROGENASE-DEFEKT DER ERYTHROZYTEN UND FAVISMUS. HAEMOLYSE HAEMOLYTISCHE ERKRANKUNGEN NOWICKI,L., MARTIN,H. AND SCHUBERT,J.C.F. ED. 147-154.. LEHMANNS, MUNICH

830. IDELSON,L.I., RUSTAMOV,R.S.H., LYSENKO,A.I.A., ABRASHKIN-ZHUCHKOV,R.G. AND GORBUNOVA,I.U.P., 1973, ATTEMPT AT PREVENTING THE HEMOLYTIC ACTION OF PRIMAQUINE IN PERSONS WITH A GLUCOSE-6-PHOSPHATE DEHYDROGENASE ACTIVITY DEFICIT IN THE ERYTHROCYTES BY THE SIMULTANEOUS ADMINISTRATION OF XYLITOL AND RIBOFLAVIN. PROBL GEMATOL PERELIV KROVI 18:24-28

831. BEUTLER,E., 1972, RED CELL METABOLISM. A. DEFECTS NOT CAUSING HEMOLYTIC DISEASE. B. ENVIRONMENTAL MODIFICATION. BIOCHIMIE 54:759-764

832. CARSON,P.E. AND TARLOV,A.R., 1962, BIOCHEMISTRY OF HEMOLYSIS. ANNU REV MED 13:105-126

833. LISKER,R., LINARES,C. AND MOTULSKY,A.G., 1972, GLUCOSE-6-PHOSPHATE DEHYDROGENASE MEXICO. A NEW VARIANT WITH ENZYME DEFICIENCY, ABNORMAL MOBILITY AND ABSENCE OF HEMOLYSIS. J LAB CLIN MED 79:788-793

PYRUVATE KINASE DEFICIENCY

3.1. History

Hereditary nonspherocytic hemolytic anemia is a relatively recently recognized entity. It was first discussed in detail by Dacie *et al.* in 1953,[1] and by 1960 over 60 cases had been reported.[2] Motulsky *et al.*[3] noted increased 2,3-DPG levels in several patients with hereditary nonspherocytic hemolytic anemia. De Gruchy *et al.*[2] described seven cases; three were designated type II according to the classification of Selwyn and Dacie[4] in that autohemolysis was increased and not corrected by glucose. Finding that the red cell ATP levels were reduced and that autohemolysis was corrected by the addition of exogenous ATP, the authors proposed:

> . . . most likely . . . the destruction of the red cells in this disorder is related to a defect in glycolysis which results in an impairment of energy production and thus in an impairment of structural integrity; this in turn results in premature destruction of the red cells by the normal mechanisms of destruction.

In a subsequent study this group of investigators[5] found that patients with type II hereditary nonspherocytic hemolytic anemia had increased red cell 2,3-DPG levels which persisted during incubation, while the already diminished ATP levels declined further. They wrote:

> These observations suggest that DPG was being synthesized, but that a block in the glycolytic cycle beyond its site of synthesis resulted in inability to utilize DPG formed. This block would result in an impairment of ATP production.

However, elucidation of the most common cause of hereditary nonspherocytic hemolytic anemia awaited the studies of Valentine, Tanaka, and Miwa.[6,7] These investigators assayed various glycolytic enzymes in seven patients with hereditary nonspherocytic hemolytic anemia which they designated as type II. The hemoglobin level of the patients varied from 6.5 to 14.2 g/100 ml and the pyruvate kinase activity from undetectable to 32% of mean normal. Numerous key observations were made in the original reports on this enzyme deficiency. Leukocyte activity was normal; heterozygotes had approximately one-half of normal enzyme activity; no inhibitors of enzyme activity were found; and glucose utilization by red cells was approximately normal but less than that of red cells from individuals with a comparable degree of reticulocytosis.

3.2.   Genetics

Hemolytic anemia due to pyruvate kinase deficiency is inherited as an autosomal recessive disorder. This is apparent from several observations. First of all, both parents of affected patients generally have diminished red cell pyruvate kinase activity, although the degree of deficiency is usually less than that found in the patient. Second, the incidence of consanguinity is increased in pyruvate kinase deficiency.[8-14] Third, the hemolytic anemia is often found in sibs of patients but not in their parents or their children. Blume *et al.*[15] found a gene frequency of 0.007 in a German population. If consanguinity were not present, this would result in a birth incidence of 1 in 20,000. Such frequencies are of an order of magnitude which may be maintained merely through the occurrence of mutations even with a marked decrease in fitness of homozygotes. The relative rarity of the gene for pyruvate kinase deficiency, its marked heterogeneity (*vide infra*), and the similar frequency of the disorder in all population groups (except for the high frequencies brought about by inbreeding in population isolates) all militate against the existence of a significant heterozygote advantage to account for the persistence of this gene in the population. If such an advantage did exist, it might be related to the capacity of heterozygotes to regulate their erythrocyte 2,3-DPG level. In point of fact, some heterozygotes for pyruvate kinase deficiency seem to have an increased concentration of 2,3-DPG in their erythrocytes (see page 171). We have examined the red cells of two such persons after a 500-ml phlebotomy to determine whether the 2,3-DPG levels reflected a greater than normal response to bleeding. In neither case was there appreciable increase in the red cell 2,3-DPG level.[16]

It has been suggested that occasionally heterozygotes may have clinical manifestations. In one family a mother and her son, both with one-half normal red cell pyruvate kinase activity, manifested evidence of hemolysis. The father had normal enzyme activity and no evidence of hemolysis. Although both osmotic fragility and hemoglobin electrophoresis were normal,[17] the possibility that an unrelated genetically dominant hemolytic disorder was present cannot be ruled out. However, the finding that the patient's 2,3-DPG level was increased to about 1.5 times normal[18] gave credence to the possibility that a cause-and-effect relationship existed between the diminished pyruvate kinase activity in these heterozygous subjects and their hemolysis. Another patient who was heterozygous for both glucose-6-phosphate dehydrogenase and pyruvate kinase deficiency showed some evidence of hemolysis.[19] In a third family evidence of hemolysis was present in two but not in three other family members heterozygous for pyruvate kinase deficiency.[20] One patient with dominantly inherited hereditary eliptocytosis and heterozygous pyruvate kinase deficiency was found to have a hemolytic anemia, but other family members with either or both defects had no evidence of increased red cell destruction.[21] Accordingly, evidence that a relationship exists in this family between these disorders and hemolytic anemia is inconclusive. Clearly, the majority of heterozygotes have no evidence of hemolytic disease, and a cause-and-effect relationship between the heterozygous status of patients and hemolysis seems doubtful. A variety of minor biochemical alterations have been described in heterozygotes. ATP levels are often decreased.[11,22,23] 2,3-DPG levels may be increased[8,11,23] but most often are normal.[11,22] The suggestion that the heterozygous state may predispose patients to cytopenias or leukemia is purely speculative.[24]

Like G-6-PD deficiency, pyruvate kinase deficiency is a heterogeneous disorder. However, much greater variability is to be expected in this disorder than is observed in G-6-PD deficiency. This is true for two reasons:(1) There is no evidence of heterozygote advantage in pyruvate kinase deficiency. A very high proportion of cases will therefore represent new mutations rather than selection of an advantageous mutation as is the case with G-6-PD A− or G-6-PD Mediterranean. (2) Two genes for pyruvate kinase are expressed in each red cell precursor. Except in families with consanguinity these are likely to represent different amino acid substitutions. The presence of the two abnormal gene products introduces further complexity by resulting in the formation of hybrid enzymes with different biochemical properties.

Pyruvate kinase deficiency ranks with glucose-6-phosphate dehydrogenase deficiency as the most common of the enzyme deficiencies leading to hereditary nonspherocytic hemolytic anemia. Occurring with a predicted frequency in excess of 5 in 100,000 births,[15] this type of hemolytic anemia should be encountered fairly often in large referral centers. In 1971 Tanaka and Paglia[25] reviewed more than 135 cases of pyruvate kinase deficiency which had been recorded in the literature. By 1974 at least

43 patients with pyruvate kinase deficiency had been studied at the Hammersmith Hospital alone,[26] and 26 cases had been collected by Blume *et al.*[27] Pyruvate kinase deficiency has been detected in virtually all major population groups.[8,9,11,12,14,25,27–34]

Pyruvate kinase deficiency is common among Basenji dogs[35–38] and has also been found in a beagle.[39] Although the clinical course in the canine form of pyruvate kinase deficiency differs somewhat from that of the human disease, terminating in myelosclerosis, this form provides the best animal model for any of the hemolytic anemias due to enzyme deficiency. Characterization of the residual enzyme has been carried out.[37,38]

3.3. Acquired Pyruvate Kinase Deficiency

The results of red cell pyruvate kinase assays indicate that "acquired" deficiency of this enzyme is relatively common among patients with a variety of hematologic disorders. Differentiation between acquired and hereditary pyruvate kinase deficiency is not always easy. It is helpful, of course, if a pyruvate kinase assay has been carried out previously or if red cell pyruvate kinase activity returns to normal when the underlying disorder is treated. In most instances, however, family studies are required to establish that the deficiency is not of hereditary origin.

Acquired pyruvate kinase deficiency has been observed most commonly in patients with acute leukemia,[40–46] various cytopenias,[24,40,41,47] and refractory anemias.[40,42,44,48] It has also been associated with smoldering leukemia and preleukemia,[42,49] dyserythropoietic anemia,[51,52] primary marrow insufficiency without aplasia,[40] erythroleukemia,[40,46] bone marrow aplasia,[40] lymphosarcoma,[43] myelomonocytic leukemia,[40] paroxysmal nocturnal hemoglobinuria,[40] Blackfan–Diamond syndrome,[40] Fanconi anemia,[40] the Chediak–Higashi anomaly,[40] Zieve's syndrome,[53] and, rarely, polycythemia vera.[40] Pyruvate kinase activity is not reduced in chronic lymphocytic leukemia,[40,43] and activity is increased in the red cells of patients with chronic granulocytic leukemia[43] and pernicious anemia.[54] In Boivin's series[40] pyruvate kinase deficiency was found in 16 of 26 patients with refractory sideroblastic anemia, in 28 of 49 patients with primary marrow insufficiency without aplasia, and in 14 of 36 patients with acute myelocytic leukemia. The degree of reduction of enzyme activity is variable but is generally in the range found in individuals heterozygous for the genetic deficiency; the level is rarely below 50% of normal.[40,42,55] However, increased concentrations of metabolites prior to the pyruvate kinase step have been observed.[47]

Levels of "pyruvate kinase antigen" are not reduced in some patients with the acquired deficiency,[50] but in others, especially those with leukemia, the quantity of antigen is diminished.[56]

Although the cause of reduced pyruvate kinase activity in various hematologic disorders remains to be elucidated, several hypotheses have been advanced to explain this phenomenon. Among these is the suggestion that the serum of patients with acquired pyruvate kinase deficiency contains an inhibitor. Arnold et al.[42] were able to restore red cell pyruvate kinase activity to normal by incubating hemolysates with β-mercaptoethanol. In some cases the addition of serum from individuals with acquired pyruvate kinase deficiency has an inhibitory effect on the pyruvate kinase activity of normal cells.[42] In other instances[50] normal enzyme activity was restored by partial purification. Kahn[57] has isolated a small protein from leukemic cells which has the capacity to inhibit G-6-PD activity, and which appears to exert a stabilizing effect on pyruvate kinase activity.[57] The possible existence of similar factors which inhibit pyruvate kinase activity remains conjectural. It has also been suggested that a positive regulatory factor is absent or sequestered in the plasma of patients with acquired pyruvate kinase deficiency. This possibility may derive support from the finding that activity of red cells with acquired pyruvate kinase deficiency was restored to normal when they were incubated in normal serum[42] or dialyzed against Krebs–Ringer's solution. Primary genetic damage has also been suggested as a possible cause of acquired pyruvate kinase deficiency, but does not take into account the reduced activity of many other glycolytic enzymes which often accompanies acquired pyruvate kinase deficiency. The significance of acquired pyruvate kinase deficiency is unclear. It appears neither to have an adverse effect on the primary disease process nor to contribute symptoms to it. Most likely it is an epiphenomenon.

Van Berkel et al.[58] have made the extraordinary suggestion that hereditary pyruvate kinase deficiency is not a primary abnormality, but rather is secondary to some other defect. This conclusion was based on the findings that treatment of normal pyruvate kinase with high concentrations of oxidized glutathione (GSSG) can simulate abnormalities found in some pyruvate kinase variants, and that treatment of a mutant pyruvate kinase with β-mercaptoethanol restored its kinetic properties toward normal. Similar changes have been observed after storage.[59] It is conceivable that some mutations involving the pyruvate kinase molecule result in changes in conformation which render its sulfhydryl groups more susceptible to oxidation, and that some of the kinetic changes which are observed represent the results of such oxidation. However, the proposal that hereditary pyruvate kinase deficiency results from in vivo oxidation of a genetically normal enzyme is totally untenable. The level of GSSG in pyruvate kinase-deficient erythrocytes is normal[60] and physiologic concentrations of GSSG exert no effect on normal or mutant kinase.[60] Levels that do produce changes are about 1000 times those encountered physiologically. Furthermore, it would be difficult to explain the intermediate levels observed in heterozygotes for the usual and hereditary types of pyruvate kinase deficiency not due to a structural gene mutation.

3.4. Pyruvate Kinase

3.4.1. The Normal Enzyme

Human tissues contain several electrophoretically, immunologically, and kinetically distinct pyruvate kinase isozymes. Two bands of pyruvate kinase have been detected in erythrocytes.[61-64] These isozymes are believed to be interconvertible; R_1 is the predominant enzyme in young red cells and R_2 the predominant enzyme in older cells. The slight kinetic differences observed by Paglia and Valentine[65] between pyruvate kinase of young and old red cells probably represent the properties of R_1 and R_2, respectively. The liver enzyme, L-type PK, was thought at one time to be identical in every respect to the red cell enzyme.[66] With the development of more discriminatory electrophoretic techniques, however, it has become apparent that the mobility of the type L enzyme differs very slightly from that of R_1 and R_2.[62,67] However, the two enzymes are closely related: the amount of L enzyme is markedly diminished in the liver of patients with pyruvate kinase deficiency,[13,17,63,68] and there is considerable immunologic cross-reactivity between the R and L isozymes.[67,69,70] It seems certain that the L and R types of enzyme are products of the same gene and that the minor electrophoretic differences observed are due to slight posttranslational modifications.[70] The M types of pyruvate kinase, in contrast, appear to be unrelated to the enzyme found in red cells.[69,71] M_1 pyruvate kinase exists as a minor component in liver and as the main component in spleen and several other tissues. The M pyruvate kinase is present in skeletal muscle, heart, and brain.[63,69,72] Forms intermediate to M_1 and M_2 have also been separated by isoelectric focusing, and were designated M_3 and M_4.[69]

The structure and properties of red cell pyruvate kinase have been investigated in numerous laboratories. Ibsen et al.[73] found that the stability of the enzyme was enhanced by phosphoenolpyruvate, magnesium, β-mercaptoethanol, and by pH levels lower than 7.4. These authors were able to achieve approximately 10,000-fold purification of the enzyme. Blume et al.,[74] utilizing the method of fructose diphosphate elution from carboxy-methyl cellulose[75] and the capacity of blue dextran to bind pyruvate kinase, achieved a similar degree of purification of the enzyme. Staal et al.[76] and Chern et al.,[77] using different methods, each succeeded in purifying the enzyme 30,000-fold with a yield of 8%. Chern et al.[77] demonstrated that the enzyme was homogeneous, and carried out amino acid analysis, but were unable to identify the amino terminal residue, suggesting that it was blocked. The purified enzyme was found to have a molecular weight of 205,000[76] and of 225,400.[77] Recently, 40,000-fold purification has been achieved with a yield of 29%.[70] The very similar L type of enzyme from liver has also been purified to homogeneity[78] and has a molecular weight estimated to be between 220,000 and 240,000. Sodium dodecyl sulfate electrophoresis demonstrated that the subunit size is approximately 60,000 daltons, indicating that the holoenzyme is a tetramer. The isoelectric point of normal red cell pyruvate kinase has been reported to be 7.36,[79] but various conformers with different pI values have also been found.[80,81]

Extensive studies of the kinetics of erythrocyte pyruvate kinase have been carried out, both in crude hemolysates and in purified preparations. The kinetic properties of the enzyme appear to change considerably during purification. This is due at least in part to the rapid changes in concentration of the substrates of the enzyme which occur in the presence of hemolysates. ADP undergoes dismutation to ATP and AMP in the presence of adenylate kinase; PEP is changed to 2- and 3-phosphoglyceric acid in the presence of enolase and monophosphoglycerate mutase. Furthermore, in crude hemolysates the 3-phosphoglyceric acid formed may be phosphorylated by ATP and phosphoglycerate kinase to 1,3-diphosphoglycerate, which in turn may serve as a substrate for the oxidation of NADH in the reverse glyceraldehyde phosphate dehydrogenase reaction.

Both in purified preparations[60,74,76,82–87] and in crude hemolysates [9,13, 28,31,33,60,83,88–90] erythrocyte pyruvate kinase has allosteric properties and the allosteric effector is fructose diphosphate (Fig. 14). The properties of the enzyme are markedly pH dependent. The fructose diphosphate effect can be demonstrated at pH 7.6 but is absent at pH 5.9. In the absence of fructose diphosphate and at pH 7.4 the $K_{1/2}$ for PEP at infinite ADP concentration was 0.63 mM, and the K_m for ADP at infinite PEP concentration was 0.60 mM.[76] The Hill constant of the purified enzyme was 1.6 at infinite ADP concentration. Similar values have been obtained with partially purified enzyme.[74,82,83,87,88,91] Fructose diphosphate is effective at astonishingly low concentrations. The $K_{1/2}$ for fructose diphosphate has been reported to be 0.06 μM,[60,74] 0.2 μM, and 0.05 μM,[86] under different experimental conditions. The binding constants obtained by equilibrium

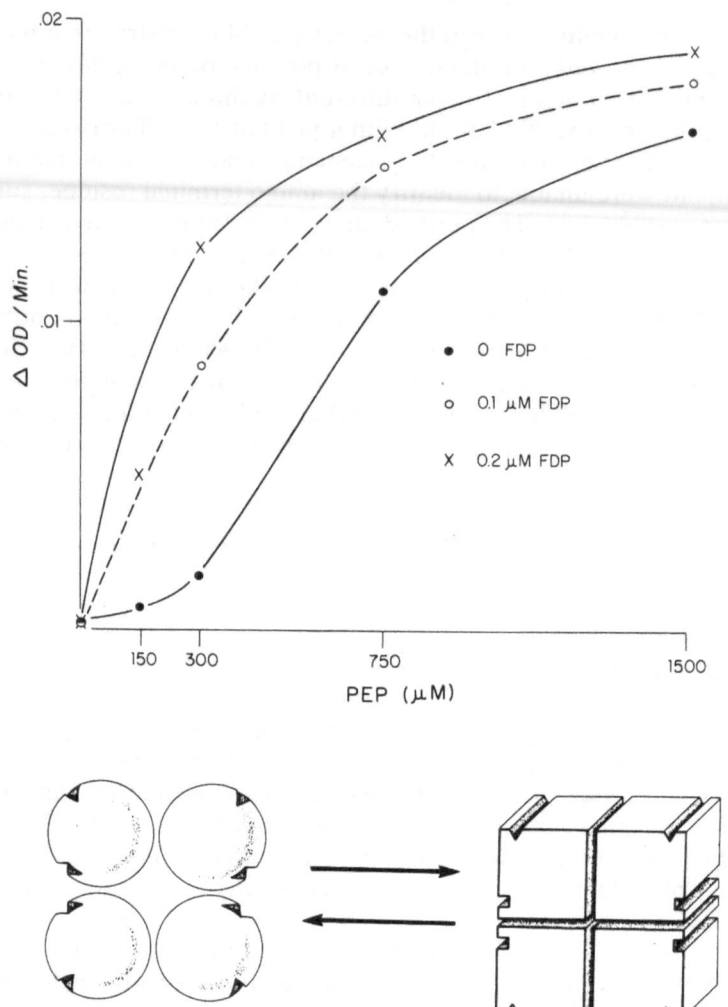

FIGURE 14.   Pyruvate kinase as an allosteric enzyme. In the presence of minute concentrations of fructose diphosphate the relationship between phosphoenolpyruvate (PEP) concentration and enzyme velocity changes from a sigmoid to a hyperbolic one. The mechanism by which this change in kinetics is achieved is schematically illustrated at the bottom of the figure. At the left side the spherical subunits depict the relaxed, or R, conformation of the enzyme which presumably has a low affinity for PEP. The cubical subunits on the right side illustrate the tense, or T, conformation of the enzyme, which has a high affinity for PEP. An equilibrium exists between these two conformations. The triangular grooves represent the fructose diphosphate binding sites, while the rectangular groove represents the PEP binding site. Binding of either of these ligands shifts the equilibrium of the enzyme from the R to the T conformation, increasing the affinity for PEP. (Reprinted from Beutler,[144] through the courtesy of Georg-Thieme Publishers, Stuttgart.)

dialysis are quite similar to the results of kinetic studies.[86] While fructose diphosphate appears to be the most potent regulator of enzyme activation, various other sugars have also been reported to stimulate enzyme activity at low PEP concentrations. Included are fructose-6-phosphate,[82] fructose-1-phosphate,[82] glucose-1,6-diphosphate,[82,92] and glucose-6-phosphate.[76,82] However, because very high concentrations of the sugars were used in these studies, the possible effects of contaminants cannot be ruled out. In other studies the stimulatory effect of glucose-1-phosphate[76] and fructose-6-phosphate[76] was insignificant. Inorganic phosphate itself stimulates activity of the enzyme,[76] and ATP[76,93] and amino acids[82] are inhibitors. Calcium stimulates the enzyme at low PEP concentrations and is inhibitory at high PEP concentrations.[84] Mn^{2+} has the capacity to substitute for Mg^{2+}, although the kinetic properties with these two divalent cations differ.[94] K^+ stimulates the enzyme by lowering its K_m for ADP–Mg.[95]

3.4.2. Mutant Pyruvate Kinase

By 1970, it was evident that considerable heterogeneity exists with respect to the kinetic properties of the residual enzyme in pyruvate kinase-deficient red cells. Enzymes with increased, normal, and decreased K_m values for PEP had been described. The results of earlier studies are reviewed in detail by Tanaka and Paglia.[25] Since 1970 an ever increasing number of variants has been investigated biochemically. Interpretation of the results is extremely difficult for the following reasons:

1. Many of the patients who have been studied are not the products of consanguineous marriages and have therefore probably inherited two different mutant genes for red cell pyruvate kinase. Since the enzyme is apparently a tetramer and mixed tetramers of two mutant subunits can presumably form five different enzyme species, the complexity of the resulting kinetic data renders them relatively meaningless.

2. Although some of the investigations have been carried out on partially purified enzyme,[28,74,85,87,96,97] the characterization of most mutant enzymes has been carried out on crude hemolysates.[9,11,17,28,29,31-33,98] Enzymes such as enolase, aldolase, and adenylate kinase which are present in abundance in crude hemolysates, change the concentration of substrates added to a system in a time-dependent fashion (see Section 3.4.1). Analysis of data is therefore very difficult. Indeed, Boivin et al.[28] have found a difference in the kinetic constants of hemolysates from pyruvate kinase-deficient patients and those obtained from partially purified enzymes. Furthermore, abnormalities observed in the crude hemolysates were not necessarily confirmed when partially purified enzyme was studied.

3. It is not always clear that leukocytes have been efficiently removed prior to the study of the red cell enzyme. The M-type enzyme in leukocytes has kinetic properties totally different from those of the R or L type. It resembles some of the fructose diphosphate-resistant variants which have been described.

4. Standardization of methods for characterization of pyruvate kinase variants has not yet been achieved. Comparison of the results obtained by different groups of investigators is therefore virtually impossible. However, several large series of kinetic studies carried out in a few laboratories in recent years[11,28,85] emphasize that the heterogeneity observed in pyruvate kinase variants is not merely a function of interlaboratory differences in methodology.

In various studies the electrophoretic mobility of pyruvate kinase from different patients has been found to be normal,[9,74] more cathodal than normal,[13,29,87,99] or more anodal than normal.[12,13,17] Measurements of the isoelectric point of some variants have also been carried out.[79,81] The K_m for PEP in residual pyruvate kinase has been found to be normal,[12,17,28,33,74,85,87,96,97] increased,[11,12,22,28,31,32,74,85,98-100] or decreased[12,28,29,96] in different patients. In contrast, the K_m value reported for ADP is almost always normal,[17,31-33,74,96] and was increased slightly in only one case.[9] The allosteric transition between the R (relaxed) and T (tense) state produced by fructose diphosphate is normal in some variants[11,12,17,28,33,85,96,97] and abnormal in others.[28,31,32,87,96,98] Accordingly, the reported K_m values for fructose diphosphate have been normal[74] or greatly increased.[9,31,74,98] The pH optimum curve may be normal[11,97] but is more often abnormal.[11,29,31,33] The heat stability of the residual enzyme is usually abnormal,[9,17,29,33,96] but may occasionally be normal.[17,98] The stability of the enzyme in urea has been studied less frequently but may be normal,[12,17] reduced,[12] or actually increased.[29] The stability of the residual enzyme in stored red cells may be normal[11] or diminished.[11,31] Abnormalities in nucleotide specificity have been found,[11,12] and abnormal susceptibility to inhibition of the enzyme by alanine and by ATP was shown in some cases.[28,98]

Evaluation by immunologic methods of the amount of pyruvate kinase antigen present in pyruvate kinase-deficient red cells has been carried out. Some cases appear to have the normal amount of PK antigen, indicating the presence of an enzyme with reduced specific activity,[12,81] while the specific activity of the residual enzyme of others appears to be normal.[12,17] In some instances the residual enzyme has been given the name of the patient's city of origin. For example, the designations Nagasaki, Sapporo, Tokyo I, Kiyose, Beppu, Osaka,[11] Tokyo II, Mabashi, Tsukiji, and Ube[12] have been assigned to a series of variants characterized by

Miwa and his collaborators. Most of these variants were the result of consanguinous marriages, and therefore represent true homozygotes. However, Tokyo II, Kiyose, Beppu, and Osaka are presumably from mixed heterozygotes.

3.5. The Pyruvate Kinase-Deficient Red Cell

The residual enzyme activity of the pyruvate kinase-deficient red cell may vary greatly. Indeed, in a few instances of hemolytic anemia due to pyruvate kinase "deficiency" elevated levels of the enzyme have been found;[11,12,28] the hemolytic anemia is presumably due to a metabolic lesion induced by altered kinetic properties of the mutant enzyme.

Because of the young mean red cell age in pyruvate kinase deficiency, the activities of other age-dependent erythrocyte enzymes are generally considerably increased.[7,8,10,22,33,97,101] Occasional reports[34,102] of normal or diminished red cell hexokinase and glucose-6-phosphate dehydrogenase activity in pyruvate kinase-deficient patients must be considered to be spurious. Although the red cell population in pyruvate kinase-deficient patients is generally very young, the expected increase in glucose utilization is usually not observed.[85,103] In a review of 32 cases glucose consumption and lactate production were within or above the normal range in 23.[103] In one case the red cells scarcely consumed any glucose at all.[104] Usually red cell ATP levels are somewhat diminished in pyruvate kinase deficiency, but cases with normal or even increased red cell ATP levels have been documented,[7,11,31,99] and these patients may manifest very severe hemolysis. In some cases red cell potassium[104,105] and the net outflow of potassium during incubation is increased.[26,101,104,105] It is obvious that the metabolic changes in pyruvate kinase-deficient cells are more complex than a simple decrease in glucose metabolism resulting from impairment of one of the enzymatic steps of the Embden–Meyerhoff pathway. Indeed, the normal red cell PEP level[106] of 12 μM is only about 25% of the K_m of the kinetically normal enzyme saturated with fructose diphosphate.[74,85] In the absence of other modulating effects it would be possible to achieve a fivefold increase in activity through the pyruvate kinase step merely as a result of a rise in the red cell PEP level to a concentration that saturates the enzyme. Secondary changes which occur in pyruvate kinase-deficient red cells may be of very great importance.[107] Levels of most metabolic intermediates are considerably increased,[10,22] but some of this increase may be due to the young mean red cell age.[108,109] Particularly striking, however, are increases in levels of phosphoenolpyruvate, 3-phosphoglyceric acid,[10,22,31,32,34,85] and 2,3-DPG.[8,11,12,22,23,31,101,110] These changes probably occur through a series of successive feedback inhibitions resulting from the pyruvate kinase deficiency. 2,3-DPG directly inhibits the activity of many key glycolytic enzymes, including hexokinase[111,112] and phosphofructokinase.[111–113] In addition it has been shown that, at least *in vitro*, 2,3-DPG can inhibit pyruvate kinase through its magnesium-chelating effect.[82,95]

Normal red cells incubated for several hours in the presence of glucose and cyanide are able to maintain ATP levels. In contrast, pyruvate kinase-deficient red cells rapidly lose their ATP in the presence of cyanide.[10,101,103,114] Since mitochondrial metabolism but not glycolysis is sensitive to cyanide, it is likely that most of the ATP in pyruvate kinase-deficient cells is derived from mitochondrial metabolism. Mitochondria are present only in young reticulocytes, and it has been suggested that it is the loss of functional mitochondria occurring with the maturation of the reticulocyte which spells the doom of the pyruvate kinase-deficient cell. Indeed, pyruvate kinase-deficient cells which are treated with cyanide lose water, increase in density, and become spiculated in appearance.[114]

Age fractionation of red cells from both pyruvate kinase-deficient and normal individuals shows that the youngest cells have highest enzyme activity.[7,114] Nonetheless, there appears to be preferential destruction in the spleen of reticulocytes from pyruvate kinase-deficient patients, as demonstrated by ^{51}Cr sequestration and ferrokinetic studies[99,114,115] and by electron microscopy.[30] There is usually less shortening of the life span of older circulating erythrocytes,[99,114] although the survival of older erythrocytes may also be severely compromised;[19,25,116] biphasic red cell survival curves are often obtained. The reason for the differential destruction of reticulocytes and mature red cells is probably that there is a considerable degree of heterogeneity among the red cells in the severity of enzyme deficiency. As red cells are released from the marrow, those that have the most residual activity have the greatest chance of surviving in the circulation. To the extent that the destruction of pyruvate kinase-deficient red cells is a function of ATP deficiency, reticulocytes are able to compensate for the lack of enzyme through mitochondrial ADP phosphorylation. However, as soon as mitochondrial function is lost, the cells may be very vulnerable to the effects of their glycolytic defect. *In vitro*, pyruvate kinase-deficient erythrocytes are more susceptible to lysis than are normal red cells.[117] Glader[118] showed that the incubation of pyruvate kinase-deficient red cells in a buffer containing salicylate appeared to aggravate their metabolic abnormality. The clinical significance of these observations, however, is doubtful.[119]

3.6. Clinical Manifestations

. Because there is considerable biochemical heterogeneity in pyruvate kinase deficiency, a great deal of clinical heterogeneity is to be expected. In a classical 1971 review Tanaka and Paglia[25] analyzed over 135 cases of pyruvate kinase deficiency. The clinical manifestations of many additional patients have been published since 1970 [8–12,22,23,26–29,31–33,87,97,98,101, 110,120,121] and several patients are mentioned in the literature without accompanying clinical data.[64,81,85,118]

Review of these cases indicates that patients with pyruvate kinase deficiency hemolytic anemia have no distinguishing or pathognomic clinical features. Jaundice of varying degree, episodes of dark urine, slight to moderate splenomegaly, and an increased incidence of gallstones are all observed. The severity of the anemia varies widely; some patients require frequent transfusions to preserve life, while others may have a mild compensated hemolytic process detected only incidentally when the patient presents with some intercurrent medical problem. In other cases the hemolytic anemia is so severe that death would result if the patient were not sustained by multiple transfusions or by splenectomy.[116,122] It is of interest that patients with pyruvate kinase deficiency appear to be able to tolerate their anemia with a paucity of symptoms; the characteristic elevation of red cell 2,3-DPG levels with the accompanying right shift in the oxygen dissociation curve helps to compensate for the lowered hemoglobin level of the blood.[123] Jaundice is usually present from the time of birth.[26] Kernicterus has been reported,[14,19,26] with death occurring in the first week of life in at least one case.[14]

Hemolysis may be exacerbated by intercurrent infection.[7,26,29,103, 117,119,124] It has been suggested that oral contraceptives increase hemolysis.[125,126] Splenomegaly is usually present, except in some infants and in older individuals with particularly mild manifestations of pyruvate kinase deficiency.[11,12,26,33,124] Gallstones are common.[26] Growth retardation may occur in severely affected children,[116] and leg ulcers,[9,127] acute pancreatitis,[124] and a biliary fistula[26] secondary to gallbladder disease have been observed. X-ray changes in the bones are not specific and resemble those of any severe anemia which results in hypertrophia of the bone marrow. The skull changes are similar to those described for thalassemia major and differ primarily in that the antra and frontal sinuses are aerated in pyruvate kinase deficiency anemia.[128]

There seems to be little relationship between the quantitative severity of the enzyme defect and the severity of anemia. Indeed, in several reported cases pyruvate kinase activity actually appears to be in-

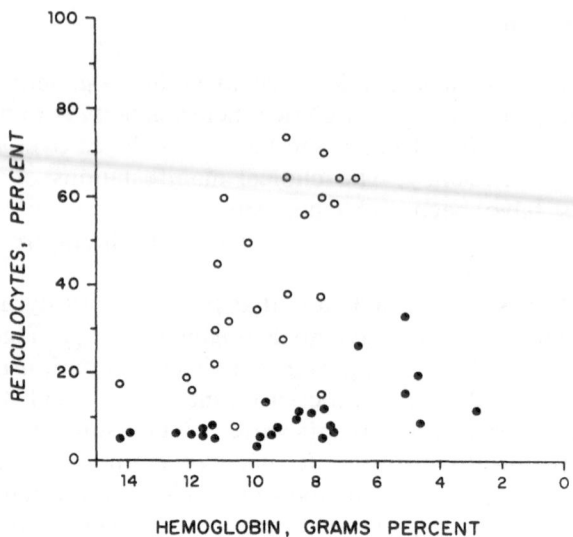

FIGURE 15.   The relationship between reticulocyte count and hemoglobin concentration of the blood in patients with pyruvate kinase deficiency. The solid circles represent unsplenectomized patients; the open circles represent splenectomized patients. (Reprinted from Keitt and Bennett,[103] through the courtesy of the author and the *American Journal of Medicine*.)

creased.[11,12,29] Presumably, kinetic abnormalities of the enzyme interfere with its normal function and result in shortened red cell life span. Schröter and Tillmann reported one case in which pyruvate kinase activity was normal in the red cell but was decreased in the membrane.[33] The anemia may be mild, moderate, or marked; in one instance the hemoglobin concentration of the blood was normal.[11] Macrocytosis is usually present, probably due to the reticulocytosis which characteristically accompanies this disorder. The reticulocytosis is usually striking, since the number of reticulocytes bears an inverse relationship to the hemoglobin level of the blood. Following splenectomy reticulocyte counts of 40 to 60% are not uncommon (Fig. 15). Marked red cell distortion and spiculation have been reported in some cases.[27,29,33] In one case in which prominent spiculation of erythrocytes was present, pyruvate kinase deficiency had been inherited together with heterozygous β-thalassemia.[129] Possibly because of the traditional interest of hematologists in morphologic changes seen on the blood film, undue emphasis seems to have been placed upon this unusual finding. However, occasional spiculated cells are commonly observed in patients with pyruvate kinase deficiency.[130] Most often no distinctive abnormalities of the blood are present (Fig. 16). Following splenectomy such cells as siderocytes, target cells, and poikilocytes of various types are seen. Erythroid hyperplasia of the bone marrow is characteristic of pyruvate kinase-deficient hemolytic anemia. Chromosome aberrations with prominent chromatid gaps have been observed in bone marrow cells.[10]

Serum bilirubin levels, mostly indirect reacting, are usually somewhat elevated, and haptoglobin levels may be decreased or absent.[25] Urobilinogen may be found in the urine. The Coombs test, the acid hemolysis test, and the Donath–Landsteiner tests are negative.[25] Osmotic fragility

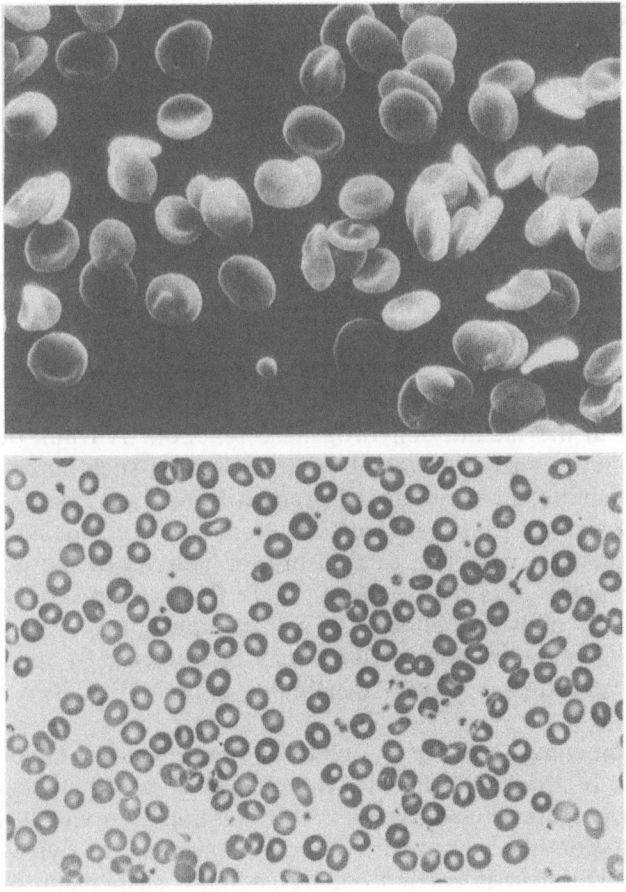

FIGURE 16.   Pyruvate kinase-deficient red cells on a standard blood film stained with Giemsa (below) and on scanning electron microscopy (above). (Electron microscopy courtesy of R. Baker.)

measured in fresh erythrocytes is usually normal,[8,22,25,32,99,131] but the incubated osmotic fragility is often abnormal.[25,26] The coexistence of pyruvate kinase deficiency and hereditary spherocytosis has been observed.[100,132] The existence of "atypical" pyruvate kinase in a family with hereditary spherocytosis has also been reported but the evidence that the abnormality was hereditary is by no means convincing.[133]

3.7. Diagnosis

The diagnosis of pyruvate kinase deficiency depends on demonstration that the activity of the enzyme is quantitatively decreased, or that well-defined qualitative abnormalities are present. It is particularly important to bear in mind that the pyruvate kinase activity of leukocytes and platelets is not compromised in pyruvate kinase deficiency because they contain the genetically distinct M type of enzyme. A hemolysate prepared from red cells which have not been meticulously freed of contaminating white cells may give the erroneous impression that enzyme activity is normal, particularly when a striking leukocytosis is present. The best means for freeing erythrocytes of contaminating leukocytes and platelets is the filtration of the blood through cotton wool or through a mixture of microcrystalline cellulose and α-cellulose.[134] The activity of the enzyme is measured in a coupled system. PEP serves as substrate for pyruvate kinase, and the pyruvate which is formed in the reaction serves as oxidant for NADH in the lactate dehydrogenase reaction. A frank decrease of pyruvate kinase activity is readily detected using such an assay procedure. More subtle abnormalities of pyruvate kinase may be missed, however, unless more sophisticated examination of the enzyme is carried out. It is particularly worthwhile to measure the activity of the enzyme in a dialyzed hemolysate at reduced levels of PEP. The responsiveness of the enzyme to the allosteric effector, fructose diphosphate, should also be measured. Qualitative abnormalities may be detected by measuring the heat stability of the enzyme,[9,23] its stability in urea,[8,12] or its activity with nucleotide analogs.[12]

Two screening tests for pyruvate kinase deficiency have been proposed. One of these depends on the change of pH that occurs in the course of pyruvate kinase reaction.[135] It has not been widely used. The fluorescent spot screening test[136] detects most cases of pyruvate kinase deficiency. This test is carried out by adding a suspension of red cells which has been partially freed of leukocytes to a hypotonic buffered system which will lyse erythrocytes but not leukocytes. The test reagent contains ADP, PEP, and NADH. The incubated blood–reagent mixture is spotted on filter paper and is examined for fluorescence produced by NADH. Normal blood causes rapid defluorescence as NADH is oxidized in the same linkaged reaction which is employed in the quantitative assay. When pyruvate kinase deficiency exists, defluorescence occurs slowly or not at all. Demonstration of elevated red cell 2,3-DPG levels, universally present in pyruvate kinase deficiency, is a useful laboratory finding in the confirmation of this disorder. By the use of more sophisticated means, it is possible to show that the level of phosphoenolpyruvate (PEP) is also elevated in pyruvate kinase-deficient red cells.

Unfortunately, the autohemolysis test enjoys an undeserved reputation in the diagnosis of pyruvate kinase deficiency. The original discovery of pyruvate kinase deficiency was an outgrowth of the investigation of patients with type II hereditary nonspherocytic hemolytic anemia. Indeed, in their original report of seven patients with pyruvate kinase deficiency, Tanaka et al.[7] wrote:

> The PK assay data to date in a variety of hematologic and nonhematologic disorders would appear to indicate that homozygosity for PK deficiency occurs only in patients conforming to type II of Dacie.

Most of the early reports of pyruvate kinase deficiency concerned cases manifesting type II autohemolysis.[19] This may have been due to the bias of ascertainment: the red cells of patients with other types of autohemolysis patterns may not have been assayed for pyruvate kinase activity. The autohemolysis data in the original seven cases revealed only minimal increase of autohemolysis in one patient, and some correction by glucose in four of the seven patients. However, perhaps as a result of the early observations, many clinicians have assumed that the type II autohemolysis pattern is characteristic of pyruvate kinase deficiency. In fact, it is not. Occasionally the type I pattern is found,[12,26] and normal autohemolysis[26,101] or mixed patterns[11,26,35] are frequent (Fig. 17). In 14 patients studied by Miwa and Nishina[11] only 6 were interpreted as showing type II autohemolysis patterns. Even in several of these patients the degree of autohemolysis was minimal, and it is questionable whether the classical criteria for type II autohemolysis were met.

3.8. Treatment

Splenectomy was originally considered to be of no value in the treatment of pyruvate kinase deficiency. This early concept was a consequence of studies carried out only in patients characterized as having type II hereditary nonspherocytic hemolytic anemia.[2,137,138] The first cases of

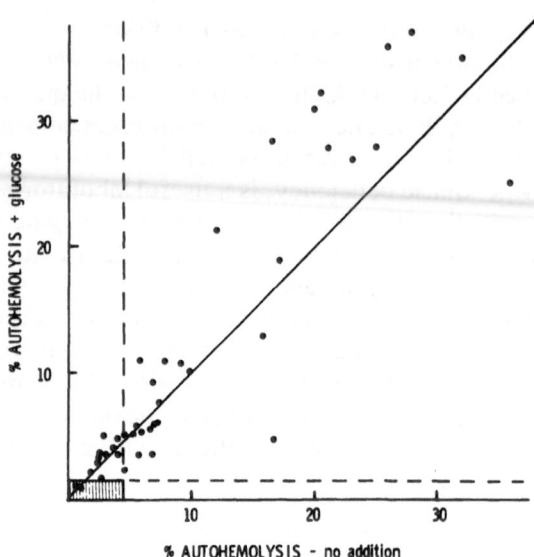

FIGURE 17.   The results of autohemolysis tests in patients with pyruvate kinase deficiency. A variety of patterns are seen; clearly, many of the patients do not have type II
autohemolysis. (Reprinted from Gordon-Smith,[26] through the courtesy of the author and the
Journal of Clinical Pathology.)

pyruvate kinase deficiency reported by Tanaka *et al.*[7] seemed to support
this concept, although two of the four patients in their series who under-
went splenectomy actually appeared to benefit from the procedure. Of the
two patients who failed to respond to splenectomy one was an asymptomatic 26-year-old man with a hemoglobin of 11.3 g/100 ml whose spleen
was not palpable; the other patient had accessory spleens. Most patients
subsequently observed appeared to improve after splenectomy.[9,11,25,26,31–33]
In severe cases splenectomy may be lifesaving.[116] Evidence of hemolysis
invariably persists following removal of the spleen. In some instances[126] it
appears that the beneficial effects of splenectomy may be temporary.

   Transfusions may be required in treatment of pyruvate kinase deficiency, particularly during the severe anemia which may follow intercurrent infection. In neonates exchange transfusions may prevent the development of kernicterus.[11,120] The use of other therapies such as steroids[19] or
immunosuppressive agents[139] has been disappointing. The administration
of AMP to one patient with pyruvate kinase deficiency yielded equivocal
results.[140] Magnesium administered to two patients with hemolytic anemia
who had slightly lowered pyruvate kinase activity produced an increase in
enzyme activity, but no change in the patients' anemia.[121] Because treat-

ment of pyruvate kinase with oxidized glutathione (GSSG) produced changes in kinetics similar to those observed in some deficient variants[141] and the activity of some deficient variants could be partially reversed by treatment with β-mercaptoethanol,[58] it was proposed that the abnormalities of pyruvate kinase, at least in some patients with pyruvate kinase deficiency hemolytic anemia, might be a "secondary effect" (see the last paragraph of Section 3.3). A patient with an abnormal pyruvate kinase and partial glutathione reductase deficiency was therefore treated with riboflavin.[142] Although there appeared to be some normalization of the kinetic properties of the mutant enzyme, and clinical improvement was claimed, a decrease in red cell pyruvate kinase activity was actually recorded. However, in the treatment of six pyruvate kinase-deficient patients with riboflavin by Blume *et al.*[143] no improvement was observed. In view of these findings it seems doubtful that riboflavin administration is of any value in the treatment of pyruvate kinase deficiency. The infusion of inosine and adenine appeared to ameliorate the anemia in one patient who had inherited a mutant enzyme which was unusually resistant to the allosteric effector fructose diphosphate.[88] The purine nucleoside apparently exerted its effect by increasing the intracellular level of fructose diphosphate to a point at which the enzyme was able to metabolize phosphoenolpyruvate more efficiently than had otherwise been the case. While theoretically of considerable interest, the infusion of inosine has not been advocated as a means for the long-term management of patients with pyruvate kinase deficiency.

References

1. DACIE,J.V., MOLLISON,P.L., RICHARDSON,N., SELWYN,J.G. AND
    SHAPIRO,L., 1953, ATYPICAL CONGENITAL HAEMOLYTIC ANAEMIA.
    Q J MED 85:79-97

2. DE GRUCHY,G.C., SANTAMARIA,J.N., PARSONS,I.C. AND CRAWFORD,H.,
    1960, NONSPHEROCYTIC CONGENITAL HEMOLYTIC ANEMIA. BLOOD
    16:1371-1397

3. MOTULSKY,A.G., GABRIO,B.W., BURKHARDT,J. AND FINCH,C.A.,
    1955, ERYTHROCYTE CARBOHYDRATE METABOLISM IN HEREDITARY
    HEMOLYTIC ANEMIAS. AM J MED 19:291

4. SELWYN,J.G. AND DACIE,J.V., 1958, AUTOHEMOLYSIS AND OTHER
    CHANGES RESULTING FROM THE INCUBATION IN VITRO OF RED CELLS
    FROM PATIENTS WITH CONGENITAL HEMOLYTIC ANEMIA. BLOOD
    9:414-438

5. ROBINSON,M.A., LODER,P.B. AND DE GRUCHY,G.C., 1961, RED-
    CELL METABOLISM IN NON-SPHEROCYTIC CONGENITAL HAEMOLYTIC
    ANAEMIA. BR J HAEMATOL 7:327-339

6. VALENTINE,W.N., TANAKA,K.R. AND MIWA,S., 1961, A SPECIFIC
    ERYTHROCYTE GLYCOLYTIC ENZYME DEFECT (PYRUVATE KINASE) IN
    THREE SUBJECTS WITH CONGENITAL NON-SPHEROCYTIC HEMOLYTIC
    ANEMIA. TRANS ASSOC AM PHYSICIANS 74:100-110

7. TANAKA,K.R., VALENTINE,W.N. AND MIWA,S., 1962, PYRUVATE
    KINASE (PK) DEFICIENCY HEREDITARY NON-SPHEROCYTIC HEMOLYTIC
    ANEMIA. BLOOD 19:267-295

8. KUBOTA,K., MOTEKI,M., OMINE,M., TSUCHIYA,J., MAEKAWA,T.
    AND MIWA,S., 1975, A NEW VARIANT OF ERYTHROCYTE PYRUVATE
    KINASE - PK 'MAEBASHI'. SCAND J HAEMATOL 14:242-248

9. MUELLER-SOYANO,A., DE ROURA,E.T., DUKE,P.-.R., DE
    ACQUATELLA,G.C., ARENDS,T., GUINTO,E. AND BEUTLER,E., 1976,
    PYRUVATE KINASE DEFICIENCY AND LEG ULCERS. BLOOD 47:807-
    813

10. MIWA,S., 1973, HEREDITARY HEMOLYTIC ANEMIA DUE TO ERYTHROCYTE
    ENZYME DEFICIENCY. ACTA HAEMATOL JAP 36:573-615

11. MIWA,S. AND NISHINA,T., 1974, STUDIES ON PYRUVATE KINASE
    (PK) DEFICIENCY. I. CLINICAL, HEMATOLOGICAL AND ERYTHROCYTE
    ENZYME STUDIES. ACTA HAEMATOL JAP 37:1-16

12. MIWA,S., NAKASHIMA,K., ARIYOSHI,K., SHINOHARA,K., ODA,E.
    AND TANAKA,T., 1975, FOUR NEW PYRUVATE KINASE (PK) VARIANTS
    AND A CLASSICAL PK DEFICIENCY. BR J HAEMATOL 29:157-169

13. NAKASHIMA,K., MIWA,S., ODA,S., TANAKA,T., IMAMURA,K. AND
    NISHINA,T., 1974, ELECTROPHORETIC AND KINETIC STUDIES OF
    MUTANT ERYTHROCYTE PYRUVATE KINASES. BLOOD 43:537-548

14. BOWMAN,H.S., MC KUSICK,V.A. AND DRUNAMRAJU,K.R., 1965,
PYRUVATE KINASE DEFICIENT HEMOLYTIC ANEMIA IN AN AMISH
ISOLATE. AM J HUM GENET 17:1-8

15. BLUME,K.G., LOEHR,G.W., PRAETSCH,O. AND HUEDIGER,H.W.,
1968, BEITRAG ZUR POPULATIONSGENETIK DER PYRUVATKINASE
MENSCHLISHER ERYTHROCYTEN. HUMANGENETIK 6:261-265

16. BEUTLER,E., 1975, UNPUBLISHED

17. KAHN,A., MARIE,J., GALAND,C. AND BOIVIN,P., 1976, CHRONIC
HAEMOLYTIC ANAEMIA IN TWO PATIENTS HETEROZYGOUS FOR
ERYTHROCYTE PYRUVATE KINASE DEFICIENCY. SCAND J HAEMATOL
16:250-257

18. KAHN,A., 1976, PERSONAL COMMUNICATION

19. OSKI,F.A., NATHAN,D.G., SIDEL,V.W. AND DIAMOND,L.K., 1964,
EXTREME HEMOLYSIS AND RED-CELL DISTORTION IN ERYTHROCYTE
PYRUVATE KINASE DEFICIENCY. N ENGL J MED 270:1023-1030

20. SACHS,J.R., WICKER,D.J., GILCHER,R.O., CONRAD,M.F. AND
COHEN,R.J., 1968, FAMILIAL HEMOLYTIC ANEMIA RESULTING FROM
AN ABNORMAL RED BLOOD CELL PYRUVATE KINASE. J LAB CLIN MED
72:359-362

21. NEUMANN,E., SCHWARZMEIER,J. AND HONETZ,H., 1972, HEREDITARY
ELLIPTOCYTOSIS AND PYRUVATE KINASE DEFICIENCY OF THE
ERYTHROCYTES. WIEN KLIN WOCHENSCHR 84:712-715

22. YAMADA,K., ADACHIBARA,A., NAKAZAWA,S., SHINKAI,A., NISHINA,T.
AND MIWA,S., 1974, ERYTHROCYTE PYRUVATE KINASE DEFICIENCY
ASSOCIATED WITH KINETICALLY ABERRANT ISOZYME. ACTA HAEMATOL
JAP 37:17-24

23. GOEBEL,K.M., GOEBEL,F.D., JANZEN,R. AND KAFFARNIK,H., 1975,
HAEMOLYTIC ANAEMIA WITH HEREDITARY PYRUVATE KINASE INSTABILITY
DEVELOPING ACUTE LEUKAEMIA. SCAND J HAEMATOL 14:249-257

24. NOWICKI,L., BEHNKEN,L. AND BISKAMP,K., 1972, PANCYTOPENIEN
MIT ERYTHROCYTAREM PYRUVATKINASE- UND GLUTATHIONREDUCTASE-
DEFEKT. KLIN WOCHENSCHR 50:566-569

25. TANAKA,K.R. AND PAGLIA,D.F., 1971, PYRUVATE KINASE DEFICIENCY.
SEMIN HEMATOL 8:367-395

26. GORDON-SMITH,E.C., 1974, ERYTHROCYTE ENZYME DEFICIENCIES.
PYRUVATE KINASE DEFICIENCY. J CLIN PATHOL 27:128-133

27. BLUME,K.G., BUSCH,D., ARNOLD,H. AND LOEHR,G.W., 1971,
KLINISCHE UNTERSUCHUNGEN ZUR HEREDITAEREN NICHTSPHAEROCYTAEREN
HAEMOLYTISCHEN ANAEMIE BEI PYRUVATKINASEMANGEL DER
ERYTHROCYTEN. KLIN WOCHENSCHR 49:228-230

28. BOIVIN,P., GALAND,C. AND DEMARTIAL,M.C., 1972, ETUDES SUR
LA PYRUVATE-KINASE ERYTHROCYTAIRE II. HETEROGENEITE
ENZYMOLOGIQUE DES DEFICITS ETUDES A PROPOS DE 28 CAS AVEC
ANEMIE HEMOLYTIQUE CONGENITALE. NOUV REV FR HEMATOL 12:569-
594

29. BRANDT,N.J. AND HANEL,H.K., 1971, ATYPICAL PYRUVATE KINASE
     IN A PATIENT WITH HAEMOLYTIC ANAEMIA. SCAND J HAEMATOL
     8:126-133

30. MATSUMOTO,N., ISHIHARA,T., NAKASHIMA,K., MIWA,S., UCHINO,F.
     AND KONDO,M., 1972, SEQUESTRATION AND DESTRUCTION OF
     RETICULOCYTE IN THE SPLEEN IN PYRUVATE KINASE DEFICIENCY
     HEREDITARY NONSPHEROCYTIC HEMOLYTIC ANEMIA. ACTA HAEMATOL
     JAP 35:525-537

31. PAGLIA,D.E., KONRAD,P.N., WOLFF,J.A. AND VALENTINE,W.N.,
     1976, BIPHASIC REACTION KINETICS IN AN ANOMALOUS ISOZYME
     OF ERYTHROCYTE PYRUVATE KINASE. CLIN CHIM ACTA 73:395-405

32. PAGLIA,D.E., VALENTINE,W.N. AND RUCKNAGEL,D.L., 1972,
     DEFECTIVE ERYTHROCYTE PYRUVATE KINASE WITH IMPAIRED KINETICS
     AND REDUCED OPTIMAL ACTIVITY. BR J HAEMATOL 22:651-665

33. SCHROETER,W. AND TILLMANN,W., 1975, MEMBRANE-LOCALIZED
     PYRUVATE KINASE OF RED BLOOD CELLS IN HEMOLYTIC ANEMIA
     ASSOCIATED WITH PYRUVATE KINASE DEFICIENCY. KLIN WOCHENSCHR
     53:1101-1106

34. MOSER,K., SCHWAZMEIER,J., DEUTSCH,E. AND ROTHMANN,W., 1967,
     NICHTSPHAEROZYTAERE HAEMOLYTISCHE ANAEMIE BEI
     PYRUVATKINASEMANGEL. KLIN WOCHENSCHR 79:542-546

35. SEARCY,G.P., MILLER,D.R. AND TASKER,J.B., 1971, CONGENITAL
     HEMOLYTIC ANEMIA IN THE BASENJI DOG DUE TO ERYTHROCYTE
     PYRUVATE KINASE DEFICIENCY. CAN J COMP MED 35:67-70

36. STANDERFER,R.J., RITTENBERG,M.B., CHERN,C.J., TEMPLETON,J.W.
     AND BLACK,J.A., 1975, CANINE ERYTHROCYTE PYRUVATE KINASE.
     II. PROPERTIES OF THE ABNORMAL ENZYME ASSOCIATED WITH
     HEMOLTIC ANEMIA IN THE BASENJI DOG. BIOCHEM GENET 13:341-
     351

37. STANDERFER,R.J., TEMPLETON,J.W. AND BLACK,J.A., 1974,
     ANOMALOUS PYRUVATE KINASE DEFICIENCY IN THE BASENJI DOG.
     AM J VET RES 35:1541-1543

38. NAKASHIMA,K., MIWA,S., SHINOHARA,K., OKA,E., TAJIRI,M.,
     ABE,S., ONO,J. AND BLACK,J.A., 1975, ELECTROPHORETIC,
     IMMUNOLOGIC AND KINETIC CHARACTERIZATION OF ERYTHROCYTE
     PYRUVATE KINASE IN THE BASENJI DOG WITH PYRUVATE KINASE
     DEFICIENCY. TOHOKU J EXP MED 117:179-185

39. PRASSE,K.W., CROUSER,D., BEUTLER,E., WALKER,M. AND
     SCHALL,W.D., 1975, PYRUVATE KINASE DEFICIENCY ANEMIA WITH
     TERMINAL MYELOFIBROSIS AND OSTEOSCLEROSIS IN THE BEAGLE.
     J AM VET MED ASSOC 166:1170-1175

40. BOIVIN,P., GALAND,C., HAKIM,J. AND KAHN,A., 1975, ACQUIRED
     RED CELL PYRUVATE KINASE DEFICIENCY IN LEUKEMIAS AND RELATED
     DISORDERS. ENZYME 19:294-299

41. KLEEBERG,U.R., HEIMPEL,H., KLEIHAUER,E. AND OLISCHLAEGER,A.,
     1971, RELATIVER GLUTATHION-UND/ODER PYRUVATKINASEMANGEL IN
     DEN ERYTHROCYTEN BEI PANMYELOPATHIEN UND AKUTEN LEUKAEMIEN.
     KLIN WOCHENSCHR 49:557-558

42. ARNOLD,H., BLUME,K.G., LOEHR,G.W., BOULARD,M. AND NAJEAN,Y.,
     1974, "ACQUIRED" RED CELL ENZYME DEFECTS IN HEMATOLOGICAL
     DISEASES. CLIN CHIM ACTA 57:187-189

43. TANPHAICHITR,V.S. AND VAN EYS,J., 1975, ERYTHROCYTE PYRUVATE
     KINASE ACTIVITY IN PATIENT WITH HAEMATOLOGICAL MALIGNANCIES.
     SCAND J HAEMATOL 15:10-16

44. BOIVIN,P., GALAND,C. AND AUDOLLENT,M., 1970,
     ERYTHROENZYMOPTHIES ACQUISES. I. ANOMALIES QUANTITATIVES
     OBSERVEES DANS 100 CAS DE'HEMOPATHIES DIVERSES. PATHOL BIOL
     (PARIS) 18:175-187

45. RAKSHIT,M.M. AND BASU,A.K., 1973, ACTIVITY OF ERYTHROCYTIC
     PYRUVATE KINASE (PK) IN LEUKAEMIA. BULL CALCUTTA SCH TROP
     MED 21:24-25

46. ABE,S., 1976, SECONDARY RED CELL PYRUVATE KINASE DEFICIENCY
     I. STUDY OF 30 SUBJECTS OF MALIGNANT HEMATOLOGICAL DISORDERS.
     ACTA HAEMATOL JAP 39:247-254

47. SCHROETER,W., 1970, TRANSITORISCHER PYRUVATKINASE- UND
     GLUTATHION-REDUCTASE-MANGEL DER ERYTHROCYTEN BEI CHRONISCHER
     IDIOPATHISCHER INFANTILER PANCYTOPENIE. KLIN WOCHENSCHR
     48:1407-1414

48. BOIVIN,P., GALAND,C. AND DREYFUS,B., 1969, ACTIVITES
     ENZYMATIQUES ERYTHROCYTAIRES AU COURS DES ANEMIES
     REFRACTAIRES. NOUV REV FR HEMATOL 9:105-112

49. DREYFUS,B., SULTAN,C., ROCHANT,H., SALMON,C.H., MANNONI,P.,
     CARTRON,J.P., BOIVIN,P. AND GALAND,C., 1969, ANOMALIES OF
     BLOOD GROUP ANTIGENS AND ERYTHROCYTE ENZYMES IN TWO TYPES
     OF CHRONIC REFRACTORY ANAEMIA. BR J HAEMATOL 16:303-312

50. KAHN,A., COTTREAU,D., BOYER,C., MARIE,J., GALAND,C. AND
     BOIVIN,P., 1976, CAUSAL MECHANISMS OF MULTIPLE ACQUIRED
     RED CELL ENZYME DEFECTS IN A PATIENT WITH ACQUIRED
     DYSERYTHROPOIESIS. BLOOD 48:653-662

51. LOWE,M.L., STELLA,A.F., MOSHER,B.S., GIN,J.B. AND
     DEMETRIOU,J.A., 1972, MICROFLUOROMETRY OF GLUCOSE-6-PHOSPHATE
     DEHYDROGENASE AND 6-PHOSPHOGLUCONATE DEHYDROGENASE IN RED
     CELLS. CLIN CHEM 18:440-445

52. VALENTINE,W.N., KONRAD,P.N. AND PAGLIA,D.E., 1973,
     DYSERYTHROPOIESIS, REFRACTORY ANEMIA, AND "PRELEUKEMIA":
     METABOLIC FEATURES OF THE ERYTHROCYTES. BLOOD 41:857-875

53. GOEBEL,K.M., GOEBEL,F.D., MUEHLFELLNER,G. AND KAFFARNIK,H.,
     1975, RED CELL METABOLISM IN TRANSIENT HAEMOLYTIC ANAEMIA
     ASSOCIATED WITH ZIEVE'S SYNDROME. EUR J CLIN INVEST 5:83-
     91

54. BOCK,H.E., WALLER,H.D., LOEHR,G.W. AND KARGES,O., 1958,
     BESONDERHEITEN IM FERMENTGEHALT VON MEGALOCYTEN. KLIN
     WOCHENSCHR 36:151-157

55. NAJMAN,A., LEROUX,J.P., TEMKINE,H., CARTIER,P. AND ANDRE,R.,
     1969, DEFICIT EN PYRUVATE-KINASE ERYTHROCYTAIRE AU COURS
     DES LEUCEMIES AIGUES. REV FRANC ETUDE CLIN BIOL 14:795-796

56.   KAHN,A., MARIE,J., BERNARD,J.-.F., COTTREAU,D. AND BOIVIN,P.,
      1976, MECHANISMS OF THE ACQUIRED ERYTHROCYTE ENZYME
      DEFICIENCIES IN BLOOD DISEASES. CLIN CHIM ACTA 71:379-387

57.   KAHN,A., BOIVIN,P., RUBINSON,H., COTTREAU,D., MARIE,J. AND
      DREYFUS,J.-.C., 1976, MODIFICATIONS OF PURIFIED GLUCOSE-6-
      PHOSPHATE DEHYDROGENASE AND OTHER ENZYMES BY A FACTOR OF
      LOW MOLECULAR WEIGHT ABUNDANT IN SOME LEUKEMIC CELLS. PROC
      NATL ACAD SCI USA 73:77-81

58.   VAN BERKEL,T.J.C., STAAL,G.E.J., KOSTER,J.F. AND NYESSEN,J.B.,
      1974, ON THE MOLECULAR BASIS OF PYRUVATE KINASE DEFICIENCY
      II. ROLE OF THIOL GROUPS IN PYRUVATE KINASE FROM PYRUVATE
      KINASE-DEFICIENT PATIENTS. BIOCHIM BIOPHYS ACTA 334:361-
      367

59.   BADWEY,J.A. AND WESTHEAD,E.W., 1977, POST-TRANSLATIONAL
      MODIFICATION OF HUMAN ERYTHROCYTE PYRUVATE KINASE. BIOCHEM
      BIOPHYS RES COMMUN 74:1326-1331

60.   BLUME,K.G., ARNOLD,H., LOEHR,G.W. AND SCHOLZ,G., 1974, ON
      THE MOLECULAR BASIS OF PYRUVATE KINASE DEFICIENCY. BIOCHIM
      BIOPHYS ACTA 370:601-604

61.   BLUME,K.G., LOEHR,G.W., RUEDIGER,H.W. AND SCHALHORN,A.,
      1968, PYRUVATE KINASE IN HUMAN ERYTHROCYTES. LANCET 1:529-
      530

62.   NAKASHIMA,K., 1974, FURTHER EVIDENCE OF MOLECULAR ALTERATION
      AND ABERRATION OF ERYTHROCYTE PYRUVATE KINASE. CLIN CHIM
      ACTA 55:245-254

63.   IMAMURA,K., TANAKA,T., NISHINA,T., NAKASHIMA,K. AND MIWA,S.,
      1973, STUDIES ON PYRUVATE KINASE (PK) DEFICIENCY II.
      ELECTROPHORETIC, KINETIC, AND IMMUNOLOGICAL STUDIES ON
      PYRUVATE KINASE OF ERYTHROCYTES AND OTHER TISSUES. J BIOCHEM
      (TOKYO) 74:1165-1175

64.   WONNEBERGER,B. AND SCHROETER,W., 1974, PYRUVATE KINASE
      ELECTROPHORESIS IN NORMAL AND PYRUVATE KINASE DEFICIENT
      HEMOLYSATES. CLIN CHIM ACTA 51:147-150

65.   PAGLIA,D.E. AND VALENTINE,W.N., 1970, EVIDENCE FOR MOLECULAR
      ALTERATION OF PYRUVATE KINASE AS A CONSEQUENCE OF ERYTHROCYTE
      AGING. J LAB CLIN MED 76:202-212

66.   BIGLEY,R.H., STENZEL,P., JONES,R.T., CAMPOS,J.O. AND
      KOLER,R.D., 1968, TISSUE DISTRIBUTION OF HUMAN PYRUVATE
      KINASE ISOZYMES. ENZYME 9:10-20

67.   KAHN,A., MARIE,J. AND BOIVIN,P., 1976, PYRUVATE KINASE
      ISOZYMES IN MAN. II. L TYPE AND ERYTHROCYTE-TYPE ISOZYMES.
      ELECTROFOCUSING AND IMMUNOLOGIC STUDIES. HUM GENET 33:35-
      46

68.   BIGLEY,R.H. AND KOLER,R.D., 1968, LIVER PYRUVATE KINASE
      (PK) ISOZYMES IN A PK-DEFICIENT PATIENT. ANN HUM GENET
      31:383-388

69. MARIE,J., KAHN,A. AND BOIVIN,P., 1976, PYRUVATE KINASE ISOZYMES IN MAN. I. M TYPE ISOZYMES IN ADULT AND FOETAL TISSUES, ELECTROFOCUSING AND IMMUNOLOGICAL STUDIES. HUM GENET 31:35-45

70. MARIE,J., KAHN,A. AND BOIVIN,P., 1977, HUMAN ERYTHROCYTE PYRUVATE KINASE. TOTAL PURIFICATION AND EVIDENCE FOR ITS ANTIGENIC IDENTITY WITH L-TYPE ENZYME. BIOCHIM BIOPHYS ACTA 481:96-104

71. LINCOLN,D.R., BLACK,J.A. AND RITTENBERG,B., 1975, IMMUNOLOGICAL PROPERTIES OF PYRUVATE KINASE. II. THE RELATIONSHIP OF THE HUMAN ERYTHROCYTE ISOZYME TO THE HUMAN LIVER ISOZYMES. BIOCHIM BIOPHYS ACTA 410:279-284

72. JANDL,J.H., ENGLE,L.K. AND ALLEN,D.W., 1960, OXIDATIVE HEMOLYSIS AND PRECIPITATION OF HEMOGLOBIN. I. HEINZ BODY ANEMIAS AS AN ACCELERATION OF RED CELL AGING. J CLIN INVEST 39:1818-1836

73. IBSEN,K.H., SCHILLER,K.W. AND VENN-WATSON,E.A., 1968, STABILIZATION, PARTIAL PURIFICATION, AND EFFECTS OF ACTIVATING CATIONS, ADP, AND PHOSPHOENOLPYRUVATE ON THE REACTION RATES OF AN ERYTHROCYTE PYRUVATE KINASE. ARCH BIOCHEM BIOPHYS 128:583-590

74. BLUME,K.G., HOFFBAUER,R.W., BUSCH,D., ARNOLD,H. AND LOEHR,G.W., 1971, PURIFICATION AND PROPERTIES OF PYRUVATE KINASE IN NORMAL AND IN PYRUVATE KINASE DEFICIENT HUMAN RED BLOOD CELLS. BIOCHIM BIOPHYS ACTA 227:364-372

75. CARMINATTI,H., ROZENGURT,E. AND JIMENEZ DE ASUA,L., 1969, ELUTION OF PYRUVATE KINASE FROM CM-CELLULOSE COLUMNS BY ITS ALLOSTERIC EFFECTOR. A NOVEL METHOD FOR ENZYME PURIFICATION. FEBS LETT 4:307-310

76. STAAL,G.E.J., KOSTER,J.F., KAMP,H., VAN MILLIGEN BOERSMA,L. AND VEEGER,C., 1971, HUMAN ERYTHROCYTE PYRUVATE KINASE. ITS PURIFICATION AND SOME PROPERTIES. BIOCHIM BIOPHYS ACTA 227:86-96

77. CHERN,C.J., RITTENBERG,M.B. AND BLACK,J.A., 1972, PURIFICATION OF HUMAN ERYTHROCYTE PYRUVATE KINASE. J BIOL CHEM 247:7173-7180

78. MARIE,J., KAHN,A. AND BOIVIN,P., 1976, L-TYPE PYRUVATE KINASE FROM HUMAN LIVER. PURIFICATION BY DOUBLE AFFINITY ELUTION, ELECTROFOCUSING AND IMMUNOLOGICAL STUDIES. BIOCHIM BIOPHYS ACTA 438:393-406

79. ODA,E., NAKASHIMA,K., SHINOHARA,K. AND MIWA,S., 1976, ISOELECTRIC FOCUSSING OF NORMAL HUMAN ERYTHROCYTE PYRUVATE KINASE (PK) AND PK VARIANTS WITH ABNORMAL ELECTROPHORETIC PATTERNS. CLIN CHIM ACTA 68:93-98

80. IBSEN,K.H. AND TRIPPET,P., 1971, HUMAN ERYTHROCYTE PYRUVATE KINASE CONFORMERS OBTAINED BY ELECTROFOCUSING. LIFE SCI 10:1021-1029

81. KAHN,A., MARIE,J., GALAND,C. AND BOIVIN,P., 1975, MOLECULAR
     MECHANISM OF ERYTHROCYTE PYRUVATE KINASE DEFICIENCY.
     HUMANGENETIK 29:271-280

82. BLACK,J.A. AND HENDERSON,M.H., 1972, ACTIVATION AND INHIBITION
     OF HUMAN ERYTHROCYTE PYRUVATE KINASE BY ORGANIC PHOSPHATES,
     AMINO ACIDS DIPEPTIDES AND ANIONS. BIOCHIM BIOPHYS ACTA
     284:115-127

83. BOIVIN,P., GALAND,C. AND DEMARTIAL,M., 1972, ETUDES SUR LA
     PYRUVATE KINASE ERYTHROCYTAIRE I. QUELQUES PROPRIETES DE
     L'ENZYME HUMAINE NORMALE. PATHOL BIOL (PARIS) 20:583-594

84. FLIKWEERT,J.P., HOORN,R.K.J. AND STAAL,G.E.J., 1975, EFFECTS
     OF CALCIUM IONS ON PYRUVATE KINASE FROM HUMAN ERYTHROCYTES.
     BIOCHIMIE 57:677-681

85. BUC,H., NAJMAN,A., COLUMELLI,S. AND CARTIER,P., 1972,
     DEFICIT EN CONGENITAL PYRUVATE KINASE ERYTHROCYTAIRE: ETUDE
     CINETIQUE DE L'ENZYME ET CONSEQUENCES METABOLIQUES. CLIN
     CHIM ACTA 38:131-140

86. GARREAU,H. AND BUC-TEMKINE,H., 1972, ALLOSTERIC ACTIVATION
     OF HUMAN ERYTHROCYTE PYRUVATE KINASE BY FRUCTOSE-1,6-
     DIPHOSPHATE. BIOCHIMIE 54:1103-1107

87. SHINOHARA,K., MIWA,S., NAKASHIMA,K., ODA,E., KAGEOKA,T.
     AND TSUJINO,G., 1976, A NEW PYRUVATE KINASE VARIANT (PK
     OSAKA) DEMONSTRATED BY PARTIAL PURIFICATION AND CONDENSATION.
     AM J HUM GENET 28:474-481

88. BLUME,K.G., BUSCH,D., HOFFBAUER,R.W., ARNOLD,H. AND
     LOEHR,G.W., 1970, THE POLYMORPHISM OF NUCLEOSID EFFECT IN
     PYRUVATE KINASE DEFICIENCY. HUMANGENETIK 9:257-259

89. FRASER,G.R., GRUNWALD,P. AND STAMATOYANNOPOULOS,G., 1966,
     GLUCOSE-6-PHOSPHATE DEHYDROGENASE (G6PD) DEFICIENCY, ABNORMAL
     HAEMOGLOBINS, AND THALASSAEMIA IN YUGOSLAVIA. J MED GENET
     3:35-41

90. ALBAUM,H.G., CAYLE,T. AND SHAPIRO,A., 1951, BLOOD LEVELS
     OF ADENINE NUCLEOTIDES. J CLIN INVEST 30:525-530

91. BOIVIN,P. AND GALAND,C., 1968, RECHERCHE D'UNE ANOMALIE
     MOLECULAIRE LORS DES DEFICITS EN PYRUVATE KINASE
     ERYTHROCYTAIRE. NOUV REV FR HEMATOL 8:201-208

92. KOSTER,J.F., SLEE,R.G., STAAL,G.E.J. AND VAN BERKEL,J.C.,
     1972, THE INFLUENCE OF GLUCOSE 1,6-DIPHOSPHATE ON THE
     ENZYMATIC ACTIVITY OF PYRUVATE KINASE. BIOCHIM BIOPHYS ACTA
     258:763-768

93. BOIVIN,P., GALAND,C. AND DEMARTIAL,M.C., 1972, COEXISTENCE
     DE DEUX TYPES DE PYRUVATE-KINASE CINETIQUEMENT DIFFERENTS
     DANS LES GLOBULES ROUGES HUMAINS NORMAUX. NOUV REV FR
     HEMATOL 12:159-169

94. LEONARD,H.A., 1972, HUMAN PYRUVATE KINASE. ROLE OF THE
     DIVALENT CATION IN THE CATALYTIC MECHANISM OF THE RED CELL
     ENZYME. BIOCHEMISTRY 11:4407-4414

95. BEUTLER,E., MATSUMOTO,F. AND GUINTO,E., 1974, THE EFFECT
     OF 2,3-DPG ON RED CELL ENZYMES. EXPERIENTIA 30:190-192

96. STAAL,G.E.J., KOSTER,J.F. AND NIJESSEN,J.G., 1972, A NEW
     VARIANT OF RED BLOOD CELL PYRUVATE KINASE DEFICIENCY.
     BIOCHIM BIOPHYS ACTA 258:685-687

97. GHERARDI,M., VERGNES,H., CORBERAND,J. AND REGNIER,C., 1974,
     DEFICIT EN PYRUVATE KINASE ERYTHROCYTAIRE ACCOMPAGNE D'UNE
     ANEMIE HEMOLYTIQUE NEONATALE SEVERE. ETUDE FAMILIALE ET
     CARACTERISATION BIOCHIMIQUE DE L'ENZYME. ACTA HAEMATOL
     52:248-256

98. STAAL,G.E.J., CEERDINK,R.P., VLUG,A.M.C. AND HAMELINK,M.L.,
     1976, DEFECTIVE ERYTHROCYTE PYRUVATE KINASE. CLIN CHIM ACTA
     68:11-15

99. GULBIS,E., WEBER,A., DECHAMPS,L., DENYS,P., SOKAL,G.,
     LOEHR,G., RUEDIGER,H., BLUME,K., PIRET,L. AND DUNJIC,A.,
     1970, CONTRIBUTION A L'ETUDE DE L'ANEMIE HEMOLYTIQUE
     CONGENITALE AVEC DEFICIT EN PYRUVATE-KINASE. ARCH FR PEDIATR
     27:31-49

100. GRIEGER,M., GUENTHER,I., JACOBASCH,G., BUSS,D. AND GERTH,C.,
     1972, STOFFWECHSELANOMALIE ROTER BLUTZELLEN MIT ATYPISCHER
     PYRUVATKINASE UND KALIUMMANGEL. HAEMATOLOGIA (BUDAP) 6:379-
     394

101. SCHROETER,W., 1972, CLINICAL HETEROGENEITY OF ERYTHROCYTE
     PYRUVATE KINASE DEFICIENCY. HELV PAEDIATR ACTA 27:471-488

102. GUMINSKA,M. AND WAZEWSKA-CZYZEWSKA,M., 1975, ENZYMATIC
     PATTERN OF GLUCOSE METABOLIC PATHWAYS IN PYRUVATE KINASE-
     DEFICIENT ERYTHROCYTES. CLIN CHIM ACTA 64:165-172

103. KEITT,A.S. AND BENNETT,D.C., 1966, PYRUVATE KINASE DEFICIENCY
     AND RELATED DISORDERS OF RED CELL GLYCOLYSIS. AM J MED
     41:762-785

104. NATHAN,D.G., OSKI,F.A., SIDEL,V.W. AND DIAMOND,L.K., 1965,
     EXTREME HEMOLYSIS AND RED-CELL DISTORTION IN ERYTHROCYTE
     PYRUVATE KINASE DEFICIENCY. II. MEASUREMENTS OF ERYTHROCYTE
     GLUCOSE CONSUMPTION, POTASSIUM FLUX AND ADENOSINE
     TRIPHOSPHATE STABILITY. N ENGL J MED 272:118-123

105. BERNARD,J.-.F., AFIFI,F. AND BOIVIN,P., 1974, NA AND K
     CATION LEVELS AND EXCHANGE ACROSS THE MEMBRANE OF THE
     ERYTHROCYTE. II. RESULTS OBTAINED IN THE ERYTHROCYTES OF
     20 PATIENTS WITH CONGENITAL HEMOLYTIC ANEMIA. PATHOL BIOL
     (PARIS) 22:51-60

106. BEUTLER,E., 1975, RED CELL METABOLISM. A MANUAL OF
     BIOCHEMICAL METHODS 2ND EDITON , GRUNE & STRATTON, NEW YORK

107. ROSE,I.A. AND WARMS,J., 1966, CONTROL OF GLYCOLYSIS IN THE
     HUMAN BLOOD CELL. J BIOL CHEM 241:4848-4854

108. OSKI,F.A., BRIGANDI,E. AND NOBLE,L., 1969, RED CELL METABOLISM
     IN THE NEWBORN INFANT. V. GLYCOLYTIC INTERMEDIATES AND
     GLYCOLYTIC ENZYMES. PEDIATRICS 44:84-91

109. NIESSNER,H. AND BEUTLER,E., 1973, FLUOROMETRIC ANALYSIS OF
      GLYCOLYTIC INTERMEDIATES IN HUMAN RED BLOOD CELLS. BIOCHEM
      MED 8:123-134

110. DACHA,M., CANESTRARI,F., BOSSU,M., ROSSI FERRINI,P.L. AND
      FORNAINI,G., 1977, INHERITED ERYTHROCYTE PYRUVATE KINASE
      DEFICIENCY: STUDIES ON 15 MEMBERS OF TWO RELATED FAMILIES.
      ACTA HAEMATOL 57:37-46

111. BEUTLER,E., 1971, 2,3-DIPHOSPHOGLYCERATE AFFECTS ENZYMES
      OF GLUCOSE METABOLISM IN RED BLOOD CELLS. NATURE (NEW
      BIOL) 232:20-21

112. SRIVASTAVA,S.K. AND BEUTLER,E., 1972, THE EFFECT OF NORMAL
      RED CELL CONSTITUENTS ON THE ACTIVITIES OF RED CELL ENZYMES.
      ARCH BIOCHEM BIOPHYS 148:249-255

113. BEUTLER,E. AND GUINTO,E., 1973, THE EFFECT OF 2,3-DPG ON
      RED CELL PHOSPHOFRUCTOKINASE. FEBS LETT 37:21-22

114. MENTZER JR,W.C., BEHNER,R.L., SCHMIDT-SCHOENBEIN,H.,
      ROBINSON,S.H. AND NATHAN,D.G., 1971, SELECTIVE RETICULOCYTE
      DESTRUCTION IN ERYTHROCYTE PYRUVATE KINASE DEFICIENCY. J
      CLIN INVEST 50:688-699

115. NATHAN,D.G., OSKI,F.A., MILLER,D.R. AND GARDNER,F.H., 1968,
      LIFE-SPAN AND ORGAN SEQUESTRATION OF THE RED CELLS IN
      PYRUVATE KINASE DEFICIENCY. N ENGL J MED 278:73-81

116. BOWMAN,H.S. AND PROCOPIO,F., 1963, HEREDITARY NON-SPHEROCYTIC
      HEMOLYTIC ANEMIA OF THE PYRUVATE-KINASE DEFICIENT TYPE.
      ANN INTERN MED 58:567-591

117. IGLEWSKI,B.H., IGLEWSKI,W.J., BIGLEY,R.H. AND KOLER,R.D.,
      1975, VIRUS-INDUCED HEMOLYSIS IN ERYTHROCYTES DEFICIENT IN
      PYRUVATE KINASE. CLINICAL RESEARCH 23:131A (ABSTRACT)

118. GLADER,B.E., 1976, SALICYLATE-INDUCED INJURY OF PYRUVATE-
      KINASE-DEFICIENT ERYTHROCYTES. N ENGL J MED 294:916-918

119. HENRY,R., 1976, LETTER: SALICYLATES AND PK-DEFICIENT
      RETICULOCYTES. N ENGL J MED 295:229-230

120. DE ACQUATELLA,G., MULLER,A. AND FRANCESCHI,A., 1971,
      DEFICIENCIA DE PIRUVATO-QUINASA EN UNA FAMILIA VENEZOLANA.
      ACTA MEDICA VENEZOLANA 1-5

121. WAZEWSKA-CZYZEWSKA,M. AND GUMINSKA,M., 1975, THE INFLUENCE
      OF MAGNESIUM IONS ON PYRUVATE KINASE-DEFICIENT RED BLOOD
      CELLS. FOLIA HAEMATOL (LEIPZ) 102:576-583

122. BOWMAN,H.S., MC KUSICK,V.A. AND DRONAMRAJU,K.R., 1965,
      PYRUVATE KINASE DEFICIENT HEMOLYTIC ANEMIA IN AN AMISH
      ISOLATE. AM J HUM GENET 17:1-8

123. DELIVORIA-PAPADOPOULOS,M., OSKI,F.A. AND GOTTLIEB,A.J.,
      1969, OXYGEN-HEMOGLOBIN DISSOCIATION CURVES: EFFECT OF
      INHERITED ENZYME DEFECTS OF THE RED CELL. SCIENCE 165:601-
      602

124. MAHOUR,G.H., LYNN,H.B. AND HILL,R.W., 1969, ACUTE PANCREATITIS WITH BILIARY DISEASE IN ERYTHROCYTE PYRUVATE-KINASE DEFICIENCY. CLIN PEDIATR 8:608-610

125. KENDALL,A.G. AND CHARLOW,G.F., 1977, RED CELL PYRUVATE KINASE DEFICIENCY: ADVERSE EFFECT OF ORAL CONTRACEPTIVES. ACTA HAEMATOL 57:116-120

126. NIXON,A.D. AND BUCHANAN,J.G., 1967, HAEMOLYTIC ANAEMIA DUE TO PYRUVATE KINASE DEFICIENCY. NZ MED J 66:859-864

127. TANAKA,K.R., VALENTINE,W.N. AND SCHNEIDER,A.S., 1963, PYRUVATE KINASE DEFICIENCY IN HEREDITARY NONSPHEROCYTIC HEMOLYTIC ANEMIA: AN INBORN ERROR OF METABOLISM. PROC 9TH CONGR EUROP SOC HAEMAT 739-744

128. BECKER,M.H., GENIESER,N.B., PIOMELLI,S., DOVE,D. AND MENDOZA,R.D., 1971, ROENTGENOGRAPHIC MANIFESTATIONS OF PYRUVATE KINASE DEFICIENCY HEMOLYTIC ANEMIA. AM J ROENTGENOL RADIUM THER NUCL MED 113:491-498

129. BAUGHAN,M.A., PAGLIA,D.E., SCHNEIDER,A.S. AND VALENTINE,W.N., 1968, AN UNUSUAL HEMATOLOGICAL SYNDROME WITH PYRUVATE-KINASE DEFICIENCY AND THALASSEMIA MINOR IN THE KINDREDS. ACTA HAEMATOL 39:345-358

130. NATHAN,D.G., OSKI,F.A., SIDEL,V.W., GARDNER,F.H. AND DIAMOND,L.K., 1966, STUDIES OF ERYTHROCYTE SPICULE FORMATION IN HAEMOLYTIC ANAEMIA. BR J HAEMATOL 12:385-395

131. VALENTINE,W.N., OSKI,F.A., PAGLIA,D.E., BAUGHAN,M.A., SCHNEIDER,A.S. AND NAIMAN,J.L., 1968, ERYTHROCYTE HEXOKINASE AND HEREDITARY HEMOLYTIC ANEMIA. HEREDITARY DISORDERS OF ERYTHROCYTE METABOLISM BEUTLER,E. ED. CITY OF HOPE SYMP. SERIES, VOL 1, GRUNE &STRATTON, NEW YORK

132. BROOK,J. AND TANAKA,K.R., 1970, COMBINATION OF PYRUVATE KINASE (PK) DEFICIENCY AND HEREDITARY SPHEROCYTOSIS (HS). CLINICAL RESEARCH 18:176 (ABSTRACT)

133. HANEL,H.K. AND PEDERSEN,J.T., 1972, ATYPICAL PYRUVATE KINASE IN A FAMILY WITH SPHEROCYTIC HAEMOLYTIC ANAEMIA. SCAND J HAEMATOL 9:557-561

134. BEUTLER,E., WEST,C. AND BLUME,K.G., 1976, THE REMOVAL OF LEUKOCYTES AND PLATELETS FROM WHOLE BLOOD. J LAB CLIN MED 88:328-333

135. BRUNETTI,P. AND NENCI,G., 1964, A SCREENING METHOD FOR THE DETECTION OF ERYTHROCYTE PYRUVATE KINASE DEFICIENCY. ENZYME 4:51-57

136. BEUTLER,E., 1966, A SERIES OF NEW SCREENING PROCEDURES FOR PYRUVATE KINASE DEFICIENCY, GLUCOSE-6-PHOSPHATE DEHYDROGENASE DEFICIENCY, AND GLUTATHIONE REDUCTASE DEFICIENCY. BLOOD 28:553-562

137. DACIE,J.V., 1964, THE HEREDITARY NON-SPHEROCYTIC HAEMOLYTIC ANAEMIAS. ACTA HAEMATOL 31:177-186

138. DE GRUCHY,G.C., 1963, RED-CELL METABOLISM IN CONGENITAL
      HAEMOLYTIC ANAEMIAS. AUST ANN MED 12:6-10

139. HANEL,H.K., HARVALD,B., MOR,G., CHRISTENSEN,N. AND DECKERT,T.,
      1967, A CASE OF HAEMOLYTIC ANAEMIA DUE TO PYRUVATE KINASE
      DEFICIENCY. SCAND J HAEMATOL 4:53-60

140. TEITEL,P., BRATU,V., XENAKIS,A. AND BUTOLIANU,E., 1965,
      FAVOURABLE THERAPEUTIC EFFECT OF ADENOSINE-5-MONOPHOSPHATE
      IN A CASE OF CHRONIC COMPENSATED HAEMOLYTIC DISEASE WITH
      AN IMPAIRED ERYTHROCYTE ENERGY METABOLISM. BIBL HAEMATOL
      23:557-560

141. VAN BERKEL,T.J.C., KOSTER,J.F. AND STAAL,G.E.J., 1973, ON
      THE MOLECULAR BASIS OF PYRUVATE KINASE DEFICIENCY. I.
      PRIMARY DEFECT OR CONSEQUENCE OF INCREASED GLUTATHIONE
      DISULFIDE CONCENTRATION. BIOCHIM BIOPHYS ACTA 321:496-502

142. STAAL,G.E.J., VAN BERKEL,T.J.C., NIJESSEN,J.G., KOSTER,J.F.
      AND WENSINK-VAN DER LOO,A., 1975, NORMALISATION OF RED
      BLOOD CELL PYRUVATE KINASE IN PYRUVATE KINASE DEFICIENCY
      BY RIBOFLAVIN TREATMENT. CLIN CHIM ACTA 60:323-327

143. BLUME,K.G., ARNOLD,H., HASSLINGER,K. AND LOEHR,G.W., 1976,
      EFFECT OF RIBOFLAVIN TREATMENT ON HUMAN RED CELL PYRUVATE
      KINASE DEFICIENCY. CLIN CHIM ACTA 71:331-334

144. BEUTLER,E., 1973, IMPORTANT RECENT ADVANCES IN THE FIELD
      OF RED CELL METABOLISM: PRACTICAL IMPLICATIONS. ERYTHROCYTES,
      THROMBOCYTES, LEUKOCYTES GERLACH,E., MOSER,K., DEUTSCH,E.
      AND WILMANNS,W. ED. 123-127, GEORG THIEME, STUTTGART

HEMOLYTIC ANEMIA
DUE TO OTHER
ENZYME
DEFICIENCIES

4.1. Hexokinase Deficiency

Hexokinase deficiency was first described by Löhr *et al.*[1] in patients with Fanconi's syndrome. In these patients the enzyme deficiency was probably a secondary phenomenon arising from chromosome breaks.[2] Hereditary deficiency of hexokinase as a primary phenomenon was described in 1967 by Valentine *et al.*[3] Only a few additional cases have been studied since that time.[4-11]

In several families hexokinase deficiency was inherited as an autosomal recessive disorder. Heterozygotes proved to have about one-half normal enzyme activity in their erythrocytes[3,7,12] but manifested no signs of hemolysis. It is of interest that the reduction of enzyme activity in hexokinase-deficient patients is often no greater than that found in heterozygotes. This is true because hexokinase is one of the most age-dependent glycolytic enzymes; the young red cell population of homozygous deficient subjects apparently masks the true severity of the enzyme deficiency. Consanguinity has not been noted in any of the reported cases. In one family, both a father and son had hemolytic anemia, suggesting autosomal dominant transmission.[4] The population origin of most patients has not been indicated, but it seems that most are of northern European origin.

Several isozymes of hexokinases can be separated by electrophoresis of erythrocytes. The major enzymes appear to correspond to the type I enzyme in liver, but a small amount of an enzyme corresponding to type III is also found. The exact relationship between red cell hexokinase enzymes and liver enzymes is not clear; although most recent studies[13-15] agree about the position of the bands that are seen, some of the earlier investigations[16] are uninterpretable. Evaluation of kinetic studies of crude red cell hexokinase preparations is complicated by the presence of several isozymes which presumably have different kinetic properties. Even from the very limited number of patients with hexokinase deficiency it is apparent that different mutations exist. Hexokinase from the patient described by Valentine et al.[3] manifested no kinetic abnormalities, but in most cases a decreased affinity of the residual enzyme for glucose[4,6,7,11] and ATP[6,7,11] has been observed, and marked decreases in the capacity to utilize glucose have been noted.[4,6,7,10] Striking instability to heating, especially in the absence of glucose, was observed in one case.[7] Leukocyte enzyme activity has been normal.[3,7] In one patient borderline reductions of platelet hexokinase activity were observed.[6] In most cases the results of hexokinase electrophoresis have not been reported. In one case, however, isozyme III was missing[4] and in the patient originally reported by Valentine et al.[3] subsequent studies[14] also demonstrated that only band I remained demonstrable on electrophoresis. The activity of age-related enzymes other than hexokinase is increased in hexokinase deficiency.[3,4,6,7,10] In spite of the young red cell population, glucose consumption by the red cells may be diminished[3,7,11] but has also been found to be slightly increased.[12] The consumption of mannose, which is also phosphorylated through the action of hexokinase, seemed to be less affected than that of glucose in one patient.[3] Methylene blue increased the consumption of glucose by hexokinase-deficient cells, but not to the same extent as was observed in normal cells.[3] Glucose-6-phosphate, 2,3-DPG, and ATP levels were diminished in the red cells of one patient, and interestingly enough also in the red cells of heterozygous relatives.[7] In other cases, normal 2,3-DPG levels have been recorded[12] and ATP levels were low.[10] Normal ATP levels have also been found.[6]

The clinical manifestations of red cell hexokinase deficiency are essentially those of nonspherocytic hemolytic anemia. It has been suggested that the symptoms of anemia are particularly severe in hexokinase deficiency because of the associated low 2,3-DPG levels,[17] and furthermore that oxygen delivery to the tissues is less than would be anticipated with the degree of anemia observed. Indeed, relatively brisk reticulocytoses have been observed in patients with relatively mild anemia.[3,7,12] In one case the results of the autohemolysis test were normal,[7] but in another case were slightly increased and partly corrected by glucose.[3] Osmotic fragility was normal.[6,7] In one patient in the postsplenectomy state, moderate anisocytosis and poikilocytosis, polychromasia, and numerous small round densely staining cells with spicule-like surface projections were observed.[3] In a patient who had not undergone splenectomy, the peripheral blood film was reported to show predominantly macrocytic red cells with sporadic microcytes, ovalocytes, and bizarre forms.[7] But in a patient we have studied, the blood film was quite unremarkable.

Although the predominant clinical effect of hexokinase deficiency has been nonspherocytic hemolytic anemia, in one family two sisters also experienced marked fatigability upon physical effort, and hypertrophy of muscles in the distal regions of the limbs. Study of the muscles showed large accumulations of glycogen.[6]

The diagnosis of hexokinase deficiency is not always simple. In most hemolytic anemias due to red cell enzyme deficiencies the level of the deficient enzyme is well below the normal range. In hexokinase deficiency this is by no means always the case. Because the level of hexokinase is so strongly dependent on red cell age, a deficiency of this enzyme may easily be masked by reticulocytosis. Normal red cell hexokinase activity in a patient with hemolytic anemia should suggest that hexokinase deficiency is actually present. Valentine et al.[3] used the ratio of hexokinase to two other age-dependent enzymes, pyruvate kinase and G-6-PD, to demonstrate that their patient was truly hexokinase-deficient. Although this patient's hexokinase activity was at the lower limit of normal, the ratio of hexokinase to these enzymes was only about one-third of the normal ratio and clearly outside the range encountered in normal controls or in patients with hemolytic anemia. Further difficulties in diagnosis may arise in detecting variants which have an elevated K_m for glucose. Such variants may appear to have normal activity when assayed in the presence of a large excess of glucose, but to be deficient at physiologic glucose levels.[4]

Experience with the treatment of hexokinase deficiency has been meager. Splenectomy produced definite improvement in two patients,[3,4] and in another patient[7] resulted in disappearance of jaundice, doubling of the reticulocyte count, but no change in hematocrit.

4.2. Glucose Phosphate Isomerase Deficiency

Although glucose phosphate isomerase deficiency is probably the third most common identified cause of hereditary nonspherocytic hemolytic anemia, the first case was not discovered until 1968. At that time Baughan et al.[18] found that the GPI activity of red cells of a patient with nonspherocytic hemolytic anemia was markedly diminished.

The parents of patients with GPI deficiency manifest enzyme levels which are intermediate between those of normal subjects and those of affected patients. It is evident that nonspherocytic hemolytic anemia due to GPI deficiency is inherited as an autosomal recessive disorder, although occasionally an acquired form of GPI deficiency may exist.[19] By 1974, Paglia and Valentine[20] had already been able to identify 20 cases of hemolytic anemia due to GPI deficiency in 16 apparently unrelated families. Since that time numerous additional patients have been reported by various investigators all over the world.[21-34] GPI deficiency has been noted in many population groups including French,[18] Irish,[18] German,[21,35-37] Spanish,[26,30] Canadian,[38] United States Caucasian,[23] Dutch,[27,28,31,32] Mexican,[24,38] and Japanese.[25,39,40]

Red cell GPI is reportedly a dimer with a molecular weight of 94,000[22] or 132,000.[41] Tissue-specific isozymes probably do not occur, since the electrophoretic mobility of enzyme derived from various tissues is in all cases very similar.[42,43] More important, in one patient with an electrophoretically abnormal GPI it was possible to conduct electrophoretic studies of the spleen, liver, and muscle as well as of leukocytes and plasma at the time of splenectomy.[44] In each tissue the electrophoretic properties of GPI were the same as those observed in the red cells. It is not surprising, then, that a decrease of leukocyte and plasma activities is regularly observed in GPI deficiency.[20,21,26,28,30,31] Decreased activity has also been found in platelets,[28,30,31] liver,[28,31] and muscle.[28,31] Although in some families consanguinity is present,[23,24,31,32,39,40,44,45] the parents of other reported patients were known to be unrelated. In the latter cases it is unlikely that the patients have inherited two identical deficient genes. Instead of being truly "homozygous" for GPI deficiency, such patients are usually heterozygous for two abnormal genes.[38] It is often possible to demonstrate this quite directly; the mutant enzymes inherited from the mother and father may show clearly distinguishable electrophoretic properties.

There appears to be considerable diversity in both deficient and nondeficient variants of GPI. An extensive polymorphism involving this enzyme has been described.[42,46] Most of the electrophoretically distinct variants which have been described have normal enzyme activity and are not known to be associated with any clinical disorder. Many deficient variants of GPI have been given geographic designations. Included among these are Seattle,[20] Whiteley County,[20] Espeln,[47] Los Angeles,[38] Winnipeg,[38] Recklinghausen,[35] Nordhorn,[21,22] Elyria,[23] Valle Hermoso,[24] Matsumoto[25,44] Narica,[44] Barcelona,[26,30] Utrecht,[28,32] Nijmegen,[27] Kentucky,[45] and Paderborn.[34] The K_m of these variants for the substrates glucose-6-phosphate and fructose-6-phosphate has in all cases been quite normal. In some instances minor deviations in the pH–activity curves have been noted,[26,30,35,44] but usually the pH optimum curve appears to be normal.[21-25,27,28,34,36,44,47] The heat stability of the residual GPI has been studied in many unrelated cases, and without exception the mutant enzyme was found to be heat labile.[21,24-28,30,34-36,38,40,44,45,47,48] In some families enzyme from only one of the two parents[21,26] or from neither[38] was found to be heat labile. These are instances in which two different abnormal alleles had apparently been inherited, and in which little or no residual abnormal enzyme activity was present in the red cells of the parents without thermolabile GPI. Limited studies of resistance of GPI variants to denaturation with urea indicate that they are labile.[30,35] Instability of red cell GPI has been noted using an ingenious in vitro "aging" system[49] and has been noted on age fractionation in red cells of one patient,[49] but not in those of another.[24] Normal GPI has a very high isoelectric point of approximately 9.65[22,30,35,47] or 9.25.[41] Electrophoresis is usually carried out using the method of Detter et al.[42] at a pH of 8.0; because the isoelectric point of the enzyme is so high, GPI moves toward the cathode. Two or three bands are ordinarily visualized. In the case of many variants only a single band is seen, and this may be due in part to the relatively low activity. Compared with the most active leading band the electrophoretic mobility of some GPI variants has been rapid,[21,22,30,34,36,37,39,44,50] slow,[23,27,35,38,50] or normal.[24,25,28,40,44,45] Except for the decrease in GPI activity, red cell enzyme activity is normal, or in the case of age-related enzymes, increased.[18,21,23,25,26,28,35,36,39,40,48,50] In one case concomitant G-6-PD deficiency was observed.[37] In those cases in which metabolic intermediates were measured, glucose-6-phosphate levels were increased. Fructose-6-phosphate levels, in contrast, are normal or only minimally increased, in spite of the young red cell population. The result, therefore, is that the ratio of glucose-6-phosphate to fructose-6-phosphate is increased.[21,23-25,28,31,35-37,39,-40,52,53] Mannose-6-phosphate levels measured in one case were found to be increased.[35] The increase of glyceraldehyde phosphate and dihydroxyacetone phosphate levels reported in one patient[39] has not been noted in others.[23,24,28,31,40] GSH levels are sometimes normal,[18,31,48,51] but in a considerable number of patients red cell GSH levels[23,25,26] or GSH stability[31] were decreased. In one case the low GSH levels may have been due to concomitant G-6-PD deficiency.[37] Levels of ATP have been judged normal[24,25,39,40] or modestly decreased when cell age is taken into account.[21,37,52] Similarly, while the rate of glucose utilization is usually increased,[18,21,24,35-37] some investigators have suggested that the increase is not commensurate with the decrease in cell age.[21,24,52] With one exception[45] a uniform finding has been the inability of GPI-deficient cells to recycle glucose through the hexose monophosphate pathway, as indicated by oxidation of the 2-carbon.[18,24,50]

The clinical manifestations of GPI deficiency vary greatly.[20] In some instances anemia is quite mild, in others very severe. Three deaths occurred in one family in which transfusion or splenectomy was refused.[45] Another patient was reported to have a hemoglobin of 2.1 g/100 ml during an aplastic crisis.[18] The ^{51}Cr $t_{1/2}$ of this patient was only 4.5 days, and even shorter red cell life spans have been recorded.[21,47] One case of neonatal jaundice necessitated exchange transfusion.[50] Most patients have had no symptoms other than those which could be related directly to nonspherocytic hemolytic anemia. However, mental retardation[28,32] and "unsatisfactory performance in school"[35] have been noted. Priapism occurred in one patient[45] and was attributed to increased blood viscosity. In one case, increased liver glycogen storage was observed.[33] The blood film generally shows anisocytosis and poikilocytosis, and darkly staining spiculated cells have been observed.[50] Ovalocytes have also been noted,[26] and in one case[52] frank spherocytosis was reported to be present.[52] In this patient a marked increase in osmotic fragility of the red cells was found; however, the vast majority of patients with GPI deficiency have normal osmotic fragility tests.[18,25,27,35,36,40,45] A slight increase in osmotic fragility,[26] particularly after incubation,[37] has been observed in isolated patients. In one case slight resistance to osmotic hemolysis was reported.[32] In most patients the white count has been normal,[21,25,32,35,36,39,40] but slight elevations of white counts have been reported occasionally,[26,45] possibly because of intercurrent infections. The platelet count is also usually normal,[21,25,26,35] but decreased platelet counts were encountered[36,37] in one instance presumably due to the development of uremia.[37] Abnormal autohemolysis tests are common in GPI deficiency. Type I autohemolysis was found in several patients,[18,26,27,35,36,50] and normal autohemolysis in another[54]; however, in most instances an atypical pattern consisting of increased autohemolysis only slightly corrected by glucose has been encountered.[21,37]

Glucose phosphate isomerase deficiency has no characteristic clinical or morphological features. Diagnosis depends on demonstration of deficiency of GPI in red cells. This can be accomplished through assay of enzyme activity[55] or through the use of a fluorescent screening test.[56]

In the management of patients with GPI deficiency the results of splenectomy have usually been quite gratifying. Only one reported patient failed to improve[28]; other patients experienced marked improvement[18,45,50] or moderate improvement.[23,35,48,52,57] Efforts to influence erythrocyte life span by bypassing the metabolic block have been unsuccessful. The administration of mannose to one patient failed to result in improvement.[9] The administration of methylene blue had no discernible effect in another patient, but the daily infusion of 500 ml of a 0.22 M sodium phosphate buffer, pH 7.4, over a period of 3 hr was associated with an increase in the hemoglobin level from approximately 13 to 14.5 g/

100 ml, and a decline in the reticulocyte count from 10 to 7%.[36] Attempts to stimulate the HMP with methylene blue and ascorbic acid failed to produce a response.[18]

4.3. Phosphofructokinase Deficiency

In 1965, Tarui et al.[58] discovered a severe deficiency of muscle phosphofructokinase (PFK) in a patient with a newly discovered type of metabolic myopathy, type VII glycogen storage disease. In their original report these authors pointed out that a partial deficiency of PFK could also be demonstrated in the erythrocytes, and subsequently noted that their patient also had a shortened red cell life span.[59] Similar kindreds were reported by Layzer et al.[60] and Serratrice et al.[61] Following the observation of shortened red cell life span in children with type VII glycogen storage disease,[58,60] several additional patients with red cell PFK deficiency have been reported,[48,62–65] all with purely hematologic clinical manifestations.

Phosphofructokinase deficiency is probably inherited as an autosomal recessive disorder. Diminished enzyme activity without hemolytic anemia has been observed in the mother and grandmother of an affected male patient,[62] and since father-to-son transmission has not been documented, a sex-linked mode of inheritance cannot be rigidly excluded.

The biochemical relationship between red cell enzyme and muscle enzyme is not entirely clear. Muscle and erythrocyte PFK are immunologically related so that approximately one-half of normal erythrocyte enzyme is inactivated when incubated with antiserum prepared against muscle PFK.[48,49,62] Electrophoresis of red cell PFK reveals an isozyme which does not appear to be present in muscle.[66,67] The red cell enzyme is more readily inhibited by ATP than is the muscle enzyme, whereas muscle PFK is more sensitive to inhibition by citrate. It seems that erythrocyte enzyme represents a composite of subunits unique to the red cell and of those in muscle.[68,70] Examination of glycolytic intermediates in PFK-deficient red cells revealed the expected increase in fructose-6-phosphate (175% of control) and decrease in fructose-1,6-diphosphate (58% of expected control) and triose phosphate (50% of control). Red cell 2,3-DPG levels were only 50% of the normal control levels, and the oxygen affinity of the red cells was increased.[69]

Nonspherocytic hemolytic anemia has been observed in association with type VII glycogen storage disease as well as in the absence of any muscle disorder. Patients with PFK deficiency with muscle glycogen storage were found to have a red cell ^{51}Cr life span of only 13 to 16 days, erythroid hyperplasia of the bone marrow, and reticulocyte counts ranging from 3.8 to 6.5%.[59]

Partial deficiency of red cell PFK was associated in five other families with nonspherocytic hemolytic anemia, but no muscle dysfunction was observed.[48,62-65] In one patient[63] an uncompensated hemolytic anemia was present with a postsplenectomy steady state hematocrit of 27 to 33, a 5 to 15% reticulocytosis, and a ^{51}Cr $t_{1/2}$ of 10 days. In three patients the residual PFK was unstable,[48,62,64] and in one of them[48] muscle enzyme had normal activity but was also markedly unstable. In another patient, muscle activity was not measured, but titration of the residual red cell enzyme with anti-human muscle enzyme suggested that no muscle component was present in the erthrocytes.[62] These investigations as well as kinetic studies of the residual red cell enzyme suggest that the defect in this patient was also in the muscle-type enzyme. The absence of muscle symptoms in these cases was probably due to the fact that the nonnucleated erythrocytes were more severely affected by a mutation affecting the enzyme stability than were the nucleated muscle cells. Red cell PFK activity in one patient with nonspherocytic hemolytic anemia was reduced to the uniquely low level of 8% of normal, whereas in all other cases the residual enzyme activity was about one-half of normal. Red cell ^{51}Cr life span was reportedly 6 days, but this rapid rate of red cell destruction seems incompatible with the apparently compensated hemolytic anemia reflected by the hemoglobin level of 12.8 g/100 ml and a reticulocyte count of 7 to 14%. Strangely, neither accumulation of glucose-6-phosphate or fructose-6-phosphate nor decrease in fructose-1,6-diphosphate could be demonstrated. No muscular symptoms were pres-

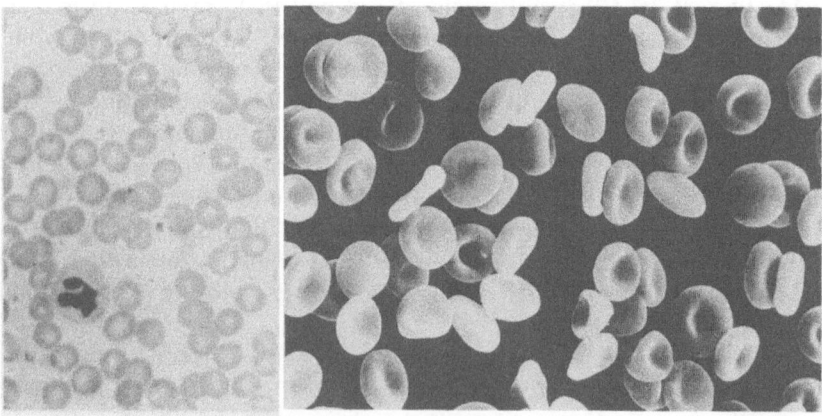

FIGURE 18.   Aldolase-deficient red cells on a standard blood film stained with Giemsa stain (left) and on scanning electron microscopy (right). (Electron microscopy courtesy of P. Klug and H. Weems.)

ent. It is possible that the deficiency in this patient was of a red cell subunit, in contrast to the other cases in which a muscle subunit appeared to be involved.

Splenectomy produced improvement in the one patient with PFK deficiency in which this procedure was carried out.[63]

4.4. Aldolase Deficiency

Aldolase deficiency has been reported only once.[71] The affected child was the offspring of first cousins, and it may therefore be assumed that inheritance was an autosomal recessive disorder. It is of interest that the enzyme activity of the red cells of both parents was normal. Aldolase is a multimeric enzyme, and it was proposed that normal subunits might have interacted with mutant subunits in such a way as to stabilize the enzyme.

Three principal types of aldolase are found in human tissues. Aldolase A is the type found in muscle and in red cells, aldolase B is found in the liver, and aldolase C occurs in the brain along with aldolase A.[72,73] A system of isozymes is found within each of these principal aldolase types, and it has been shown that deamidation of the subunits with the formation of the five possible tetrameric arrangements is responsible for the isozymes of aldolase A.[74] The residual enzyme in the homozygous aldolase A-deficient patient had normal electrophoretic mobility and normal kinetic properties, and was normally inactivated by heat. All isozymes were diminished, but the greatest decrease in activity was in the more basic isozymes, those which had not been deamidated. This suggested the possibility that the mutant enzyme might be deamidated more rapidly than normal.

The aldolase-deficient patient was moderately mentally retarded and had been shown to have increased deposition of glycogen in the liver. A mild nonspherocytic hemolytic anemia was present (Fig. 18). The activities of all glycolytic enzymes other than aldolase were increased or normal. Determination of red cell intermediates showed increased concentration of substrates proximal to the metabolic block in aldolase, a finding consistent with this enzyme deficiency.[75] The patient was not splenectomized, and no effort was made to treat the hemolytic anemia.

4.5. Triose Phosphate Isomerase Deficiency

Triose phosphate isomerase (TPI) deficiency was first reported by Schneider et al. in 1965.[76] A marked decrease in the activity of this enzyme was noted in a 13-month-old child of French–African ancestry. In

addition to nonspherocytic hemolytic anemia, the child manifested neuromuscular abnormalities involving the flexor of the hips, knees, and
calves, and the pronators of the arms. Several additional kindreds with
triose phosphate isomerase deficiency have been observed.[77-81] One additional patient with possible Fanconi anemia was observed to have TPI
activity which was about 30% of mean normal.[10] The patient's mother had
normal red cell TPI activity, and the father's enzyme activity was only
slightly reduced. Moreover, the child had no neurologic symptoms but
moderately severe thrombocytopenia. It seems unlikely that this patient
had genetically determined TPI-deficient nonspherocytic hemolytic
anemia.

Hemolytic anemia due to triose phosphate isomerase deficiency is
inherited as an autosomal recessive disorder.[76] Heterozygotes manifest
approximately one-half normal enzyme activity, and consanguinity has
probably been present in families of some of the affected patients.[76]

Triose phosphate isomerase has a molecular weight of 56,000 daltons
and is a dimer.[82] On electrophoresis three bands of enzyme activity are
present in erythrocytes and an additional band is found in other tissues.[83]
However, since all bands appear to be affected by mutations, it seems
most likely that they represent various posttranscriptional modifications
of a single gene product. In addition to red cells the following tissues have
been examined during life or at autopsy: leukocytes[77-79,81]; plasma[81]; cultured skin fibroblasts,[80] brain stem,[80] occipital lobe,[80] and temporal lobe[80];
skeletal muscle[80,81]; pancreas,[80] heart,[80] cerebellum,[80] diaphragm,[80] liver,[80]
lung,[80] kidney,[80] spleen,[80] tongue,[80] intestine,[80] testes,[80] and thymus.[80] All
were found to be deficient in TPI activity. Age-dependent enzymes other
than TPI are increased.[81] TPI-deficient red cells utilize glucose at a rapid
rate and show the expected accumulation of dihydroxyacetone phosphate.[78,84] The rate of glucose utilization was more rapid than that of
control red cells with a similarly elevated reticulocyte count, and it was
suggested that the increase was due to accelerated HMP metabolism. In
one patient the ATP level was normal; in a second patient it was
decreased.

The clinical manifestations of triose phosphate isomerase deficiency
are those of chronic hemolytic anemia and in most cases neurologic dysfunction and death in early childhood. Some affected infants were jaundiced in the immediate neonatal period and died in the first few days of
life; in other patients, jaundice did not become apparent but severe anemia was noted at 4 or 5 weeks of age.[79] Infections appear to have been
particularly common in TPI-deficient children. Neurologic impairment
was generally not present in the immediate neonatal period, but those
infants who survived the first half-year of life developed progressive

neuromuscular deterioration. For example, one child who had been able to sit up and ambulate in a "walker" at age 6 months subsequently lost the ability to sit and even to hold the head erect.[79] A variety of neurologic deficits have been noted. These have included elasticity,[77,79] hypotonia,[77,79] and opisthotonos.[77] One patient who survived to the age of 21 was described as manifesting muscle weakness, unintelligible speech, absent limb reflexes, frog position with fixed deformities of the feet and hands, and bilateral hand tremors with accentuation during tension.[78] Severe anemia with hemoglobin levels of 5 g/100 ml or less is encountered.[76,77,80] Slight macrocytosis with small numbers of target cells and occasional nucleated red cells have been observed.[76] Osmotic fragility of fresh erythrocytes is normal, but some flattening of the fragility curve was noted after 24 hr incubation.[79] Autohemolysis was markedly increased, with correction by glucose, adenosine, or ATP.[79] In one subject Heinz body formation in red cells was markedly increased when they were incubated with acetylphenylhydrazine.[79] The leukocyte count is commonly elevated,[76,77] possibly because of the propensity to infection that these patients may exhibit. Phagocytosis by leukocytes in the presence of normal serum was normal,[77,79] and a borderline decrease in the number of B lymphocytes and increase in T lymphocytes has been reported.[77] Electroencephalogram, electromyogram, and nerve biopsy have all been found to be normal.[80] The spinal fluid is normal.[79] Respiratory impairment and repeated respiratory infections or sudden cardiac arrest have led to death of most of the patients.[77,79,80,85] TPI deficiency is diagnosed by carrying out an enzyme assay on a red cell hemolysate.[55] A fluorescent screening test for TPI deficiency has also been devised.[86,87]

Splenectomy was carried out in one patient, without apparent benefit.[78]

4.6. Phosphoglycerate Kinase Deficiency

The first cases of phosphoglycerate kinase (PGK) deficiency were reported independently by Valentine et al.[88] and Kraus et al.[89] in 1968. The pedigree studied by Valentine and co-workers strongly suggested a sex-linked mode of inheritance. With the development of an electrophoretic method for the detection of phosphoglycerate kinase[90] normally active electrophoretically distinguishable variants of PGK were soon found, and the sex-linked nature of this structural gene was established.[91] Moreover, the results of density fractionation of the red cells of women with partial PGK activity were consistent with the existence of two separate red cell populations—enzyme-deficient and normal cells—as predicted by the X-inactivation hypothesis.[88] PGK deficiency has been reported in families of Chinese,[88] United States Caucasian,[89,92] Swedish,[93] Italian,[94] French,[95,96] and Japanese[97] ancestry.

PGK deficiency has been shown to affect not only the red cells but also leukocytes.[88,92,95,98] Leukocyte function has been found to be normal,[96,98] except in one case.[99] Because neurologic disturbances are common in patients with PGK deficiency (*vide infra*), it may be presumed that other tissues, particularly the central nervous system, are affected. Normal red cell PGK has been crystallized and fingerprinted.[100,101] It appears to be a monomer with a molecular weight of 50,000 daltons. The amino acid substitution of a normally active, electrophoretically abnormal variant has been determined.[101] A few studies of the characteristics of the residual enzyme in PGK-deficient males have been carried out. The electrophoretic mobility,[95,96] K_m for 3-PGA and ATP,[96] pH optimum,[96] and thermal stability[96] of the residual enzyme have been found to be normal. Immunologic studies demonstrated that normal quantities of PGK antigen were present in the red cells of one patient, indicating that the specific activity of the enzyme was drastically reduced.[102] The enzyme had a slightly increased isoelectric point,[102] although its electrophoretic mobility had previously been reported to be normal.[96] In one case the mutant enzyme was more stable than normal to heat and urea.[102]

Red cell ATP levels have been reported to be low[95] or normal,[94,96,97,179] but less than that expected with a similar degree of reticulocytosis.[88,96] Levels of red cell 2,3-DPG were elevated[88,94,95] or normal.[97] Spectacular[92,97,98] and more modest[94,95] increases in triose phosphate and fructose-1,6-diphosphate have been found. The activity of glycolytic enzymes other than PGK has generally been increased[88,89,95-97] but in one case[94] a decrease in hexokinase and pyruvate kinase activity was documented.

The onset of symptoms has generally been early in the case of male hemizygotes[88,92,95-97] and late in heterozygous females.[89,94] In males, neonatal jaundice is often present[92,95,97] and convulsions have been observed in the neonatal period.[96] Splenomegaly is present in most patients. Neurologic symptoms have been a constant feature of all reported males with phosphoglycerate kinase deficiency. A moderate degree of mental retardation with slowed ability to learn has been noted.[88,92,95-97] A particularly lucid description of the neurologic changes in one patient has been presented by Konrad *et al.*[92]:

> Development appeared normal until 3 years of age when speech difficulties were first noted. He was in kindergarten for two years because of mild retardation and emotional immaturity after which he was transferred to a special school. Detailed evaluation at 8 years revealed mild retardation with poor eye–hand coordination and expressive aphasia. . . . The electro-

encephalogram was abnormal with generalized brief sequences of slow irregular activity and occasional random fast sharp waves in the left occipital area. The urinary amino acids were normal. At 12 years a fine tremor was first noted. . . . At 16 years . . . the facial expression was dull, almost mask-like with mouth open. An almost constant generalized fine tremor was present. He was responsive and cooperative, but there was no spontaneous speech. Articulation was poor and connected speech was unintelligible. Posturing of the hands with the wrists in metacarpal phalangeal joints in flexion and the fingers in extension was noted. . . . When walking he threw out the right leg from the knee while rotating the foot clockwise in the air. He was able to walk a straight line slowly. He could hop but not skip, and maintained the Romberg position. The tremor increased with tension. Finger to nose and heel to shin tests were performed well. Muscle mass and tone, sensation, and deep tendon reflexes were normal. There was no clonus or abnormal superficial reflexes. The Wexler intelligence scale for children full scale IQ was 60. . . . For the past four years he has been treated with artane and L-Dopa without objective improvement. He has never had a seizure.

The degree of anemia has been variable, ranging from a level of 3 to 4 g/100 ml in one patient to as high as 13.7 g/100 ml in another.[92] Mild jaundice has been the rule although in one heterozygous patient the total bilirubin level was only 1.2 mg/100 ml.[89] Reticulocytosis has been present in all reported cases, and reported red cell life spans have varied from a ^{51}Cr $t_{1/2}$ of 11 days[96] to one of 16 days.[94] Autohemolysis has been increased in all patients; in some it was corrected by glucose,[88,92] in others increased. Neurologic abnormalities have usually been observed in affected males, but were absent in one case.[95] Phosphoglycerate kinase activity of red cells is readily detected by spectrophotometric assay of the enzyme in hemolysates.[55] As in other sex-linked disorders, marked variation in the enzyme activity of the red cells of heterozygotes may occur, and therefore enzymatic assay cannot be relied upon for the detection of all carriers.

In three patients who were splenectomized, the response appeared to be favorable.[88,95,97] In a fourth splenectomized patient no improvement was noted.[89]

4.7.   Glyceraldehyde Phosphate Dehydrogenase Deficiency

Partial deficiency of red cell glyceraldehyde phosphate dehydrogenase (GAPD) has been associated in several families with hemolytic states. In most instances, hemolysis was attributed to the enzyme deficiency.[103-105] However, careful examination of the data concerning a number of these families suggests that hemolysis was frequently dissociated from the GAPD deficiency and that no cause-and-effect relationship exists between partial GAPD deficiency and hemolysis.

In the first case to be reported[105] a father and son with 20 to 30% of normal GAPD activity presented with compensated hemolytic disease. Osmotic fragility was normal. There was accumulation of fructose diphosphate and decreased levels of ATP and phosphoglyceric acid in the red cells. However, findings in a large kindred with GAPD deficiency (coexistent with hereditary spherocytosis and G-6-PD deficiency) cast serious doubt on the role of the enzyme deficiency in the etiology of the hemolytic anemia.[106] Affected family members showed a 50% reduction in red cell GAPD activity and a decrease in intensity of band 6 on polyacrylamide gel SDS electrophoresis of red cell membranes. Of the individuals investigated, four were normal, two had hereditary spherocytosis with normal GAPD activity, three had reduced GAPD activity and did not have hereditary spherocytosis, and four inherited both hereditary spherocytosis and GAPD deficiency. The hemoglobin concentration of the blood was normal in the group that had inherited only GAPD deficiency, and the results of autohemolysis tests were normal. The residual GAPD had a normal kinetic property.[106] In another family[104] two sibs with hemolytic disease which had been responsive to splenectomy had red cell GAPD levels approximately 50% of normal. The younger child had anemia in the neonatal period with a hemoglobin of only 5.7 g/100 ml. Osmotic fragility of the red cells was normal. After splenectomy a compensated hemolytic state with a hemoglobin of 12.5 g/100 ml and a reticulocyte count of 10% was documented. Although the authors concluded that the hemolytic anemia was due to GAPD deficiency, the family history suggests that this was not the case. GAPD activity was normal in the mother, and in the father was only 40% of normal, a level somewhat lower than that encountered in the children. Yet, he did not have hemolytic disease. Accordingly, it seems most likely that the children had an autosomal recessive hemolytic anemia of undetermined etiology, and that the decreased GAPD activity was an unrelated finding.

Glyceraldehyde phosphate dehydrogenase activity of red cells is readily measured by a direct spectrophotometric assay.[55]

4.8. Diphosphoglycerate Mutase Deficiency

The possibility that 2,3-diphosphoglycerate mutase (DPGM) deficiency of red cells might cause nonspherocytic hemolytic anemia was first suggested before a quantitative assay for this enzyme had been developed. The validity of early reports is therefore very difficult to evaluate. In one family[107] low red cell 2,3-DPG levels in the patient and his father and failure of 2,3-DPG to accumulate when the terminal portion of the glycolytic pathway was inhibited with fluoride were interpreted as indicating that the mutase was defective. Alagille et al.[108] presented two cases under the possibly misleading title "Congenital Deficiency in 2,3-Diphosphoglyceromutase." One of these patients had been reported previously by Löhr and Waller[109] and was also the subject of a subsequent report.[110] These cases may be the same patients discussed in two additional publications.[111,112] It is apparent that the deficiency which was actually demonstrated was not one of DPGM, but rather of monophosphoglyceromutase. The "deficiency" of this enzyme was corrected by addition of the necessary cofactor, 2,3-DPG. It was suggested[109] that the red cells were deficient in 2,3-DPG and that this led to secondary underactivity of monophosphyoglyceromutase. Whether an actual deficiency of 2,3-DPG existed was not clear, and no direct assays of DPGM were carried out. Moser[10] also reported a patient with diminished red cell 2,3-DPG levels and assumed, but did not demonstrate, that DPGM deficiency existed.

On the basis of the fragmentary data which were available the clinical consequences of DPGM deficiency could not be considered clearly defined. The early reports of putative DPGM deficiency[10,107,108,110] all lack documentation that a deficiency of this enzyme actually existed in the patients studied. Indeed, even if a partial deficiency was present, a cause-and-effect relationship between the deficiency and the clinical state observed has not been clearly demonstrated. The patients described all had nonspherocytic hemolytic anemia. In one case, mesobilifuchsinuria was present, and there was marked benefit from splenectomy.[110] This patient antedated the discovery of the unstable hemoglobins and may, in point of fact, have had a hemoglobinopathy.

Only a few families with DPGM deficiency have been described since quantitative assay for this enzyme has been available. In one of these families, probable homozygosity was associated with a severe hemolytic anemia with a fatal outcome at 3 months of age. This child required almost 80 blood transfusions. Strangely, the bilirubin concentration of the serum did not rise over 1 mg/100 ml. Death was due to bronchopneumonia. Although the erythrocytes of the propositus were not examined, assay of the enzyme of the parents, who were cousins, was carried out and subnormal DPGM activity was demonstrated. It is of interest, however, that the monophosphoglyceromutase activity in these family members was found to be normal. The essentially benign nature of partial DPGM deficiency is emphasized by a fortuitous observation reported by Cartier et al.[114] In the process of verifying a new technique for measurement of red cell 2,3-DPG levels, a normal 36-year-old woman used as a control was found to have 2,3-DPG levels which were only about 30% of mean normal. A similar decrease in 2,3-DPG levels was discovered in the red cells of her father. Quantitation of DPGM activity in the erythrocytes disclosed an approximately 50% reduction in the enzyme activity. As expected, with subnormal 2,3-DPG levels there was a leftward displacement of the oxygen dissociation curve and the hemoglobin concentration of the blood was at the upper limit of normal. However, there was suggestive evidence that a mild hemolytic state existed: a borderline increase in the reticulocyte count and an increase in activity of age-related enzymes such as hexokinase and glucose-6-phosphate dehydrogenase was documented. The levels of the red cell intermediates were determined and a "crossover plot" showed a decrease in hexose monophosphate but a marked elevation of triose phosphates and fructose diphosphate, findings which are quite consistent with a block at the DPGM step of metabolism. ATP, ADP, and AMP levels were normal. Glucose consumption with or without methylene blue was normal. Very recently, total deficiency of DPGM was observed in a clinically healthy 42-year-old male.[225] 2,3-DPG was absent, there was marked increase in oxygen affinity of the red cells, and there was a moderate degree of polycythemia. Diphosphoglycerate phosphatase activity was absent, confirming the identity between this enzyme and DPGM. The clinical picture in this patient was very different from that of the possible case presented by Schröter,[113] suggesting either that Schröter's patient had a defect other than or in addition to DPGM deficiency, or that there is marked variability in expression of total DPGM deficiency. The heterozygous defect seems to be quite benign as indicated by the apparent normalcy of the parents of the child[113] and the heterozygotes detected by Cartier et al.[114]

It is noteworthy that the activity of monophosphoglycerate mutase (MPGM) has been reported to be normal in most patients with putative DPGM deficiency, even those in which DPGM was actually measured. This is somewhat surprising in view of the demonstration by Sasaki et al.[115] that each of these activities is a function of the same enzyme proteins. It is possible that an active site involved in DPGM activity has been affected by a mutation while the active site in monophosphoglyceromutase activity has been left unscathed. Moreover, the distribution of the various enzyme activities among the isozymes is not equal, so that one of the fractions has the highest proportion of MPGM but a smaller proportion of the total DPGM activity. The diagnosis of DPGM deficiency can now be clearly demonstrated by the direct spectrophotometric assay devised by Schröter and Kalinowsky.[55,116]

4.9. Diphosphoglycerate Phosphatase Deficiency

Two infants with cerebral dysgenesis, retarded development, hypertonia of musculature, very light hair, hyperlipidemia, and mild compensated hemolytic state have been studied by Jacobasch *et al.*[117] Hemolysates from these infants did not have the capacity to release inorganic phosphate from 2,3-DPG, suggesting that they were deficient in diphosphoglycerate phosphatase. The ATP content of the red cells was modestly increased to 159 and 140% of normal. Quantitative measurements of phosphoglycerate phosphatase were not carried out, and no additional patients with this syndrome appear to have been reported.

The diagnosis of 2,3-diphosphoglycerate phosphatase deficiency would be difficult because of the very low activity of this enzyme in normal red cells (Table 2). The reaction may be markedly accelerated by the addition of phosphoglycolate,[118] and the rate of decomposition of 2,3-DPG by hemolysates in the presence of phosphoglycolate can be used as a means for the estimation of the activity of this enzyme. However, it is conceivable that mutant forms of the enzyme may exist which are relatively inactive in their native state, but which assume normal activity in the presence of phosphoglycolate. Accordingly, it is probably preferable to attempt to measure this enzyme by incubating 2,3-DPG with crude hemolysates for several hours at 37°C, and measuring the gradual decline of 2,3-DPG levels.

4.10. Enolase Deficiency

The case of a patient studied in 1959 after developing hemolytic anemia following administration of nitrofurantoin was reported in 1972.[119] It was claimed that the patient and her sister were deficient in red cell enolase activity and suggested that there was a cause-and-effect relationship between the enolase deficiency and the hemolytic disorder. Several circumstances cast serious doubt upon the validity of this report. First of all, the putative decrease in enolase activity was very great, so that the patient would be expected to be homozygous for the deficiency state. No other homozygotes or even heterozygotes for enolase deficiency have ever been reported, even from laboratories which carry out hundreds of assays of this enzyme. More disturbing is the fact that the methods which were alleged to have been used to assay the red cell enzymes in this patient in 1959 were techniques developed long *after* the studies were done. Thus, it is reported that in 1959 assays for hexokinase were carried out by a method published in 1967, pyruvate kinase by a method published in 1962, and glucose-6-phosphate dehydrogenase by a screening method reported in 1966—a method which does not provide quantitative results of the type reported in the paper. Moreover, values are given for glutathione synthetase, an enzyme for which no assay method had been described at the time that this patient was studied.

In view of the serious weaknesses and discrepancies in this report, one is compelled to conclude that the existence of enolase deficiency has not been convincingly demonstrated, and the relationship between such a disorder and hemolytic anemia is totally unknown. Reliable enolase assays are carried out readily by a spectrophotometric technique.[55]

4.11. Defects in Glutathione Synthesis

Profound deficiency of red cell reduced glutathione was first reported by Oort et al. in 1961.[120] Additional details concerning their case were described in later publications[121,122] and additional reports of patients with severe deficiencies of red cell GSH appeared subsequently.[123–127] More moderate decreases in GSH levels have also been reported,[128–132] but the significance of the lowering of GSH levels in these patients is not clear; in most instances the change in GSH level was probably secondary to some other defect. Prins et al.[122] established that a defect in the synthesis of GSH existed in the patient originally reported by Oort and co-workers but the defective step was not identified. Since GSH synthesis is the result of two sequential enzymatic reactions, one catalyzed by γ-glutamyl cysteine synthetase (GC-S) and the other by glutathione synthetase (GSH-S), a deficiency in either of these two enzymes might have been responsible for inadequate glutathione synthesis. Identification of the defect responsible for GSH deficiency was first achieved by Boivin et al.[123,133] who demonstrated the lack of GSH-S activity in the red cells of their first patient. Subsequently, Boivin presented two patients with severe GSH-S deficiency, one patient with enzyme activity which was about one-third normal, and a fourth patient with GC-S deficiency whose red cell GSH levels varied from one-third to two-thirds normal.[132] Somewhat strangely, this patient is not mentioned in a subsequent review[134] and the credit for detecting the first case of γ-glutamyl cysteine synthetase deficiency is accorded to Konrad et al.[126] In 1970, Jellum et al.[135] reported a case of a mentally retarded and partially paralyzed 19-year-old boy who excreted large amounts of 5-oxoproline (pyroglutamic acid) in the urine. Although further studies of the metabolism of 5-oxoproline by the subject were reported in 1972,[136] it was not until 1974 that it was recognized that the patient's red cells lacked GSH.[137] The basic defect was established to be a deficiency in GSH-S,[138] and with the publication of additional, similar cases[127,139] it has become apparent that there are two types of GSH-S deficiency: some of the patients suffer from a neurologic defect and excrete large quantities of 5-oxoproline whereas others show only the presence of nonspherocytic hemolytic anemia.

Glutathione synthetase deficiency and GC-S deficiency both appear to be inherited as autosomal recessive disorders. Consanguinity is present in several families.[122,124] Heterozygotes for both types of defect were shown to have one-half normal enzyme activity.[124,126] In the case of both defects sex linkage is ruled out by pedigrees showing the father-to-son transmission.[124,126] Heterozygotes for defects in GSH synthesis are able to maintain normal GSH levels in their erythrocytes.[120,124,126] An animal model for glutathione deficiency exists: the red cells of low GSH sheep have been shown to be deficient in GC-S.[140] In the patients with GC-S deficiency the concentration of acid-soluble sulfhydryl compounds was decreased in leukocytes (42% of mean normal) and muscle (25% of mean normal).[125] In patients with glutathione synthetase deficiency, enzyme levels of cultured fibroblasts and placenta were found to be decreased.[138]

In addition to hereditary defects in the enzymes of glutathione synthesis, moderate degrees of GSH deficiency may exist as secondary manifestations of other red cell defects. The most common cause of modestly reduced red cell GSH level is G-6-PD deficiency.[141] Red cell GSH levels also appear to be diminished in the red cells of patients with unstable hemoglobins,[129,142] after drug intoxication,[128] in GPI deficiency,[23,25,26] and have been observed in association with abnormalities in cation homeostasis of red cells.[130]

The red cells in glutathione deficiency generally contain very little GSH. Red cells of members of a family studied by Prins et al.[122] contained 2 to 8 mg/100 ml GSH measured as acid-soluble sulfhydryl compounds, approximately 3 to 12% of normal. The fact that the red cells of these individuals contained glyoxylase activity, an activity which has an absolute requirement for GSH, indicates that some residual GSH was present. The red cells of a GSH synthetase-deficient patient reported by Mohler et al.[124] contain 8 to 15 mg/100 ml GSH, and those reported by Boivin[132] 0 to 21 mg/100 ml GSH. The red cells of the two sibs with GC-S deficiency contained 2 to 3% of normal GSH levels. In these patients, too, some glyoxylase activity was present, indicating that some GSH was actually present in the erythrocytes. The activity of other enzymes in GSH-deficient cells has generally been normal or somewhat increased.[122,124,126] Prins et al. observed a decrease in glutathione peroxidase (GSHPx) activity in the red cells of their patient,[122] but in the other reported cases[124,126] the activity of glutathione peroxidase was normal. Lactate production by GSH-deficient red cells is normal,[122] and minor abnormalities in cation fluxes have been described.[134] Study of the residual GSH-S in patients from two families with 5-oxoprolinuria showed no kinetic abnormalities with respect to glycine, γ-glutamyl-α-aminobutyrate, or ATP–magnesium. The temperature of activation appeared to be normal and there was no evidence of an inhibitor.[143]

All but one of the reported patients with hereditary glutathione defiency of the red cells have manifested a mild hemolytic anemia or compensated hemolysis with intermittent icterus. The single reported exception was a patient with 5-oxoprolinuria due to GSH-S deficiency. This patient unaccountably manifested no evidence of shortening of red cell life span.[127] Another such case also appears to exist.[143] Hemolysis seems to be exacerbated by the ingestion of "oxidant" drugs,[122,125] and an attack of favism has been observed in a GSH-deficient subject.[122,144] Cholelithiasis has been present in most of the patients with GSH deficiency. The two sibs with GC-S deficiency suffered from spinocerebellar degeneration.[125,126] One of these patients manifested psychotic behavior at age 29 and at age 35 was noted to have mild ataxia, impairment of coordination, and dysmetria in both upper and lower extremities. Her brother had slowed speech and a pes cavus deformity. Patients with 5-oxoprolinuria present with a severe metabolic acidosis. Neurologic symptoms were present in three out of the seven known cases. They included mental retardation, spastic tetraparesis, cerebellar disturbances with intentional tremor and atactic gait, increased resistance to passive movements predominantly of the pyramidal type, impaired coordination, and dysarthric speech.[135] Splenomegaly has been present in approximately half of the reported cases of GSH-S deficiency.

In one case, slight anisocytosis and hypochromia of the erythrocytes were noted on the blood film.[122] Moderate anisocytosis, poikilocytosis, and polychromatophilia were noted in another case.[126] The osmotic fragility of the erythrocytes is normal.[122,124,126] Autohemolysis has been slightly to moderately increased and not corrected by glucose.[123,124,126] The ascorbate–cyanide test has been reported to be positive[122] and negative.[125] When incubated with acetylphenylhydrazine[145] the red cells form many small Heinz bodies—even larger numbers than are found in G-6-PD-deficient cells.[122,124] Chromium-51 red cell survival studies are unreliable because GSH-deficient red cells are exquisitely sensitive to the damaging effect of chromium.[122] Leukocyte and platelet counts have been normal. In the patients with GC-S deficiency dibasic and monobasic monocarboxylic aminoaciduria was observed.[125] In these patients EEG and peripheral nerve conduction abnormalities were also documented and cerebrospinal fluid examination was normal.[125] Leukocyte oxygen consumption and phagocytosis were found to be normal.[125]

Treatment of the hematologic disease consists of avoidance of fava beans and drugs of the type that produce hemolysis and G-6-PD deficiency. Splenectomy was carried out in one patient and resulted in considerable improvement.[124] Detection of GSH deficiency of the erythrocytes is readily achieved using the 5,5'-dithiobis-(2-nitrobenzoic acid) reaction for nonprotein sulfhydryl compounds.[55,146] Definition of the underlying enzymatic defect is much more difficult. Assays for GSH-S and GC-S have been described,[147] and while technically difficult, are quite suitable for the definition of the enzymatic defect.

4.12. Glutathione Reductase Deficiency

In 1959 DesForges et al.[148] noted that the red cells of the patient who had undergone hemolysis after the administration of sulfoxone contained adequate amounts of G-6-PD, but that the red cell glutathione reductase activity was only approximately 60% of normal. Moderately decreased glutathione reductase activity was subsequently noted in patients with hemolytic anemia by Carson et al.[149] and by Löhr and Waller.[150] Subsequently, glutathione reductase deficiency was found in association not only with hereditary nonspherocytic hemolytic anemia, but also in patients with thrombocytopenia, leukopenia, pancytopenia, acute leukemia, hemophilia B, and a variety of nonhematologic disorders.[151] Moreover, screening of normal populations revealed a relatively high percentage of individuals with low red cell glutathione reductase activity.[152] It was initially believed that glutathione reductase deficiency, like some of the other recently discovered red cell enzyme deficiencies, was a hereditary abnormality, and it was proposed that it was an autosomal dominant trait.[152] The poorly defined clinical effects of the putative deficiency and the unconvincing nature of the family studies led to the suggestion that glutathione reductase deficiency was a secondary manifestation of a poorly understood basic disorder.[153] The nature of this disorder became evident when it was demonstrated that the hemolysates of riboflavin-deficient rats and humans were activated by small amounts of flavine adenine dinucleotide (FAD). Even normal human hemolysates were activated by traces of FAD, and the hemolysates of glutathione reductase-deficient patients could be restored to normal by incubation with FAD. Furthermore, the administration of physiologic quantities of riboflavin restored the glutathione reductase levels of the red cells of "deficient" individuals to normal within a few days.[154-156] The fact that red cell glutathione reductase activity can be manipulated by the administration of riboflavin made it possible to examine critically the putative cause-and-effect relationship between glutathione reductase deficiency and disease states. The production of glutathione reductase deficiency in rats through dietary riboflavin deprivation demonstrated that decreasing enzyme activity by about one-half, the degree commonly encountered in "glutathione reductase-deficient" patients, failed to render the red cells sensitive to drug-induced hemolysis.[157] A glutathione reductase-deficient woman was shown not to be sensitive to the hemolytic effect of primaquine when her red cell survival was monitored with the ^{51}Cr technique. No change in red cell survival occurred when the glutathione reductase deficiency was corrected by the administration of riboflavin[157] (Fig. 19). Correction of glutathione reductase deficiency by the administration of riboflavin has failed to affect the associated hematologic disorders. Restoration to normal of the glutathione reductase activity of the red cells of patients with hypoplastic anemia did not influence erythropoiesis.[158–161] It is quite apparent from these observations that the association between glutathione reductase and various disease states has been a fortuitous one; the glutathione reductase deficiency presumably was due to suboptimal riboflavin intake in ill patients. Many of the patients previously reported to be glutathione reductase-deficient have been reexamined. Assay of the red cell enzyme with and without activation by FAD or stimulation of riboflavin administration suggests that occasionally a partial deficiency of glutathione reductase unrelated to riboflavin nutrition may, indeed, exist.[162–165] The genetics of this less common type of glutathione reductase deficiency have not been established, although it is probably an autosomal dominant disorder. In no case has any cause-and-effect relationship between partial glutathione reductase deficiency and a disease state been demonstrated.

The fact that partial glutathione reductase deficiency is unlikely to produce any clinical consequences is emphasized by the unique observation of a patient with virtually total glutathione reductase deficiency.[166] Three sibs, offspring of a consanguinous marriage, were found to have no detectable glutathione reductase in their red cells. Neither riboflavin administration nor incubation of hemolysates with FAD restored any detectable enzyme activity. The glutathione reductase-deficient homozygotes were apparently hematologically normal (although details were not presented), except that a severe hemolytic episode was observed in one of the deficient subjects after ingestion of fava beans. G-6-PD deficiency was not present and the fact that G-6-PD activity was not increased suggests that in the steady state red cell life span was normal. One, and possibly two, of the sibs had cataracts.

It is interesting to note that although relatively sensitive methods did

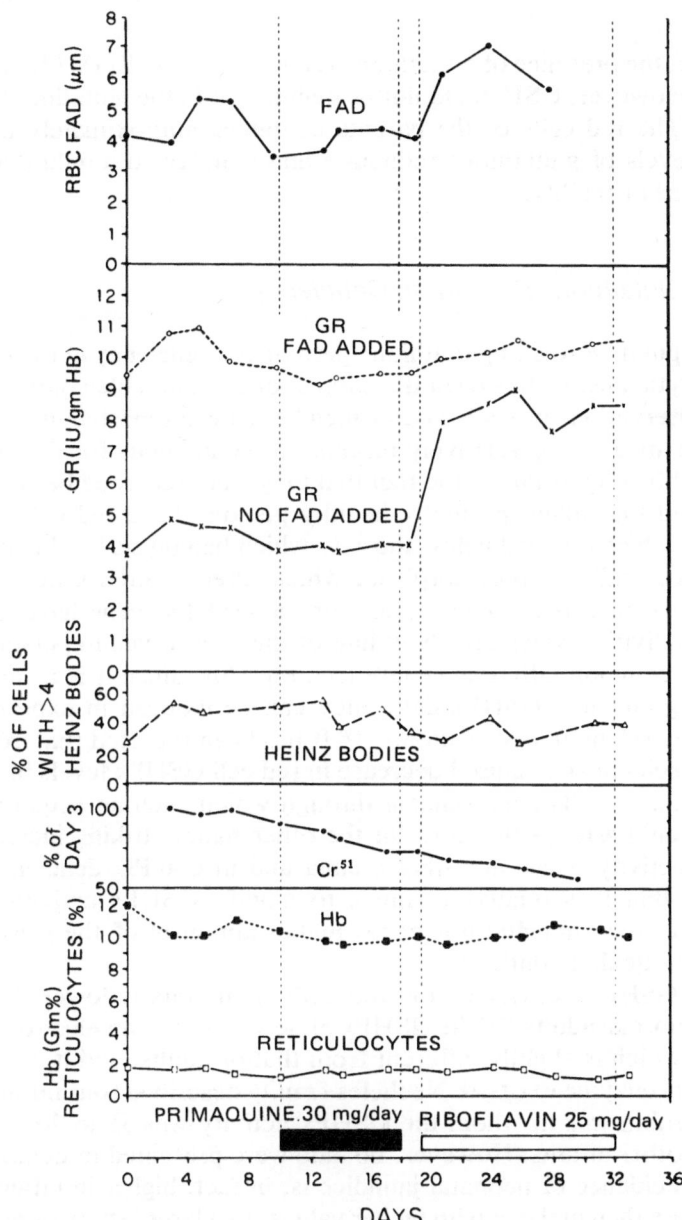

FIGURE 19. The effect of primaquine and of riboflavin administration on a patient with glutathione reductase (GR) deficiency. Although this subject's red cell GR activity was only approximately one-half of normal, administration of 30 mg of primaquine daily produced no evidence of hemolysis. Neither was red cell life span affected by the administration of riboflavin, which quickly normalized red cell glutathione reductase activity. (Reprinted from Beutler and Srivastava,[157] through the courtesy of *Nature*.)

not detect the presence of glutathione reductase, red cell GSH levels were normal. However, GSH could not be maintained in the glutathione stability test. The red cells of the parents contained approximately one-half normal levels of glutathione reductase and manifested a mild degree of glutathione instability.

4.13. Glutathione Peroxidase Deficiency

The putative role of glutathione peroxidase deficiency in the etiology of hemolytic anemia has been the subject of considerable confusion. All of the observations of such cases which have been reported in the literature were made using relatively unsatisfactory methods for the assay of GSHPx. Most important is the fact that they were recorded before it was recognized that many perfectly healthy persons have red cell GSHPx activities which are well below those to which hemolysis has been attributed. Specifically, a polymorphism which affects GSHPx activity has been shown to exist. Homozygotes for the GSHPx[L] gene have average GSHPx activities which are about half of those observed in persons with the more common GSHPx[H] gene[167] (see Fig. 20). Since it is a selenium-containing enzyme, GSHPx deficiency can be induced in experimental animals by selenium deprivation.[168,169] It has been reported that iron deficiency results in an acquired decrease in red cell GSHPx levels in rabbits and in man.[170-172] The mechanism through which such an acquired deficiency would arise is unclear. On the other hand, striking increases in GSHPx activity occur in α-thalassemia and in G-6-PD deficiency.[173,174] The fact that it is relatively simple to modify GSHPx activities by a variety of environmental influences makes appraisal of the genetics of GSHPx particularly difficult.

The GSHPx activity of the red cells of infants is lower than that found in normal adults.[175] The GSHPx of newborns has an electrophoretic mobility which is slightly different from that of adults, and it is possible that a fetal enzyme exists.[176] Necheles et al.[177] described four infants with hyperbilirubinemia in whom the GSHPx activity was 55 to 70% of that found in other infants. However, no data were presented to demonstrate that the incidence of neonatal jaundice is, in fact, higher in infants with low GSHPx than in those with higher values. In a larger study of newborn infants, no impressive relationship was observed between bilirubinemia and GSHPx activity. Only if the GSHPx activities of the infants with the highest and the lowest bilirubin levels were compared was any difference observed, and this difference was of borderline statistical significance.[178]

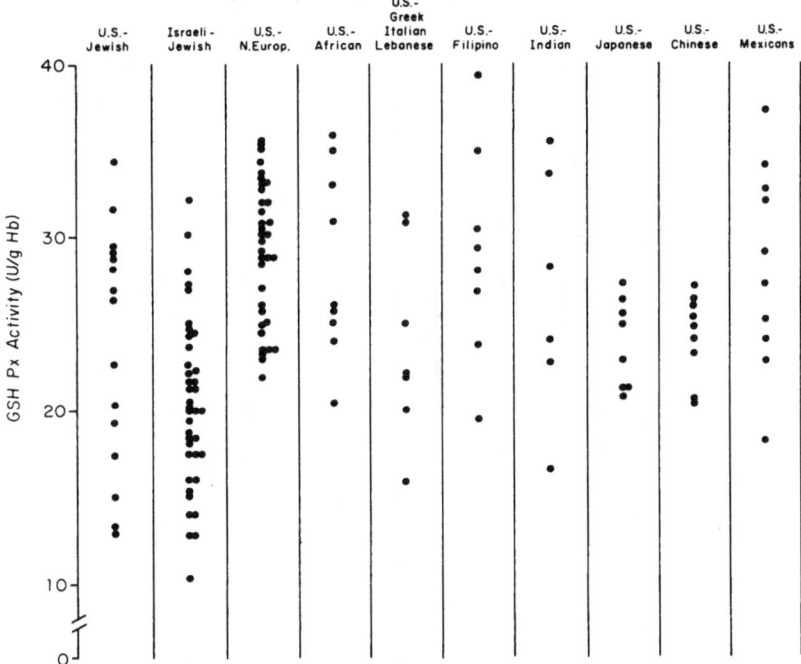

FIGURE 20.   Glutathione peroxidase (GSHPx) activities of the red cells of subjects from different ethnic groups. It is apparent that the red cell GSHPx activity of Jews and others of Mediterranean origin is substantially lower than that from those who are of northern European or African origin. Intermediate values are found in Orientals but there is a significant decrease in the extent of variability. (Reprinted from Beutler and Matsumato,[167] through the courtesy of Grune and Stratton.)

Figure 21 compares the reported cases with diminished GSHPx activity and hemolytic anemia with the GSHPx activities in healthy Jewish populations from the United States and a hospital population from Israel. It is apparent that in the vast majority of patients in whom a cause-and-effect relationship was assumed to exist between lowered GSHPx activity and hemolytic anemia the activity of the enzyme was in the same range as is encountered in unselected asymptomatic persons. In view of the very limited number of patients in whom an association was found between hemolysis and GSHPx activity and the very high frequency of the benign GSHPx[L] gene, not only in Jewish but in non-Jewish populations,[167] it does not seem valid to conclude that hemolysis in the subjects with "GSHPx deficiency" was, in point of fact, related to the lowered levels of this enzyme. Indeed, in one family in which severe anemia was ascribed to

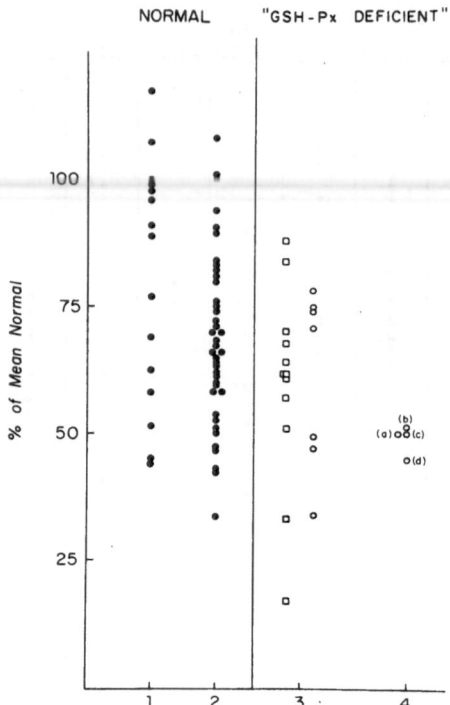

FIGURE 21. Comparison of glutathione peroxidase (GSHPx) activities in normal Jewish–
American (column 1) and Jewish–Israeli (column 2)[167] subjects with those which have been
reported in the literature to be diminished in infants (open squares) and adults (open circles).
Cases shown in column 3 are from Necheles *et al.*,[179] and in column 4 from (a) Miwa *et
al.*[180]; (b) Boivin *et al.*[181]; (c) Steinberg *et al.*[182]; and (d) Boivin *et al.*[183] Mean normal
values are those of non-Jewish U.S. adults.

GSHPx deficiency, the father of the patient whose GSHPx activity was
lower than that of the propositus had a hemoglobin of 17.0 g/100 ml, with
a reticulocyte count of 1%.[180]

   Although it is recognized that functional defects of an enzyme may
exist which are not reflected in absolute enzyme activity, kinetic characterization of the enzyme and thermal stability have been quite normal
when they were studied.[180,183] It is also possible that GSHPx deficiency,
like the common variants of G-6-PD deficiency, is not enough alone to
produce hemolysis. Perhaps GSHPx deficiency plus some other stress is
needed to precipitate hemolysis; no evidence has been presented to indicate that this is the case. Glutathione peroxidase deficiency has also been
observed with toxic sulfhemoglobinemia[184] and far advanced cirrhosis of

the liver.[185] The GSHPx activity of the red cells of the patient with sulfhemoglobinemia remained reduced to about 50% of normal, several months after the discontinuation of the drug which had caused the sulfhemoglobinemia. It seems unlikely that the GSHPx deficiency had any relationship to this drug-induced disorder. Examinations of the blood of the patient with liver failure were carried out shortly before death, and no relationship between GSHPx and the disease process could be demonstrated.

4.14. Phosphogluconate Dehydrogenase Deficiency

Although it has been suggested[186] that a deficiency of 6-phosphogluconate dehydrogenase (6-PGD) may cause hemolytic anemia, the weight of the evidence suggests that the association was a coincidental one. Lausecker et al.[186] observed that the 6-PGD activity of the red cells of a jaundiced newborn was only about one-half of normal. No other cause of newborn jaundice was found, but a variety of other metabolic disturbances of the red cells appeared to be present. Included were a marked decrease of red cell GSH levels to only 28% of mean normal with glutathione instability and a reduction of red cell ATP levels. Heinz body formation on incubation with acetylphenylhydrazine was altered with the formation of increased numbers of Heinz bodies, and the total of $NADP^+$ and NADPH was reported to be diminished. In view of these varied findings, it is difficult to determine the cause of the hemolytic anemia, but it seems unlikely that the decreased 6-PGD activity was an etiologic factor, since the well-documented genetic occurrence of much lower levels of 6-PGD has not been associated with significant hemolytic disease. In the course of a population survey Parr and Fitch[187] identified a mutant 6-phosphogluconate dehydrogenase which they designated the "Whitechapel" variant. The red cells of two subjects who were apparently homozygous for this variant contained only 2.4 and 4.5% of the mean normal 6-PGD activity. Unfortunately, no clinical description of these subjects was provided, but it is stated that neither of these two individuals showed any obvious clinical manifestations that could be attributed to red cell 6-PGD deficiency. Moreover, their red cell G-6-PD activity was only very slightly elevated, suggesting that minimal shortening of red cell life span might be present. A more extensive study[188] of individuals with partial 6-PGD deficiency indicated that these persons were heterozygous for a gene, very likely similar to the Whitechapel variant, and that their red cell life span was normal. Even when challenged with 60 mg of primaquine daily, little shortening of red cell survival was observed, and this was clearly attributable to partial G-6-PD deficiency.

4.15. Disorders of Nucleotide Metabolism

Because of the central role that ATP plays in red cell energy metabolism, numerous efforts have been made to implicate changes in ATP metabolism in the clinical occurrence of hemolysis. Only in the case of pyrimidine 5'-nucleotidase deficiency and increased adenosine deaminase activity, to be described later, is a cause-and-effect relationship between the enzymatic lesion and hemolytic anemia clear.

4.15.1. ATPase Deficiency

Adenosine triphosphatase (ATPase) deficiency was first described by Harvald et al. in 1964.[189] Additional cases were subsequently reported by Cotte et al.[190] and Löhr.[191] Harvald et al. reported occurrence of low red cell ATPase activity in some family members with hemolytic anemia, but other family members with similarly reduced ATPase levels manifested no evidence of hemolysis. Furthermore, in several family members who were reported to have had reduced ATPase activities in 1963 and 1964,[189] the total enzyme activity was normal in 1970 and the abnormality consisted only of failure of ATPase to be inhibited by digoxin.[192] The patient described by Cotte et al.[190] had a severely hypochromic microcytic anemia with a plasma iron decreased to 41 µg/100 ml and an iron binding capacity of 320 g/100 ml. Although the ^{51}Cr half-life of the red cells was reported to be decreased to 22$^{1}/_{2}$ days there were a few stigmata of hemolysis. The reticulocyte count was normal, or actually somewhat diminished; the serum bilirubin was only 0.2 mg/100 ml. It seems quite possible that the anemia of this patient was due to iron deficiency, and that the mild deficiency of ATPase which was observed was unrelated to the hematologic abnormality. Löhr's patient was a 9-year-old child with nonspherocytic hemolytic anemia and a 59% reduction in red cell ATPase activity. The potassium content of this patient's red cells was only 42% of normal while the sodium concentration was only about twice normal, leaving a large, unexplained deficit in total red cell cation content. There are a considerable number of other inconsistencies in the data presented. For example, the child's grandfather, whose red cell ATPase was normal, or nearly so, was reported to have a red cell potassium of 40 mEq/liter and a sodium of 14.4 mEq/liter. This would suggest that this apparently healthy male had only one-half of the normal cation content in his red cells.

ATPase activity seems to be sporadically decreased in a number of diverse red cell abnormalities, such as membrane lipid disturbances,[193] and in some patients with hereditary spherocytosis.[194-196] The fact that secondary changes in ATPase do occur and the marked inconsistencies in all the reports of ATPase deficiency cast serious doubt on the role of this enzyme deficiency in hemolytic anemia. While it is possible that partial ATPase deficiency may exist on a hereditary basis, its etiologic role in a disease state cannot be considered to be established.

4.15.2. Adenylate Kinase Deficiency

Adenylate kinase (AK) deficiency was first described by Szeinberg *et al.*[197,198] Like the electrophoretic variants of AK it is apparently transmitted as an autosomal recessive disorder: consanguinity was present in the parents, and their red cells contained approximately one-half normal AK activity.

Interpretation of findings in the family reported by Szeinberg *et al.* was complicated by the fact that the propositus was also severely G-6-PD deficient. The G-6-PD variant was not fully identified but was not of the common Mediterranean type. The propositus had a severe hemolytic anemia with a hemoglobin of 5.1 to 5.6 g/100 ml. A sister of the propositus, on the other hand, manifested more severe AK deficiency than her brother, but had only a relatively mild hemolytic anemia with a hemoglobin of 8.5 to 9 g/100 ml and a reticulocyte count of 2 to 3.2%. It seemed likely, therefore, that the relatively severe hemolysis observed in the propositus represented in large part the effect of a class 1 variant of G-6-PD. Hematologic data from six sibs with partial AK deficiency were, unfortunately, not presented. Although some doubt remains regarding a cause-and-effect relationship between AK deficiency and hemolysis in this family, this possibility is strengthened by a report of another case by Boivin *et al.*[199,200] A 14-year-old boy, known to be anemic since the age of 3 months, was found to have between 1 and 13% of normal AK activity in his red cells. Although hemoglobin levels were very slightly reduced during infancy, by the time the child was 7 years old a compensated hemolytic state was present with a hemoglobin level of 13.7 g/100 ml and 3.5% reticulocytes. Also present were thrombocytopenia with 31,000 platelets/mm³, 1 cm splenomegaly, and mild mental retardation. The parents had half-normal adenylate kinase activity, but were hematologically normal. Other family members, heterozygous and normal, were also hematologically normal. In the cases reported by Szeinberg et al.[198] the activity of age-related enzymes was slightly increased; in the case reported by Boivin it was normal—a surprising finding in view of the putative reticulocytosis. Levels of ATP were minimally elevated in the patients reported by Szeinberg et al.[198] and normal in the case reported by Boivin et al.[200]

4.15.3. "High ATP" Syndromes

An ill-defined group of disorders designated as "high ATP syndromes" has been described. Unexplained hereditary elevation of red cell ATP levels has been reported as a benign finding, unassociated with hemolytic disease.[201] When first studied, it was claimed that the original family described was different from that reported by Zürcher et al.[202] (vide infra) in that activity of red cell pyruvate kinase was normal. Restudy of the same family several years later[203] revealed a pattern of red cell intermediates which suggested that, in point of fact, the red cell pyruvate kinase activity was increased. Although the V_{max} of the enzyme appeared to be normal or actually somewhat decreased in vitro, the K_m for PEP also seemed to be decreased. This might impart a greater velocity to the enzyme reactions in vivo. In the family described by Zürcher et al.,[202] a dominantly inherited increase in ATP levels to about twice normal was associated with a moderately shortened ^{51}Cr red cell life span. However, probably as a result of a marked decrease in 2,3-DPG levels, hemoglobin levels were actually increased. An elevated red cell pyruvate kinase activity was believed to be responsible for the metabolic aberration.[202] In a similar family subsequently reported,[204] both parents and all three children had increased red cell ATP levels, making it difficult to ascertain the mode of inheritance.

Slightly elevated pyruvate kinase levels were documented in the two children whose red cells were examined for the activity of this enzyme. The elevated ATP levels observed in the two infants believed to have a deficiency in diphosphoglycerate phosphatase activity is discussed in Section 4.9.

In contrast with the findings in these families, a 37-year-old woman with long-standing hemolytic anemia was found to have red cell ATP and ADP levels which were aproximately twice normal. Pyruvate kinase activity was also elevated, and 2,3-DPG levels were about 1.5 times normal. The rate of glycolysis was not increased as might have been expected in a young red cell population. When the cells were incubated in the absence of substrate, the rate at which ATP levels fell was only about one-fifth of the rate observed in normal erythrocytes. It is not clear whether this patient suffered, in reality, from pyrimidine 5'-nucleotidase deficiency.

We have found that the method of ATP estimation which was employed by the authors measures cytidine and uridine triphosphates to only a very limited extent.[205] Furthermore, neither the illustration of the blood cell nor its relatively detailed description which reports the presence of poikilocytosis with bizarre cells, "spike cells," anisocytosis and polychromasia, occasional target cells, and Howell–Jolly bodies, gives any indication of the presence of stippled cells, which have been found in all cases of pyrimidine 5'-nucleotidase deficiency.

4.15.4. Pyrimidine 5'-Nucleotidase Deficiency

A new type of hemolytic anemia associated with ribose phosphate pyrophosphokinase (RPK) deficiency and what was thought initially to be an elevated red cell ATP level was described by Valentine et al.[206] The findings clearly differed from those previously described as "high ATP syndrome," in that striking basophilic stippling of the erythrocytes was present. Other features of the hemolytic disorder included type II autohemolysis, normal osmotic fragility, and moderately elevated GSH levels. In evaluating the potential relationship between high ATP levels and shortened red cell life span on the one hand, and RPK deficiency on the other, Valentine et al. concluded:

> It remains to be determined if RPK deficiency observed here is an epiphenomenon or is primary and causative. . . .

They soon detected second and third kindreds with the same disorder,[207] with clinical and biochemical findings very similar to those described in their first case. RPK activity was diminished to about 25% of normal in the red cells of one proband and to 35% of normal for the other. The GSH content of the red cells was increased. No RPK deficiency was observed in nonanemic family members, and the authors cautiously wrote:

> an etiologic role for RPK deficiency remains in doubt, though certainly not excluded.

Such a conservative approach to the possible relationship between the enzyme deficiency and the hemolytic anemia soon proved to be entirely warranted. With remarkable serendipity Valentine and co-workers demonstrated that the underlying defect was not RPK deficiency at all, but a deficiency of a hitherto undescribed enzyme, pyrimidine 5'-nucleotidase. Valentine et al.[208] noted that in the assay of ATP, carried out using the phosphoglycerate kinase reaction, the progress curves for ATP were consistently slower in red cell extracts from these patients than with those from other erythrocytes. This suggested that the substance being measured was not actually ATP, but rather an ATP analog which could react,

albeit slowly, with phosphoglycerate kinase. Enzymatic, chromatographic, and spectroscopic studies showed that large amounts of pyrimidine nucleotides were present in the erythrocytes. This led to the discovery of an enzymatic activity in normal hemolysates which had the
capacity to cleave phosphate from uridine monophosphate (UMP) or cytidine monophosphate (CMP). It was this activity, designated pyrimidine
5'-nucleotidase, which was lacking in the red cells of the affected
patients.

Pyrimidine 5'-nucleotidase deficiency is inherited as an autosomal
recessive disorder. The parents of patients as well as other nonanemic
relatives manifest a partial deficiency, and consanguinity was present in
two cases.[208,209] It has become clear that it is one of the more common
identified causes of nonspherocytic hemolytic anemia. In addition to the
two kindreds originally observed by Valentine *et al.*,[206,207] cases have been
reported from Israel,[210] Spain,[209] the United States,[211] France,[212] and Japan,[213] and we have examined deficient samples referred to us from Can-
ada[214] and from an Ashkenazi Jewish patient living in South Africa.[215,216]

Pyrimidine 5'-nucleotidase deficiency not only exists in a hereditary
form but can also be acquired as a result of lead poisoning. The enzyme is
strongly inhibited by lead,[217] and marked diminution of enzyme activity
has been observed in patients with lead poisoning.[218] Basophilic stippling
appears to be a consequence of pyrimidine 5'-nucleotidase deficiency,
whether hereditary or induced by lead intoxication.

The enzyme has recently been purified 250,000-fold from normal
human hemolysates. Its molecular weight is 45,000, its K_m for CMP is
10^{-5} M, and its pI is 5.0.[219]

The clinical manifestations of pyrimidine 5'-nucleotidase deficiency
are remarkably uniform in the 12 cases which have been detected to date.
The degree of anemia has been relatively mild, varying from a low of 7.5
g/100 ml[215] to a high of 10 g/100 ml.[207,208,220] In some instances the disorder
was first noted in early infancy,[207,210,214–216] in some cases in early childhood,[64,208] and in others not until late childhood or adult life.[207,220] Severe
neonatal jaundice was noted in two cases[215,216] in which the serum bilirubin level increased to about 15 mg/100 ml. Splenomegaly has been present
in all but two cases.[214,216] Basophilic stippling of the erythrocytes has been
the hallmark of this enzyme defect; it has been noted in all reported cases.
However, if blood is collected in EDTA and stored for 3 hr prior to
preparation of films, the stippling is no longer discernible. In contrast, the
stippling is easily seen in heparinized blood even after 24 hr of storage.[210]
Presumably the aggregation of RNA which forms the biochemical basis
for the appearance of stippling on stained blood films requires the presence of a divalent cation. A similar observation has been made in the case

of lead poisoning.[221] Type II autohemolysis[207,220] or atypical autohemolysis with a moderately increased hemolysis partially corrected by glucose[210,216] have been reported. The osmotic fragility has been normal[207,208,216,220] or minimally increased.[207,220] The red cells have shown increased activities of the age-related enzymes,[207,209,210,214,215,220,222] elevation of GSH levels,[207,209,215,220] decreased RPK activity,[207,209,220] and increased levels of glucose-6-P and fructose-6-P.[222] In one case increased Heinz body formation was noted after incubation with acetylphenylhydrazine,[207] but in other cases Heinz body formation was normal.[209] Splenectomy produced slight improvement in one case[220] and had no effect in another.[208]

4.15.5. Increased Adenosine Deaminase Activity

In 1972 Giblett *et al.* demonstrated that a marked decrease in the red cell adenosine deaminase (ADA) activity was associated with a combined immunodeficiency syndrome.[223] Deficiency of this enzyme did not appear to significantly influence erythrocyte function or survival. However, an increase in the activity of this enzyme has recently been shown to be the cause of an unusual type of hereditary hemolytic anemia.[224] Eleven members of three generations in one family were found to be affected. Transmission was as an autosomal dominant disorder. The anemia was mild, and in some instances fully compensated. In affected individuals, the reticulocyte count ranged from 3.3 to 11.7%. Splenomegaly was present. Red cell ATP levels in affected individuals averaged about 60% of normal controls and about 50% of controls with elevated reticulocyte counts. The activity of adenosine deaminase was 45 to 70 times the normal level. The ADA seemed to be normal in its electrophoretic mobility, displaying the common 1–1 phenotype. The possibility exists that this hemolytic disorder may represent the result of a regulatory mutation. It was suggested that increased activity of this enzyme may lead to lower red cell ATP levels by competing with adenosine kinase for adenosine which might be used by red cells to replenish adenine nucleotides.

References

1. LOEHR,G.W., WALLER,H.D., ANSCHUETZ,F. AND KNOPP,A., 1965,
    BIOCHEMISCHE DEFEKTE IN DEN BLUTZELLEN BEI FAMILIAERER
    PANMYELOPATHIE (TYP FANCONI). HUMANGENETIK 1:383-387

2. SCHROEDER,T.M., 1966, CYTOGENETISCHE UND CYTOLOGISCHE
    BEFUNDE BEI ENZYMOPENISCHEN PANMYELOPATHIEN UND PANCYTOPENIEN.
    HUMANGENETIK 2:287-316

3. VALENTINE,W.N., OSKI,F.A., PAGLIA,D.E., BAUGHAN,M.A.,
    SCHNEIDER,A.S. AND NAIMAN,J.L., 1967, HEREDITARY HEMOLYTIC
    ANEMIA WITH HEXOKINASE DEFICIENCY. ROLE OF HEXOKINASE IN
    ERYTHROCYTE AGING. N ENGL J MED 276:1-11

4. NECHELES,T.F., RAI,U.S. AND CAMERON,D., 1970, CONGENITAL
    NONSPHEROCYTIC HEMOLYTIC ANEMIA ASSOCIATED WITH AN UNUSUAL
    ERYTHROCYTE HEXOKINASE ABNORMALITY. J LAB CLIN MED 76:593-
    602

5. BADALYAN,L.O., BONDARENKO,E.S. AND ERMILCHENKO,G.V., 1970,
    HEREDITARY NONSPECIFIC HEMOLYTIC ANEMIA ASSOCIATED WITH A
    DEFICIENCY OF ERYTHROCYTE HEXOKINASE IN COMBINATION WITH
    GLYCOGENOSIS OF THE MUSCLES (RUSSIAN). KLIN MED (MOSK)
    48:156-163 (EXCERPTA MEDICA 5:420)

6. GOEBEL,K.M., GASSEL,W.D., GOEBEL,F.D. AND KAFFARNIK,H.,
    1972, HEMOLYTIC ANEMIA AND HEXOKINASE DEFICIENCY ASSOCIATED
    WITH MALFORMATIONS. KLIN WOCHENSCHR 50:349-851

7. KEITT,A.S., 1969, HEMOLTIC ANEMIA WITH IMPAIRED HEXOKINASE
    ACTIVITY. J CLIN INVEST 48:1997-2007

8. SEMENUK,M., WICKS,P., TOEWS,C.J. AND BRAIN,M.C., 1975,
    HEXOKINASE HAMILTON: AN ENZYME VARIANT WITH ABNORMAL KM
    FOR ADENOSINE TRIPHOSPHATE (ATP) IN NON-SPHEROCYTIC HEMOLYTIC
    ANEMIA. CLINICAL RESEARCH 23:628A (ABSTRACT)

9. BEUTLER,E., 1975, UNPUBLISHED

10. MOSER,K., 1969, DIE KONGENITALEN ENZYMOPENISCHEN
    HAEMOLYTISCHEN ANAEMIEN. WIEN KLIN WOCHENSCHR 14:249-258

11. MOSER,K., CIRESA,M. AND SCHWARZMEIER,J., 1970,
    HEXOKINASEMANGEL BEI HAEMOLYTISCHER ANAEMIE. MED WELT
    21:1976-1981

12. BEUTLER,E., DYMENT,P.G. AND MATSUMOTO,F., 1978, HEREDITARY
    NONSPHEROCYTIC HEMOLYTIC ANEMIA AND HEXOKINASE DEFICIENCY.
    BLOOD IN PRESS

13. KAPLAN,J.C. AND BEUTLER,E., 1968, HEXOKINASE ISOENZYMES IN
    HUMAN ERYTHROCYTES. SCIENCE 159:215-216

14. ALTAY,C., ALPER,C.A. AND NATHAN,D.G., 1970, NORMAL AND
    VARIANT ISOENZYMES OF HUMAN BLOOD CELL HEXOKINASE AND THE
    ISOENZYME PATTERNS IN HEMOLYTIC ANEMIA. BLOOD 36:219-227

15. SPENCER,N., HOPKINSON,D.A. AND HARRIS,H., 1964, AN
    ELECTROPHORETIC STUDY OF THE DISTRIBUTION AND PROPERTIES
    OF HUMAN HEXOKINASES. NATURE 204:742-745

16. MALONE,J.I., WINEGRAD,A.I., OSKI,F.A. AND HOLMES JR,E.W.,
    1968, ERYTHROCYTE HEXOKINASE ISOENZYME PATTERNS IN HEREDITARY
    HEMOGLOBINOPATHIES. N ENGL J MED 279:1071-1077

17. DELIVORIA-PAPADOPOULOS,M., OSKI,F.A. AND GOTTLIEB,A.J.,
    1969, OXYGEN-HEMOGLOBIN DISSOCIATION CURVES: EFFECT OF
    INHERITED ENZYME DEFECTS OF THE RED CELL. SCIENCE 165:601-
    602

18. BAUGHAN,M.A., VALENTINE,W.N., PAGLIA,D.E., WAYS,P.O.,
    SIMON,E.R. AND DE MARSH,Q.B., 1968, HEREDITARY HEMOLYTIC
    ANEMIA ASSOCIATED WITH GLUCOSEPHOSPHATE ISOMERASE (GPI)
    DEFICIENCY - A NEW ENZYME DEFECT OF HUMAN ERYTHROCYTES.
    BLOOD 32:236-249

19. KAHN,A., COTTREAU,D., BOYER,C., MARIE,J., GALAND,C. AND
    BOIVIN,P., 1976, CAUSAL MECHANISMS OF MULTIPLE ACQUIRED
    RED CELL ENZYME DEFECTS IN A PATIENT WITH ACQUIRED
    DYSERYTHROPOIESIS. BLOOD 48:653-662

20. PAGLIA,D.E. AND VALENTINE,W.N., 1974, HEREDITARY
    GLUCOSEPHOSPHATE ISOMERASE DEFICIENCY. A REVIEW. AM J CLIN
    PATHOL 62:740-751

21. SCHROETER,W., KOCH,H.H., WONNEBERGER,B. AND KALINOWSKY,W.,
    1974, GLUCOSE PHOSPHATE ISOMERASE DEFICIENCY WITH CONGENITAL
    NONSPHEROCYTIC HEMOLYTIC ANEMIA: A NEW VARIANT (TYPE
    NORDHORN) I. CLINICAL AND GENETIC STUDIES. PEDIATR RES
    8:18-25

22. ARNOLD,H., BLUME,K.G. AND LOEHR,G.W., 1974, GLUCOSE PHOSPHATE
    ISOMERASE DEFICIENCY WITH CONGENITAL NONSPHEROCYTIC HEMOLYTIC
    ANEMIA: A NEW VARIANT (TYPE NORDHORN). II. PURIFICATION
    AND BIOCHEMICAL PROPERTIES OF THE DEFECTIVE ENZYME. PEDIATR
    RES 8:26-30

23. BEUTLER,E., SIGALOVE,W.H., MUIR,W.A., MATSUMOTO,F. AND
    WEST,C., 1974, GLUCOSEPHOSPHATE-ISOMERASE (GPI) DEFICIENCY:GPI
    ELYRIA. ANN INTERN MED 80:730-732

24. PAGLIA,D.E., PAREDES,R., VALENTINE,W.N., DORANTES,S. AND
    KONRAD,P.N., 1975, UNIQUE PHENOTYPIC EXPRESSION OF
    GLUCOSEPHOSPHATE ISOMERASE DEFICIENCY. AM J HUM GENET 27:62-
    70

25. MIWA,S., NAKASHIMA,K., TAJIRI,M., ONO,J., ABE,S., ODA,E.,
    NONAKA,H., MATSUOKA,I., SHIMOYAMA,S., HIRATA,Y., AMAKI,I.,
    HORIUCHI,A., YAMAGUCHI,H. AND NISHINA,T., 1975, THREE CASES
    IN TWO FAMILIES WITH CONGENITAL NONSPHEROCYTIC HEMOLYTIC
    ANEMIA DUE TO DEFECTIVE GLUCOSEPHOSPHATE ISOMERASE: GPI
    MATSUMOTO. ACTA HAEMATOL JAP 38:238-247

26. VIVES-CORRONS,J.L., ROZMAN,C., KAHN,A., CARRERA,A. AND
    TRIGINER,J., 1975, GLUCOSE PHOSPHATE ISOMERASE DEFICIENCY
    WITH HEREDITARY HEMOLYTIC ANEMIA IN A SPANISH FAMILY:
    CLINICAL AND FAMILIAL STUDIES. HUMANGENETIK 29:291-297

27.   VAN BIERVLIET,J.P., VLUG,A., BARTSTRA,H., ROTTEVEEL,J.J.,
      DE VAAN,G.A.M. AND STAAL,G.E.J., 1975, A NEW VARIANT OF
      GLUCOSEPHOSPHATE ISOMERASE DEFICIENCY. HUMANGENETIK 30:35-
      40

28.   VAN BIERVLIET,J.P.G., VAN MILLIGEN-BOERSMA,L. AND
      STAAL,G.E.J., 1975, A NEW VARIANT OF GLUCOSEPHOSPHATE
      ISOMERASE DEFICIENCY (GPI-UTRECHT). CLIN CHIM ACTA 65:157-
      165

29.   ARNOLD,H., SEIBERLING,M., BLUME,K.G. AND LOEHR,G.W., 1975,
      IMMUNOLOGICAL STUDIES ON GLUCOSEPHOSPHATE ISOMERASE
      DEFICIENCY: INSTABILITY AND IMPAIRED SYNTHESIS OF THE
      DEFECTIVE ENZYME. KLIN WOCHENSCHR 53:1135-1136

30.   KAHN,A., VIVES,J.-.L., BERTRAND,O., COTTREAU,D., MARIE,J.
      AND BOIVIN,P., 1976, GLUCOSE-PHOSPHATE ISOMERASE DEFICIENCY
      DUE TO A NEW VARIANT (GP I BARCELONA) AND TO A SILENT GENE:
      BIOCHEMICAL, IMMUNOLOGICAL AND GENETIC STUDIES. CLIN CHIM
      ACTA 66:145-155

31.   VAN BIERVLIET,J.P.G., 1975, GLUCOSEPHOSPHATE ISOMERASE
      DEFICIENCY IN A DUTCH FAMILY. ACTA PAEDIATR SCAND 64:868-
      872

32.   HELLEMAN,P.W. AND VAN BIERVLIET,J.P.M., 1975, HAEMATOLOGICAL
      STUDIES IN A NEW VARIANT OF GLUCOSEPHOSPHATE ISOMERASE
      DEFICIENCY (GPI UTRECHT). HELV PAEDIATR ACTA 30:525-536

33.   VAN BIERVLIET J-P,G.M. AND STAAL,G.E.J., 1977, EXCESSIVE
      HEPATIC GLYCOGEN STORAGE IN GLUCOSEPHOSPHATE ISOMERASE
      DEFICIENCY. ACTA PAEDIATR SCAND 66:311-315

34.   SCHROETER,W. AND TILLMANN,W., 1977, CONGENITAL NONSPHEROCYTIC
      HEMOLYTIC ANEMIA ASSOCIATED WITH GLUCOSEPHOSPHATE ISOMERASE
      DEFICIENCY: VARIANT PADERBORN. KLIN WOCHENSCHR 55:393-396

35.   ARNOLD,H., ENGELHARDT,R. AND LOEHR,G.W., 1973,
      GLUCOSEPHOSPHAT-ISOMERASE TP RECKLINGHAUSEN- EINE NEUE
      DEFEKTVARIANTE MIT HAEMOLYTISCHER AENAMIE. KLIN WOCHENSCHR
      51:1198-1204

36.   ARNOLD,H., BLUME,K.G., BUSCH,D., LENKEIT,U., LOEHR,G.W.
      AND LUEBS,E., 1970, KLINISCHE UND BIOCHEMISCHE UNTERSUCHUNGEN
      ZUR GLUCOSEPHOSPHATISOMERASE NORMALER MENCHLICHER ERYTHROCYTEN
      UND BEI GLUCOSEPHOSPHATIOSMERASE- MANGEL. KLIN WOCHENSCHR
      48:1299-1308

37.   SCHROETER,W., BRITTINGER,G., ZIMMERSCHMITT,E., KOENIG,E.
      AND SCHRADER,D., 1971, COMBINED GLUCOSEPHOSPHATE ISOMERASE
      AND GLUCOSE-6-PHOSPHATE DEHYDROGENASE DEFICIENCY OF THE
      ERYTHROCYTES: A NEW HAEMOLYTIC SYNDROME. BR J HAEMATOL
      20:249-261

38.   BLUME,K.G., HRYNIUK,W., POWARS,D., TRINIDAD,F., WEST,C.
      AND BEUTLER,E., 1972, CHARACTERIZATION OF TWO NEW VARIANTS
      OF GLUCOSE-PHOSPHATE-ISOMERASE DEFICIENCY WITH HEREDITARY
      NONSPHEROCYTIC HEMOLYTIC ANEMIA. J LAB CLIN MED 79:942-949

39. MIWA,S., NAKASHIMA,K., ODA,S., ODA,E., MATSUMOTO,N., OGAWA,H. AND FUKUMOTO,Y., 1973, GLUCOSEPHOSPHATE ISOMERASE (GPI) DEFICIENCY. HEREDITARY NONSPHEROCYTIC HEMOLYTIC ANEMIA. REPORT OF THE FIRST CASE FOUND IN JAPANESE. ACTA HAEMATOL JAP 36:65-69

40. MIWA,S., NAKASHIMA,K., ODA,S., MATSUMOTO,N., OGAWA,H., KOBAYASHI,R., KOTANI,M., HARATA,A., ONAYA,T. AND YAMADA,T., 1973, GLUCOSEPHOSPHATE ISOMERASE (GPI) DEFICIENCY HEREDITARY NONSPHEROCYTIC HEMOLYTIC ANEMIA. REPORT OF SECOND CASE FOUND IN JAPANESE. ACTA HAEMATOL JAP 36:70-73

41. TILLEY,B.E., GRACY,R.W. AND WELCH,S.G., 1974, A POINT MUTATION INCREASING THE STABILITY OF HUMAN PHOSPHOGLUCOSE ISOMERASE. J BIOL CHEM 249:4571-4579

42. DETTER,J.C., WAYS,P.O., GIBLETT,E.R., BAUGHAN,M.A., HOPKINSON,D.A., POVEY,S. AND HARRIS,H., 1968, INHERITED VARIATIONS IN HUMAN PHOSPHOHEXOSE ISOMERASE. ANN HUM GENET 31:329-338

43. PAYNE,D.M., PORTER,D.W. AND GRACY,R.W., 1972, EVIDENCE AGAINST THE OCCURRENCE OF TISSUE-SPECIFIC VARIANTS AND ISOENZYMES OF PHOSPHOGLUCOSE ISOMERASE. ARCH BIOCHEM BIOPHYS 151:122-127

44. NAKASHIMA,K., MIWA,S., ODA,S., ODA,E., MATSUMOTO,N., FUKUMOTO,Y. AND YAMADA,T., 1973, ELECTROPHORETIC AND KINETIC STUDIES OF GLUCOSEPHOSPHATE ISOMERASE (GPI) IN TWO DIFFERENT JAPANESE FAMILIES WITH GPI DEFICIENCY. AM J HUM GENET 25:294-301

45. HUTTON,J.J. AND CHILCOTE,R.R., 1974, GLUCOSE PHOSPHATE ISOMERASE DEFICIENCY WITH HEREDITARY NONSPHEROCYTIC HEMOLYTIC ANEMIA. J PEDIATR 85:494-497

46. GIBLETT,E.R., 1969, GENETIC MARKERS IN HUMAN BLOOD FA DAVIS CO, PHILADELPHIA

47. LOEHR,G.W., ARNOLD,H., BLUME,K.G., ENGELHARDT,R. AND BEUTLER,E., 1973, HEREDITARY DEFICIENCY OF GLUCOSEPHOPHATE ISOMERASE AS A CAUSE OF NONSPHEROCYTIC HEMOLYTIC ANEMIA. BLUT 26:393-398

48. KAHN,A., ETIEMBLE,J., MEIENHOFER,M.C., BOIVIN,P., GALAND,C., COTTREAU,D. AND MARIE,J., 1975, ERYTHROCYTE PHOSPHOFRUCTOKINASE DEFICIENCY ASSOCIATED WITH AN UNSTABLE VARIANT OF MUSCLE PHOSPHOFRUCTOKINASE. CLIN CHIM ACTA 61:415-419

49. ARNOLD,H., BLUME,K.G., ENGELHARDT,R. AND LOEHR,G.W., 1973, GLUCOSEPHOSPHATE ISOMERASE DEFICIENCY: EVIDENCE FOR IN VIVO INSTABILITY OF AN ENZYME VARIANT WITH HEMOLYSIS. BLOOD 41:691-699

50. PAGLIA,D.E., HOLLAND,P., BAUGHAN,M.A. AND VALENTINE,W.N., 1969, OCCURRENCE OF DEFECTIVE HEXOSEPHOSPHATE ISOMERIZATION IN HUMAN ERYTHROCYTES AND LEUKOCYTES. N ENGL J MED 280:66-71

51.   MUELLER,E., MARTI,H.R., BACH,J., MICHELI,J.L. AND GASSER,C.,
      1974, HEREDITAERE NICHT-SPHAEROZYTAERE HAEMOLYTISCHE ANAEMIE
      DURCH GLUKOSEPHOSPHATISOMERASE-MANGEL: DER ERSTE IN DER
      SCHWEIZ BEOBACHTETE FALL. SCHWEIZ MED WOCHENSCHR 104:1379-
      1381

52.   OSKI,F. AND FULLER,E., 1971, GLUCOSE-PHOSPHATE ISOMERASE
      (GPI) DEFICIENCY ASSOCIATED WITH ABNORMAL OSMOTIC FRAGILITY
      AND SPHEROCYTES. CLINICAL RESEARCH 19:427 (ABSTRACT)

53.   VAN BIERVLIET,J.P.G., 1975, GLUCOSEPHOSPHATE ISOMERASE
      DEFICIENCY DRUKKERIJ ELINKWIJK BV, UTRECHT

54.   CHILCOTE,R.R. AND BAEHNER,R.L., 1974, RED CELL (RBC) GLUCOSE
      PHOSPHATE-ISOMERASE DEFICIENCY (GPI): CLINICAL AND LABORATORY
      EVIDENCE OF INCREASED BLOOD VISCOSITY. PEDIATR RES 8:398
      (ABSTRACT)

55.   BEUTLER,E., 1975, RED CELL METABOLISM. A MANUAL OF
      BIOCHEMICAL METHODS 2ND EDITON , GRUNE & STRATTON, NEW YORK

56.   BLUME,K.G. AND BEUTLER,E., 1972, DETECTION OF GLUCOSE-
      PHOSPHATE ISOMERASE DEFICIENCY BY A SCREENING PROCEDURE.
      BLOOD 39:685-687

57.   MATSUMOTO,N., ISHIHARA,T., ODA,E., MIWA,S., NAKASHIMA,K.,
      UCHINO,F. AND FUKUMOTO,Y., 1973, FINE STRUCTURE OF THE
      SPLEEN AND LIVER IN GLUCOSE-PHOSPHATE ISOMERASE (GPI)
      DEFICIENCY. HEREDITARY NONSPHEROCYTIC HEMOLYTIC ANEMIA--
      SELECTIVE RETICULOCYTE DESTRUCTION AS A MECHANISM OF
      HEMOLYSIS. ACTA HAEMATOL JAP 36:46-54

58.   TARUI,S., OKUNO,G., IKURA,Y., TANAKA,T., SUDA,M. AND
      NISHIKAWA,M., 1965, PHOSPHOFRUCTOKINASE DEFICIENCY IN
      SKELETAL MUSCLE. A NEW TYPE OF GLYCOGENOSIS. BIOCHEM BIOPHYS
      RES COMMUN 19:517-523

59.   TARUI,S., KONO,N., NASU,T. AND NISHIKAWA,M., 1969, ENZYMATIC
      BASIS FOR THE COEXISTENCE OF MYOPATHY AND HEMOLYTIC DISEASE
      IN INHERITED MUSCLE PHOSPHOFRUCTOKINASE DEFICIENCY. BIOCHEM
      BIOPHYS RES COMMUN 34:77-83

60.   LAYZER,R.B., ROWLAND,L.P. AND RANNEY,H.M., 1967, MUSCLE
      PHOSPHOFRUCTOKINASE DEFICIENCY. ARCH NEUROL 17:512-523

61.   SERRATRICE,G., MONGES,A., ROUX,H., AQUARON,R. AND
      GAMBARELLI,D., 1969, FORME MYOPATHIQUE DU DEFICIT EN
      PHOSPHOFRUCTOKINASE. REV NEUROL (PARIS) 120:271-277

62.   WATERBURY,L. AND FRENKEL,E.P., 1972, HEREDITARY NONSPHEROCYTIC
      HEMOLYSIS WITH ERYTHROCYTE PHOSPHOFRUCTOKINASE DEFICIENCY.
      BLOOD 39:415-425

63.   LUTCHER,C.L. AND BIGLEY,R.L., 1974, HEMOLYTIC ANEMIA DUE
      TO PHOSPHOFRUCTOKINASE (PFK) DEFICIENCY. CLINICAL RESEARCH
      22:66A (ABSTRACT)

64.   ODA,S., ODA,E. AND TANAKA,K.R., 1977, ERYTHROCYTE
      PHOSPHOFRUCTOKINASE (PFK) DEFICIENCY: CHARACTERIZATION AND
      METABOLIC STUDIES. CLINICAL RESEARCH 25:344A (ABSTRACT)

65. MIWA,S., SATO,T., MURAO,H., KOZURU,M. AND IBAYASHI,H., 1972, A NEW TYPE OF PHOSPHOFRUCTOKINASE DEFICIENCY HEREDITARY NONSPHEROCYTIC HEMOLYTIC ANEMIA. ACTA HAEMATOL JAP 35:113-118

66. NIESSNER,H. AND BEUTLER,E., 1974, STARCH GEL ELECTROPHORESIS OF PHOSPHOFRUCTOKINASE IN RED CELLS. BIOCHEM MED 9:73-76

67. LAYZER,R.B., ROWLAND,L.P. AND BANK,W.J., 1969, PHYSICAL AND KINETIC PROPERTIES OF HUMAN PHOSPHOFRUCTOKINASE FROM SKELETAL MUSCLE AND ERYTHROCYTES. J BIOL CHEM 244:3823-3831

68. ETIEMBLE,J., KAHN,A., BOIVIN,P., BERNARD,J.F. AND GOUDEMAND,M., 1976, HEREDITARY HEMOLYTIC ANEMIA WITH ERYTHROCYTE PHOSPHOFRUCTOKINASE DEFICIENCY. HUM GENET 31:83-91

69. TARUI,S., KONO,N. AND KUMAJIMA,M., 1976, INTERRELATION BETWEEN PHOSPHOFRUCTOKINASE ACTIVITY AND 2,3-DIPHOSPHOGLYCERATE LEVEL IN ERYTHROCYTES: STUDIES ON HERDITARY PHOSPHOFRUCTOKINASE DEFICIENCY AND DIABETIC KEOTACIDOSIS. 16TH CONGRESS INTERNATIONAL SOCIETY OF HEMATOLOGY, KYOTO ABSTRACT 2-68

70. KARADSHEH,N.S., UYEDA,K. AND OLIVER,R.M., 1977, STUDIES ON STRUCTURE OF HUMAN ERYTHROCYTE PHOSPHOFRUCTOKINASE. J BIOL CHEM 252:3515-3524

71. BEUTLER,E., SCOTT,S., BISHOP,A., MARGOLIS,N., MATSUMOTU,F. AND KUHL,W., 1974, RED CELL ALDOLASE DEFICIENCY AND HEMOLYTIC ANEMIA: A NEW SYNDROME. TRANS ASSOC AM PHYSICIANS 86:154-166

72. PENHOET,E., RAJKUMAR,T. AND RUTTER,W.J., 1966, MULTIPLE FORMS OF FRUCTOSE DIPHOSPHATE ALDOLASE IN MAMMALIAN TISSUES. PROC NATL ACAD SCI USA 56:1275-1282

73. LEBHERZ,H.G. AND RUTTER,W.J., 1969, DISTRIBUTION OF FRUCTOSE DIPHOSPHATE ALDOLASE VARIANTS IN BIOLOGICAL SYSTEMS. BIOCHEMISTRY 8:109-121

74. MIDELFORT,C.F. AND MEHLER,A.H., 1972, DEAMIDATION IN VIVO OF AN ASPARAGINE RESIDUE OF RABBIT MUSCLE ALDOLASE. PROC NATL ACAD SCI USA 69:1816-1819

75. BEUTLER,E., 1977, COMMENT ON " 'ALDOLASE A' DEFICIENCY WITH SYNDROME OF GROWTH AND DEVELOPMENTAL RETARDATION, MIDFACIAL HYPOPLASIA, HEPATOMEGALY, AND CONSANGUINEOUS PARENTS" BY R.B. LOWRY AND J.W. HANSON. BIRTH DEFECTS: ORIGINAL ARTICLE SERIES ALDOLA,S.E. ED. 13:227-228

76. SCHNEIDER,A.S., VALENTINE,W.N., HATTORI,M. AND HEINS JR,H.L., 1965, HEREDITARY HEMOLYTIC ANEMIA WITH TRIOSEPHOSPHATE ISOMERASE DEFICIENCY. N ENGL J MED 272:229-235

77. FREYCON,F., LAURAS,B. AND BOVIER-LAPIERRE,F., 1975, HEREDITARY HEMOLYTIC ANEMIA WITH TRIOSE PHOSPHATE ISOMERASE DEFICIENCY. PEDIATRIE 30:55-65

78. HARRIS,S.R., PAGLIA,D.E., JAFFE,E.R., VALENTINE,W.N. AND
     KLEIN,R.L., 1970, TRIOSEPHOSPHATE ISOMERASE DEFICIENCY IN
     AN ADULT. CLINICAL RESEARCH 18:529

79. VALENTINE,W.N., SCHNEIDER,A.S., BAUGHAN,M.A., PAGLIA,D.E.
     AND HEINS JR,H.L., 1966, HEREDITARY HEMOLYTIC ANEMIA WITH
     TRIOSEPHOSPHATE ISOMERASE DEFICIENCY. AM J MED 41:27-41

80. BEUTLER,E. AND BATTLES,N., 1977, UNPUBLISHED

81. SCHNEIDER,A.S., VALENTINE,W.N., BAUGHAN,M.A., PAGLIA,D.E.,
     SHORE,N.A. AND HEINS JR,H.L., 1968, TRIOSEPHOSPHATE ISOMERASE
     DEFICIENCY. A MULTI-SYSTEM INHERITED ENZYME DISORDER:
     CLINICAL AND GENETIC ASPECTS. HEREDITARY DISORDERS OF
     ERYTHROCYTE METABOLISM BEUTLER,E. ED. 265-272, CITY OF HOPE
     SYMP. SERIES, VOL. I, GRUNE & STRATTON, N.Y.

82. ROZACKY,E.E., SAWYER,T.H., BARTON,R.A. AND GRACY,R.W.,
     1971, STUDIES ON HUMAN TRIOSEPHOSPHATE ISOMERASE. 1.
     ISOLATION AND PROPERTIES OF THE ENZYME FROM ERYTHROCYTES.
     ARCH BIOCHEM BIOPHYS 146:312-320

83. KAPLAN,J.C., TEEPLE,L., SHORE,N. AND BEUTLER,E., 1968,
     ELECTROPHORETIC ABNORMALITY IN TRIOSEPHOSPHATE ISOMERASE
     DEFICIENCY. BIOCHEM BIOPHYS RES COMMUN 31:768-773

84. SCHNEIDER,A.S., DUNN,I., IBSEN,K.H. AND WEINSTEIN,I.M.,
     1968, TRIOSEPHOSPHATE ISOMERASE DEFICIENCY. B. INHERITED
     TRIOSEPHOSPHATE ISOMERASE DEFICIENCY. ERYTHROCYTE
     CARBOHYDRATE METABOLISM AND PRELIMINARY STUDIES. HEREDITARY
     DISORDERS OF ERYTHROCYTE METABOLISM BEUTLER,E. ED. 273-279,
     CITY OF HOPE SYMP. SERIES, VOL. I, GRUNE & STRATTON, N.Y.

85. ANGELMAN,H., BRAIN,M.C. AND MAC IVER,J.E., 1970, A CASE OF
     TRIOSEPHOSPHATE ISOMERASE DEFICIENCY WITH SUDDEN DEATH.
     XIII INTERNATIONAL CONGRESS OF HEMATOLOGY, MUNICH 122
     (ABSTRACT)

86. KAPLAN,J.C., SHORE,N. AND BEUTLER,E., 1968, THE RAPID
     DETECTION OF TRIOSE PHOSPHATE ISOMERASE DEFICIENCY. AM J
     CLIN PATHOL 50:656-658

87. LOWE,M.L. AND GIN,J.B., 1972, MODIFICATION IN A SCREENING
     TEST FOR TRIOSEPHOSPHATE ISOMERASE DEFICIENCY. CLIN CHEM
     18:1551 (LETTER TO THE EDITOR)

88. VALENTINE,W.N., HSIEH,H., PAGLIA,D.E., ANDERSON,H.M.,
     BAUGHAN,M.A., JAFFE,E.R. AND GARSON,O.M., 1969, HEREDITARY
     HEMOLYTIC ANEMIA ASSOCIATED WITH PHOSPHOGLYCERATE KINASE
     DEFICIENCY IN ERYTHROCYTES AND LEUKOCYTES. N ENGL J MED
     280:528-534

89. KRAUS,A.P., LANGSTON JR,M.F. AND LYNCH,B.L., 1968, RED CELL
     PHOSPHOGLYCERATE KINASE DEFICIENCY. BIOCHEM BIOPHYS RES
     COMMUN 30:173-177

90. BEUTLER,E., 1969, ELECTROPHORESIS OF PHOSPHOGLYCERATE
     KINASE. BIOCHEM GENET 3:189-195

91. CHEN,S.-.H., MALCOLM,L.A., YOSHIDA,A. AND GIBLETT,E.R., 1971, PHOSPHOGLYCERATE KINASE: AN X-LINKED POLYMORPHISM IN MAN. AM J HUM GENET 23:87-91

92. KONRAD,P.N., MC CARTHY,D.J., MAUER,A.M., VALENTINE,W.N. AND PAGLIA,D.E., 1973, ERYTHROCYTE AND LEUKOCYTE PHOSPHOGLYCERATE KINASE DEFICIENCY WITH NEUROLOGIC DISEASE. J PEDIATR 82:456-460

93. HJELM,M. AND WADMAN,B., 1970, NONSPHEROCYTIC HAEMOLYTIC ANAEMIA WITH PHOSPHOGLYCERATE KINASE DEFICIENCY. 13TH INTERNATIONAL CONGRESS HEMATOLOGY, MUNICH, P. 121

94. ARESE,P., BOSIA,A., GALLO,E., MAZZA,U. AND PESCARMONA,G.P., 1973, RED CELL GLYCOLYSIS IN A CASE OF 3-PHOSPHOGLYCERATE KINASE DEFICIENCY. EUR J CLIN INVEST 3:86-92

95. CARTIER,P., HABIBI,B., LEROUX,J.P. AND MARCHAND,J.C., 1971, ANEMIE HEMOLYTIQUE CONGENITALE ASSOCIEE A UN DEFICIT EN PHOSPHOGLYCERATE-KINASE DANS LES GLOBULES ROUGES, LES POLYNUCLEAIRES ET LES LYMPHOCYTES. NOUV REV FR HEMATOL 11:565-578

96. BOIVIN,P., HAKIM,J., MANDEREAU,J., GALAND,C., DEGOS,F. AND SCHAISON,G., 1974, ERYTHROCYTE AND LEUCOCYTE 3- PHOSPHOGLYCERATE KINASE DEFICIENCY. STUDIES OF PROPERTIES OF THE ENZYME, PHAGOCYTIC ACTIVITY OF THE POLYMORPHONUCLEAR LEUCOCYTES AND A REVIEW OF THE LITERATURE. NOUV REV FR HEMATOL 14:496-508

97. MIWA,S., NAKASHIMA,K., ODA,S., OGAWA,H., NAGAFUJI,H., ARIMA,M., OKUNA,T. AND NAKASHIMA,T., 1972, PHOSPHOGLYCERATE KINASE (PGK) DEFICIENCY HEREDITARY NONSPHEROCYTIC HEMOLYTIC ANEMIA: REPORT OF A CASE FOUND IN A JAPANESE FAMILY. ACTA HAEMATOL JAP 35:571-574

98. STRAUSS,R.G., MC CARTHY,D.J. AND MAUER,A.M., 1974, NEUTROPHIL FUNCTION IN CONGENITAL PHOSPHOGLYCERATE KINASE DEFICIENCY. J PEDIATR 85:341-344

99. BAEHNER,R.L., FEIG,S.A., SEGEL,G.B., ANDERSON,H.N. AND JAFFE,E.R., 1971, METABOLIC PHAGOCYTIC AND BACTERIOCIDAL PROPERTIES OF PHOSPHOGLYCERATE KINASE DEFICIENT (PGK) POLYMORPHONUCLEAR LEUKOCYTES (PMN). BLOOD 38:833 (ABSTRACT)

100. YOSHIDA,A. AND WATANABE,S., 1972, HUMAN PHOSPHOGLYCERATE KINASE I. CRYSTALLIZATION AND CHARACTERIZATION OF NORMAL ENZYME. J BIOL CHEM 247:440-445

101. YOSHIDA,A., WATANABE,S., CHEN,S.-.H., GIBLETT,E.R. AND MALCOLM,L.A., 1972, HUMAN PHOSPHOGLYCERATE KINASE II. STRUCTURE OF A VARIANT ENZYME. J BIOL CHEM 247:446-449

102. KAHN,A., COTTREAU,D., GALAND,C. AND BOIVIN,P., 1976, HUMAN ERYTHROCYTE PHOSPHOGLYCERATE KINASE DEFICIENCY: PRESENCE IN A DEFICIENT PATIENT OF A STABLE VARIANT WITH LOWERED CATALYTIC ACTIVITY. CLIN CHIM ACTA 69:21-28

103. OSKI,F. AND WHAUN,J., 1969, HEMOLYTIC ANEMIA AND RED CELL GLYCERALDEHYDE-3-PHOSPHATE DEHYDROGENASE (G-3-PD) DEFICIENCY. CLINICAL RESEARCH 17:601 (ABSTRACT)

104. PEZNIK,B.I.A. AND SOROKA,I.U.A., 1972, RARE CASE OF HEREDITARY NONSPHEROCYTIC ANEMIA CAUSED BY GLYCERALDEHYDE-PHOSPHATE DEHYDROGENASE DEFICIENCY IN ERYTHROCYTES. PROBL GEMATOL PERELIV KROVI 17:53-54

105. HARKNESS,D.R., 1966, A NEW ERYTHROCYTIC ENZYME DEFECT WITH HEMOLYTIC ANEMIA: GLYCERALDEHYDE-3-PHOSPHATE DEHYDROGENASE DEFICIENCY. J LAB CLIN MED 68:879-880 (ABSTRACT)

106. MC CANN,S.R., FINKEL,B., CADMAN,S. AND ALLEN,D.W., 1976, STUDY OF A KINDRED WITH HEREDITARY SPHEROCYTOSIS AND GLYCERALDEHYDE-3- PHOSPHATE DEHYDROGENASE DEFICIENCY. BLOOD 47:171-181

107. BOWDLER,A.J. AND PRANKERD,T.A.J., 1964, STUDIES IN CONGENITAL NON-SPHEROCYTIC HAEMOLYTIC ANAEMIAS WITH SPECIFIC ENZYME DEFECTS. ACTA HAEMATOL 31:65-78

108. ALAGILLE,D., FLEURY,J. AND ODIEVRE,M., 1964, DEFICIT CONGENITAL EN 2-3-DIPHOSPHOGLYCEROMUTASE. SOCIETE MEDICALE DES HOPITAUX DE PARIS 115:493-499

109. LOEHR,G.W. AND WALLER,H.D., 1963, ZUR BIOCHEMIE EINIGER ANGEBORENER HAEMOLYTISCHER ANAEMIEN. FOLIA HAEMATOL (LEIPZ) 8:377-397

110. LELONG,M., FLEURY,J., ALAGILLE,D., MALASSENET,R., LORTHOLARY,P. AND PARA,M., 1961, L'ANEMIE HEMOLYTIQUE CONSTITUTIONNNELLE NON SPHEROCYTAIRE AVEC PIGMENTURIE. NOUV REV FR HEMATOL 1:819-831

111. LOEHR,G.W., 1962, NICHTSPHAEROZYTAERE HAEMOLYTISCHE ANAEMIEN. ERBLICHE STOFFWECHSELKRANKHEITEN LINNEWEH,F. ED. 328-332, URBAN & SCHWARZENBERG, MUNICH/BERLIN

112. WALLER,H.D., 1962, HEREDITAERE ENZYMOPATHIEN DER ROTEN BLUTKOERPERCHEN. PROC 8TH CONG EUROP SOC HAEMATOL

113. SCHROETER,W., 1965, KONGENITALE NICHTSPHAEROCYTAERE HAEMOLYTISCHE ANAEMIE BEI 2,3-DIPHOSPHO- GLYCERATMUTASE- MANGEL DER ERYTHROCYTEN IM FRUEHEN SAUGLINGSALTER. KLIN WOCHENSCHR 43:1147-1153

114. CARTIER,P., LABIE,D., LEROUX,J.P., NAJMAN,A. AND DEMAUGRE,F., 1972, DEFICIT FAMILIAL EN DIPHOSPHOGLYCERATE-MUTASE: ETUDE HEMATOLOGIQUE ET BIOCHIMIQUE. NOUV REV FR HEMATOL 12:269-288

115. SASAKI,R., IKURA,K., SUGIMOTO,E. AND CHIBA,H., 1975, PURIFICATION OF BISPHOSPHOGLYCEROMUTASE, 2,3- BISPHOSPHOGLYCERATE PHOSPHATASE AND PHOSPHOGLYCEROMUTASE FROM HUMAN ERYTHROCYTES. EUR J BIOCHEM 50:581-593

116. SCHROETER,W. AND KALINOWSKY,W., 1969, ERYTHROCYTE 2,3- DIPHOSPHOGLYCERATE MUTASE: AN OPTICAL TEST IN HEMOLYSATES. CLIN CHIM ACTA 25:283-285

117. JACOBASCH,G., SYLLM-RAPOPORT,I., ROIGAS,H. AND RAPOPORT,S., 1964, 2,3-PGASE-MANGEL ALS MOEGLICHE URSACHE ERHOEHTEN ATP- GEHALTES. CLIN CHIM ACTA 10:477-478

118. ROSE,Z. AND LIEBOWITZ,J., 1970, 2,3-DIPHOSPHOGLYCERATE PHOSPHATASE FROM HUMAN ERYTHROCYTES. GENERAL PROPERTIES AND ACTIVATION BY ANIONS. J BIOL CHEM 245:3232-3241

119. STEFANINI,M., 1972, CHRONIC HEMOLYTIC ANEMIA ASSOCIATED WITH ERYTHROCYTE ENOLASE DEFICIENCY EXACERBATED BY INGESTION OF NITROFURANTOIN. AM J CLIN PATHOL 58:408-414

120. OORT,M., LOOS,J.A. AND PRINS,H.K., 1961, HEREDITARY ABSENCE OF REDUCED GLUTATHIONE IN THE ERYTHROCYTES - A NEW CLINICAL AND BIOCHEMICAL ENTITY?. VOX SANG 6:370-373

121. PRINS,H.K., OORT,M., LOOS,J.A., ZUERCHER,C. AND BECKERS,T., 1963, HEREDITARY ABSENCE OF GLUTATHIONE IN THE ERYTHROCYTES; BIOCHEMICAL, HAEMATOLOGICAL, AND GENETICAL STUDIES. PROC. 9TH CONG. EUROP. SOC. HAEMAT., LISBON PART II/I: 721-728

122. PRINS,H.K., OORT,M., LOOS,J.A., ZUERCHER,C. AND BECKERS,T., 1966, CONGENITAL NONSPHEROCYTIC HEMOLYTIC ANEMIA, ASSOCIATED WITH GLUTATHIONE DEFICIENCY OF THE ERYTHROCYTES. BLOOD 27:145-166

123. BOIVIN,P., GALAND,C., ANDRE,R. AND DEBRAY,J., 1966, ANEMIES HEMOLYTIQUES CONGENITALES AVEC DEFICIT ISOLE EN GLUTATHION REDUIT PAR DEFICIT EN GLUTATHION SYNTHETASE. NOUV REV FR HEMATOL 6:859-866

124. MOHLER,D.N., MAJERUS,P.W., MINNICH,V., HESS,C.E. AND GARRICK,M.D., 1970, GLUTATHIONE SYNTHETASE DEFICIENCY AS A CAUSE OF HEREDITARY HEMOLYTIC DISEASE. N ENGL J MED 283:1253-1257

125. RICHARDS II,F., COOPER,M.R., PEARCE,L.A., COWAN,R.J. AND SPURR,C.L., 1974, FAMILIAL SPINOCEREBELLAR DEGENERATION, HEMOLYTIC ANEMIA, AND GLUTATHIONE DEFICIENCY. ARCH INTERN MED 134:534-537

126. KONRAD,P.N., RICHARDS II,F., VALENTINE,W.N. AND PAGLIA,D.E., 1972, GAMMA-GLUTAMYL-CYSTEINE SYNTHETASE DEFICIENCY. N ENGL J MED 286:557-561

127. MARSTEIN,S., JELLUM,E., HALPERN,B., ELDJARN,L. AND PERRY,T.L., 1976, BIOCHEMICAL STUDIES OF ERYTHROCYTES IN A PATIENT WITH PYROGLUTAMIC ACIDEMIA (5-OXOPROLINEMIA). N ENGL J MED 295:406-412

128. LOEHR,G.W., BAUM,P. AND KAMM,G., 1963, TOXISCHE HAEMOLYTISCHE ANAEMIEN. MED KLIN 58:2111-2120

129. ZINKHAM,W.H. AND LENHARD,R.E., 1959, METABOLIC ABNORMALITIES OF ERYTHROCYTES FROM PATIENTS WITH CONGENITAL NONSPHEROCYTIC HEMOLYTIC ANEMIA. J PEDIATR 55:319-336

130. LO,S.S., MARTI,H.R. AND HITZIG,W.H., 1971, HEMOLYTIC ANEMIA ASSOCIATED WITH DECREASED CONCENTRATION OF REDUCED GLUTATHIONE IN RED CELLS. ACTA HAEMATOL 46:14-23

131. WALLER,H.D. AND GEROK,W., 1964, SCHWERE STAHLENINDUZIERTE HAEMOLYSE BEI HEREDITAEREM MANGEL AN REDUZIERTEM GLUTATHION IN BLUTZELLEN. KLIN WOCHENSCHR 42:948-954

132. BOIVIN,P., 1968, ANEMIES HEMOLYTIQUES CONGENITALES AVEC
      TROUBLES DU GLUTATHION (A L'EXCLUSION DU DEFICT EN GLUCOSE-
      6-PHOSPHATE-DEHYDROGENASE). MINERVA PEDIATR 20:2659-2666

133. BOIVIN,P. AND GALAND,C., 1965, LA SYNTHESE DU GLUTATHION
      AU COURS DE L'ANEMIE HEMOLYTIQUE CONGENITALE AVEC DEFICIT
      EN GLUTATHION REDUIT. DEFICIT CONGENITAL EN GLUTATHION-
      SYNTHETASE ERYTHROCYTAIRE?. NOUV REV FR HEMATOL 5:707-720

134. BOIVIN,P., GALAND,C. AND BERNARD,J.F., 1974, DEFICIENCIES
      IN G-SH BIOSYNTHESIS. GLUTATHIONE FLOHE,L., BENOEHR,H.C.,
      SIES,H., WALLER,H.D. AND WENDEL,A. ED. 146-157, ACADEMIC
      PRESS, INC., NEW YORK

135. JELLUM,E., KLUGE,T., BOERRESEN,H.C., STOKKE,O. AND ELDJARN,L.,
      1970, PYROGLUTAMIC ACIDURIA - A NEW INBORN ERROR OF
      METABOLISM. SCAND J CLIN LAB INVEST 26:327-335

136. ELDJARN,L., JELLUM,E. AND STOKKE,O., 1972, PYROGLUTAMIC
      ACIDURIA: STUDIES ON THE ENZYMIC BLOCK AND ON THE METABOLIC
      ORIGIN OF PYROGLUTAMIC ACID. CLIN CHIM ACTA 40:461-476

137. LARSSON,A. AND ZETTERSTROEM,R., 1974, PYROGLUTAMIC ACIDURIA
      (5-OXOPROLINURIA), AN INBORN ERROR IN GLUTATHIONE METABOLISM.
      PEDIATR RES 8:852-856

138. WELLNER,V.P., SEKURA,R., MEISTER,A. AND LARSSON,A., 1974,
      GLUTATHIONE SYNTHETASE DEFICIENCY, AN INBORN ERROR OF
      METABOLISM INVOLVING THE GAMMA-GLUTAMYL CYCLE IN PATIENTS
      WITH 5-OXOPROLINURIA (PYROGLUTAMIC ACIDURIA). PROC NATL
      ACAD SCI USA 71:2505-2509

139. HAGENFELDT,L., LARSSON,A. AND ZETTERSTROEM,R., 1974,
      PYROGLUTAMIC ACIDURIA. STUDIES IN AN INFANT WITH CHRONIC
      METABOLIC ACIDOSIS. ACTA PAEDIATR SCAND 63:1-8

140. SMITH,J.E., LEE,M.S. AND MIA,A.S., 1973, DECREASED GAMMA-
      GLUTAMYLCYSTEINE SYNTHETASE: THE PROBABLE CAUSE OF GLUTATHIONE
      DEFICIENCY IN SHEEP ERYTHROCYTES. J LAB CLIN MED 82:713-
      718

141. BEUTLER,E., DERN,R.J., FLANAGAN,C.L. AND ALVING,A.S., 1955,
      THE HEMOLYTIC EFFECT OF PRIMAQUINE. VII. BIOCHEMICAL STUDIES
      OF DRUG-SENSITIVE ERYTHROCYTES. J LAB CLIN MED 45:286-295

142. BEUTLER,E., LANG,A. AND LEHMANN,H., 1974, HEMOGLOBIN DUARTE:
      (ALPHA 2 BETA 2 62 ALA PRO): A NEW UNSTABLE HEMOGLOBIN WITH
      INCREASED OXYGEN AFFINITY. BLOOD 43:527-535

143. LARSSON,A., ZETTERSTROEM,R., HOERNELL,H. AND PORATH,U.,
      1976, ERYTHROCYTE GLUTATHIONE SYNTHETASE IN 5-OXOPROLINURIA:
      KINETIC STUDIES OF THE MUTANT ENZYME AND DETECTION OF
      HETEROZYGOTES. CLIN CHIM ACTA 73:19-23

144. PRINS,H.K., LOOS,J.A. AND ZUERCHER,C., 1968, GLUTATHIONE
      DEFICIENCY. HEREDITARY DISORDERS OF ERYTHROCYTE METABOLISM
      BEUTLER,E. ED. 165-184, CITY OF HOPE SYMP. SERIES, VOL. I,
      GRUNE & STRATTON, N.Y.

145. BEUTLER,E., DERN,R.J. AND ALVING,A.S., 1955, THE HEMOLYTIC
      EFFECT OF PRIMAQUINE. VI. AN IN VITRO TEST FOR SENSITIVITY
      OF ERYTHROCYTES TO PRIMAQUINE. J LAB CLIN MED 45:40-50

146. BEUTLER,E., DURON,O. AND KELLY,B.M., 1963, IMPROVED METHOD
      FOR THE DETERMINATION OF BLOOD GLUTATHIONE. J LAB CLIN MED
      61:882-890

147. MINNICH,V., SMITH,M.B., BRAUNER,M.J. AND MAJERUS,P.W.,
      1971, GLUTATHIONE BIOSYNTHESIS IN HUMAN ERYTHROCYTES I.
      IDENTIFICATION OF THE ENZYMES OF GLUTATHIONE SYNTHESIS IN
      HEMOLYSATES. J CLIN INVEST 50:507-513

148. DESFORGES,J.F., THAYER,W.W. AND DAWSON,J.P., 1959, HEMOLYTIC
      ANEMIA INDUCED BY SULFOXONE THERAPY, WITH INVESTIGATIONS
      INTO THE MECHANISMS OF ITS PRODUCTION. AM J MED 27:132-136

149. CARSON,P.E., BREWER,G.J. AND ICKES,C., 1961, DECREASED
      GLUTATHIONE REDUCTASE WITH SUSCEPTIBILITY TO HEMOLYSIS. J
      LAB CLIN MED 58:804 (ABSTRACT)

150. LOEHR,G.W. AND WALLER,H.D., 1962, EINE NEUE ENZYMOPENISCHE
      HAEMOLYTISCHE ANAEMIE MIT GLUTATHIONREDUKTASE-MANGEL. MED
      KLIN 57:1521-1525

151. WALLER,H.D., 1968, GLUTATHIONE REDUCTASE DEFICIENCY.
      HEREDITARY DISORDERS OF ERYTHROCYTE METABOLISM BEUTLER,E.
      ED. 185-208, CITY OF HOPE SYMP. SERIES, VOL. I, GRUNE &
      STRATTON, N.Y.

152. BLUME,K.G., GOTTWIK,M., LOEHR,G.W. AND RUEDIGER,H.W., 1968,
      FAMILIENUNTERSUCHUNGEN ZUM GLUTATHIONREDUKTASE-MANGEL
      MENSCHLICHER ERYTHROCYTEN. HUMANGENETIK 6:163-170

153. BEUTLER,E., 1969, DRUG-INDUCED HEMOLYTIC ANEMIA. PHARMACOL
      REV 21:73-103

154. BEUTLER,E., 1969, EFFECT OF FLAVIN COMPOUNDS ON GLUTATHIONE
      REDUCTASE ACTIVITY: IN VIVO AND IN VITRO STUDIES. J CLIN
      INVEST 48:1957-1966

155. BEUTLER,E., 1969, GLUTATHIONE REDUCTASE: STIMULATION IN
      NORMAL SUBJECTS BY RIBOFLAVIN SUPPLEMENTATION. SCIENCE
      165:613-615

156. BAMJI,M.S., 1969, GLUTATHIONE REDUCTASE ACTIVITY IN RED
      BLOOD CELLS AND RIBOFLAVIN NUTRITIONAL STATUS IN HUMANS.
      CLIN CHIM ACTA 26:263-269

157. BEUTLER,E. AND SRIVASTAVA,S.K., 1970, RELATIONSHIP BETWEEN
      GLUTATHIONE REDUCTASE ACTIVITY AND DRUG-INDUCED HAEMOLYTIC
      ANAEMIA. NATURE 226:759-760

158. SCHROETER,W., 1969, GLUTATHIONE REDUCTASE AND RIBOFLAVIN
      IN HYPOPLASTIC ANEMIA. N ENGL J MED 281:851-852

159. KLEEBERG,U.R., HEIMPEL,H., KLEIHAUER,E. AND OLISCHLAEGER,A.,
      1971, RELATIVER GLUTATHION-UND/ODER PYRUVATKINASEMANGEL IN
      DEN ERYTHROCYTEN BEI PANMYELOPATHIEN UND AKUTEN LEUKAEMIEN.
      KLIN WOCHENSCHR 49:557-558

160. GOEBEL,K.M., HAUSMANN,L. AND KAFFARNIK,H., 1971, PANCYTOPENIA
     WITH HEMOLYTIC ANEMIA IN GLUTATHIONE REDUCTASE DEFICIENCY.
     IN VIVO AND IN VITRO STUDIES WITH RIBOFLAVIN/FAD ENZYME.
     ENZYME 12:375-381

161. GOEBEL,K.M. AND GOEBEL,F.D., 1972, HEMOLYTIC ANEMIA AND
     PANCYTOPENIA IN GLUTATHIONE REDUCTASE DEFICIENCY:FURTHER
     EXPERIENCE WITH RIBOFLAVIN. ACTA HAEMATOL 47:292-296

162. LOEHR,G.W., BLUME,K.G., RUEDIGER,H.W. AND ARNOLD,H., 1974,
     GENETIC VARIABILITY IN THE ENZYMATIC REDUCTION OF OXIDIZED
     GLUTATHIONE. GLUTATHIONE FLOHE,L., BENOEHR,H.C., SIES,H.,
     WALLER,H.D. AND WENDEL,A. ED. 165-173, ACADEMIC PRESS, NEW
     YORK

163. BENOEHR,H.C. AND WALLER,H.D., 1970, ACTIVATION OF GLUTATHIONE
     REDUCTASE WITH FLAVIN ADENINE DINUCLEOTIDE (FAD). 13TH
     INTERNATIONAL CONGRESS HEMATOLOGY, MUNICH P. 120

164. FLATZ,G., 1971, POPULATION STUDY OF ERYTHROCYTE GLUTATHIONE
     REDUCTASE ACTIVITY. II. HEMATOLOGICAL DATA OF SUBJECTS WITH
     LOW ENZYME ACTIVITY AND STIMULATION CHARACTERISTICS IN
     THEIR FAMILIES. HUMANGENETIK 11:278-285

165. FLATZ,G., 1971, POPULATION STUDY OF ERYTHROCYTE GLUTATHIONE
     REDUCTASE ACTIVITY. I. STIMULATION OF THE ENZYME BY FLAVIN
     ADENINE DINUCLEOTIDE AND BY RIBOFLAVIN SUPPLEMENTATION.
     HUMANGENETIK 11:269-277

166. LOOS,H., ROOS,D., WEENING,R. AND HOUWERZIJL,J., 1976,
     FAMILIAL DEFICIENCY OF GLUTATHIONE REDUCTASE IN HUMAN BLOOD
     CELLS. BLOOD 48:53-62

167. BEUTLER,E. AND MATSUMOTO,F., 1975, ETHNIC VARIATION IN RED
     CELL GLUTATHIONE PEROXIDASE ACTIVITY. BLOOD 46:103-110

168. SCOTT,D.L., KELLEHER,J. AND LOSOWSKY,M.S., 1976, THE EFFECT
     OF DIETARY SELENIUM AND VITAMIN E ON GLUTATHIONE PEROXIDASE
     AND GLUTATHIONE IN THE RAT. BIOCHEM SOC TRANS 4:295-296

169. SMITH,P.J., TAPPEL,A.L. AND CHOW,C.K., 1974, GLUTATHIONE
     PEROXIDASE ACTIVITY AS A FUNCTION OF DIETARY SELENOMETHIONINE.
     NATURE 247:392-393

170. CELLERINO,R., GUIDI,G. AND PERONA,G., 1976, PLASMA IRON
     AND ERYTHROCYTIC GLUTATHIONE PEROXIDASE ACTIVITY. A POSSIBLE
     MECHANISM FOR OXIDATIVE HAEMOLYSIS IN IRON DEFICIENCY
     ANAEMIA. SCAND J HAEMATOL 17:111-116

171. RODVIEN,R., GILLUM,A. AND WEINTRAUB,L.R., 1974, DECREASED
     GLUTATHIONE PEROXIDASE ACTIVITY SECONDARY TO SEVERE IRON
     DEFICIENCY: A POSSIBLE MECHANISM RESPONSIBLE FOR THE
     SHORTENED LIFE SPAN OF THE IRON-DEFICIENT RED CELL. BLOOD
     43:281-289

172. MAC DOUGALL,L., 1972, RED CELL METABOLISM IN IRON DEFICIENCY
     ANEMIA. III. THE RELATIONSHIP BETWEEN GLUTATHIONE PEROXIDASE,
     CATALASE, SERUM VITAMIN E, AND SUSCEPTIBILITY OF IRON-
     DEFICIENT RED CELLS TO OXIDATIVE HEMOLYSIS. J PEDIATR
     80:775-782

173. BEUTLER,E., MATSUMOTO,F., POWARS,D. AND WARNER,J., 1977,
      INCREASED GLUTATHIONE PEROXIDASE ACTIVITY IN ALPHA-
      THALASSEMIA. BLOOD 50:647-655

174. BEUTLER,E., 1977, GLUCOSE-6-PHOSPHATE DEHYDROGENASE DEFICIENCY
      AND RED CELL GLUTATHIONE PEROXIDASE. BLOOD 49:467-469

175. GROSS,R.T., BRACCI,R., RUDOLPH,N., SCHROEDER,E. AND
      KOCHEN,J.A., 1967, HYDROGEN PEROXIDE TOXICITY AND
      DETOXIFICATION IN THE ERYTHROCYTES OF NEW-BORN INFANTS.
      BLOOD 29:481-493

176. BEUTLER,E., WEST,C. AND BEUTLER,B., 1974, ELECTROPHORETIC
      POLYMORPHISM OF GLUTATHIONE PEROXIDASE. ANN HUM GENET
      38:163-169

177. NECHELES,T.F., BOLES,T.A. AND ALLEN,D.M., 1968, ERYTHROCYTE
      GLUTATHIONE-PEROXIDASE DEFICIENCY AND HEMOLYTIC DISEASE OF
      THE NEWBORN INFANT. J PEDIATR 72:319-324

178. WHAUN,J.M. AND OSKI,F.A., 1970, RELATION OF RED BLOOD CELL
      GLUTATHIONE PEROXIDASE TO NEONATAL JAUNDICE. J PEDIATR
      76:555-560

179. NECHELES,T.F., STEINBERG,M.H. AND CAMERON,D., 1970,
      ERYTHROCYTE GLUTATHIONE-PEROXIDASE DEFICIENCY. BR J HAEMATOL
      19:605-612

180. MIWA,S., NAKASHIMA,K., ARIYOSHI,K., UEMURA,M., MURASHIMA,N.
      AND EMI,I., 1974, HETEROZYGOUS ERYTHROCYTE GLUTATHIONE
      PEROXIDASE DEFICIENCY ASSOCIATED WITH NEONATAL
      HYPERBILIRUBINEMIA FOUND IN A JAPANESE FAMILY. ACTA HAEMATOL
      JAP 37:266-270

181. BOIVIN,P., GALAND,C., HAKIM,J. AND BLERY,M., 1970, DEFICIT
      EN GLUTATHION-PEROXYDASE ERYTHROCYTAIRE ET ANEMIE HEMOLYTIQUE
      MEDICAMENTEUSE. UNE NOUVELLE OBSERVATION. LA PRESSE MEDICALE
      78:171-178

182. STEINBERG,M., BRAUER,M.J. AND NECHELES,T.F., 1970, ACUTE
      HEMOLYTIC ANEMIA ASSOCIATED WITH ERYTHROCYTE GLUTATHIONE-
      PEROXIDASE DEFICIENCY. ARCH INTERN MED 125:302-303

183. BOIVIN,P., GALAND,C., HAKIM,J., ROGE,J. AND GUEROULT,N.,
      1969, ANEMIE HEMOLYTIQUE AVEC DEFICIT EN GLUTATHION-PEROXYDASE
      CHEZ UN ADULTE. ENZYME 10:68-80

184. TURSZ,T., BERNARD,J.-.F., VERDIER,F. AND BOIVIN,P., 1974,
      SULFHEMOGLOBINE ET DEFICIT EN GLUTATHION PEROXYDASE. NOUV
      PRESSE MED 3:1487-1490

185. GHARIB,H., FAIRBANKS,V.F. AND BARTHOLOMEW,L.G., 1969,
      HEPATIC FAILURE WITH ACANTHOCYTOSIS: ASSOCIATION WITH
      HEMOLYTIC ANEMIA AND DEFICIENCY OF ERYTHROCYTE GLUTATHIONE
      PEROXIDASE. MAYO CLIN PROC 44:96-101

186. LAUSECKER,C., HEIDT,P., FISCHER,D., HARTLEYB,H. AND
      LOEHR,G.W., 1965, ANEMIE HEMOLYTIQUE CONSTITUTIONNELLE AVEC
      DEFICIT EN 6-PHOSPHO-GLUCONATE- DESHYDROGENASE. ARCH FR
      PEDIATR 21:789-797

187. PARR,C.W. AND FITCH,L.I., 1967, INHERITED QUANTITATIVE
      VARIATIONS OF HUMAN PHOSPHOGLUCONATE DEHYDROGENASE. ANN
      HUM GENET 30:339-353

188. DERN,R.J., BREWER,G.J., TASHIAN,R.E. AND SHOWS,T.B., 1966,
      HEREDITARY VARIATION OF ERYTHROCYTIC 6-PHOSPHOGLUCONATE
      DEHYDROGENASE. J LAB CLIN MED 67:255-264

189. HARVALD,B., HANEL,K.H., SQUIRES,R. AND TRAP-JENSEN,J.,
      1964, ADENOSINE-TRIPHOSPHATASE DEFICIENCY IN PATIENTS WITH
      NON-SPHEROCYTIC HAEMOLYTIC ANAEMIA. LANCET 2:18-19

190. COTTE,J., KISSIN,C., MATHIEU,M., PONCET,J., MONNET,P.,
      SALLE,B. AND GERMAIN,D., 1968, OBSERVATIONS ON A CASE OF
      PARTIAL DEFICIENCY OF ERYTHROCYTIC ATPASE. REV FRANC ETUDE
      CLIN BIOL 13:284

191. LOEHR,G.W., 1969, GENETISCHE ENZYMDEFEKTE DER HEXOKINASE
      UND DER TRANSPORT-ADENOSIN- TRIPHOSPHAT-PHOSPHOHYDROLASE
      DER ERYTHROZYTEN. FOLIA HAEMATOL (LEIPZ) 91:28-38

192. HANEL,H.K., COHN,J. AND HARVALD,B., 1971, ADENOSINE-
      TRIPHOSPHATASE DEFICIENCY IN A FAMILY WITH NON SPHEROCYTIC
      HAEMOLYTIC ANEMIA. HUM HERED 21:313-319

193. GOTTFRIED,E.L. AND MILLER,D.R., 1975, DECREASED ATPASE
      ACTIVITY IN HEREDITARY HEMOLYTIC ANEMIA WITH INCREASED
      MEMBRANE PHOSPHATIDYLCHOLINE. AMERICAN SOCIETY OF HEMATOLOGY
      18TH ANNUAL MEETING (ABSTRACT #183)

194. FEIG,S.A. AND GUIDOTTI,G., 1974, RELATIVE DEFICIENCY OF
      CA2+-DEPENDENT ADENOSINE TRIPHOSPHATASE ACTIVITY OF RED
      CELL MEMBRANES IN HEREDITARY SPHEROCYTOSIS. BIOCHEM BIOPHYS
      RES COMMUN 58:487-494

195. KIRKPATRICK,F.H., WOODS,G.M. AND LA CELLE,P.L., 1975,
      ABSENCE OF ONE COMPONENT OF SPECTRIN ADENOSINE TRIPHOSPHATASE
      IN HEREDITARY SPHEROCYTOSIS. BLOOD 46:945-954

196. NAKAO,K., KURASHINA,S. AND NAKAO,M., 1967,
      ADENOSINETRIPHOSPHATASE ACTIVITY OF ERYTHROCYTE MEMBRANE
      IN HEREDITARY SPHEROCYTOSIS. LIFE SCI 6:595-600

197. SZEINBERG,A., GAVENDO,S. AND CAHANE,D., 1969, ERYTHROCYTE
      ADENYLATE-KINASE DEFICIENCY. LANCET 1:315-316

198. SZEINBERG,A., KAHANA,D., GAVENDO,S., ZAIDMAN,J. AND
      BEN-EZZER,J., 1969, HEREDITARY DEFICIENCY OF ADENYLATE
      KINASE IN RED BLOOD CELLS. ACTA HAEMATOL 42:111-126

199. BOIVIN,P., GALAND,C., HAKIM,J., SIMONY,D. AND SELIGMAN,M.,
      1970, DEFICIT CONGENITAL EN ADENYLATE-KINASE ERYTHROCYTAIRE.
      LA PRESSE MEDICALE 78:1443

200. BOIVIN,P., GALAND,C., HAKIM,J., SIMONY,D. AND SELIGMAN,M.,
      1971, ANEMIE HEMOLYTIQUE CONGENITALE NON SPHEROCYTAIRE ET
      DEFICIT HEREDITAIRE EN ADENYLATE-KINASE ERYTHROCYTAIRE. LA
      PRESSE MEDICALE 79:215-218

201. BREWER,G.J., 1965, A NEW INHERITED ABNORMALITY OF HUMAN
      ERYTHROCYTES - ELEVATED ERYTHROCYTIC ADENOSINE TRIPHOSPHATE.
      BIOCHEM BIOPHYS RES COMMUN 18:430-434

202. ZUERCHER,C., LOOS,J.A. AND PRINS,H.K., 1965, HEREDITARY
      HIGH ATP CONTENT OF HUMAN ERYTHROCYTES. PROC 10TH CONGR
      INT SOC BLOOD TRANSF, STOCKHOLM 549-556

203. OELSHLEGEL,F.J., SANDER,B.J. AND BREWER,G.J., 1975, ROLE
      OF IN VIVO PYRUVATE KINASE ACTIVITY: A. INHERITANCE OF
      ELEVATED RED CELL ATP LEVELS B. RED CELL MALARIAL PARASITE
      INTERACTIONS. PROG CLIN BIOL RES 1:199-218

204. BUSCH,D., 1970, UEBERHOHTER ERYTHROCYTEN-ATP-SPIEGEL-MERKMAL
      EINER HEREDITAEREN NICHTSPHAERO CYTAEREN HAEMOLYTISCHEN
      ANAMIE BEI GESTOERTER ATP-UTILISATION UND EINER
      STOFFWECHSELANOMALIE ROTER ZELLEN OHNE KRANKHEITSWERT. KLIN
      WOCHENSCHR 48:543-550

205. BEUTLER,E. AND MATSUMOTO,F., 1975, UNPUBLISHED

206. VALENTINE,W.N., ANDERSON,H.M., PAGLIA,D.E., JAFFE,E.R.,
      KONRAD,P.N. AND HARRIS,S.R., 1972, STUDIES ON HUMAN
      ERYTHROCYTE NUCLEOTIDE METABOLISM. II. NONSPHEROCYTIC
      HEMOLYTIC ANEMIA, HIGH RED CELL ATP AND RIBOSEPHOSPHATE
      PYROPHOSPHOKINASE (RPK, E.C. 2.7.6.1) DEFICIENCY. BLOOD
      39:675-684

207. VALENTINE,W.N., BENNETT,J.M., KRIVIT,W., KONRAD,P.N.,
      LOWMAN,J.T., PAGLIA,D.E. AND WAKEM,C.J., 1973, NONSPHEROCYTIC
      HAEMOLYTIC ANAEMIA WITH INCREASED RED CELL ADENINE
      NUCLEOTIDES, GLUTATHIONE AND BASOPHILIC STIPPLING AND
      RIBOSEPHOSPHATE PYROPHOSPHOKINASE (RPK) DEFICIENCY: STUDIES
      ON TWO NEW KINDREDS. BR J HAEMATOL 24:157-167

208. VALENTINE,W.N., FINK,K., PAGLIA,D.E., HARRIS,S.R. AND
      ADAMS,W.S., 1974, HEREDITARY HEMOLYTIC ANEMIA WITH HUMAN
      ERYTHROCYTE PYRIMIDINE 5'- NUCLEOTIDASE DEFICIENCY. J CLIN
      INVEST 54:866-879

209. VIVES-CORRONS,J.L., MONTSERRAT-COSTA,E. AND ROZMAN,C.,
      1976, HEREDITARY HEMOLYTIC ANEMIA WITH ERYTHROCYTE PYRIMIDINE
      5'-NUCLEOTIDASE DEFICIENCY IN SPAIN. HUM GENET 34:285-292

210. BEN-BASSAT,I., BROK-SIMONI,F., KENDE,G., HOLTZMANN,F. AND
      RAMOT,B., 1976, A FAMILY WITH RED CELL PYRIMIDINE 5'-
      NUCLEOTIDASE DEFICIENCY. BLOOD 47:919-922

211. ODA,S. AND TANAKA,K.R., 1976, METABOLIC STUDIES IN ERYTHROCYTE
      PRIMIDINE 5'-NUCLEOTIDASE DEFICIENCY. CLINICAL RESEARCH
      24:149A

212. ROCHANT,H., DREYFUS,B., ROSA,R. AND BOIRON,M., 1975, FIRST
      CASE OF PYRIMIDINE 5'NUCLEOTIDASE DEFICIENCY IN A MALE.
      3RD MEETING OF THE EUROPEAN & AFRICAN DIV (INT SOC HAEMATOL)
      LONDON, AUGUST 1975 VOL. 1, ABSTRACT, 1:19

213. MIWA,S., NAKASHIMA,K., FUJII,H., MATSUMOTO,M. AND NOMURA,K.,
      1977, THREE CASES OF HEREDITARY HEMOLYTIC ANEMIA WITH
      PYRIMIDINE 5' NUCLEOTIDASE DEFICIENCY IN A JAPANESE FAMILY.
      HUM GENET 37:361-364

214. SELBY,G. AND BEUTLER,E., 1975, PERSONAL COMMUNICATION

215. KATZ,J., 1976, PERSONAL COMMUNICATION

216. TORRANCE,J.D., KARABUS,C., SHNIER,M., MELTZER,M., KATZ,J.
      AND JENKINS,T., 1977, HAEMOLYTIC ANAEMIA DUE TO RED CELL
      PYRIMIDINE 5' NUCLEOTIDASE DEFICIENCY: FIRST SOUTH AFRICAN
      FAMILY. UNPUBLISHED

217. PAGLIA,D.E., VALENTINE,W.N. AND DAHLGREN,J.G., 1975, EFFECTS
      OF LOW-LEVEL LEAD EXPOSURE ON PYRIMIDINE 5'-NUCLEOTIDASE
      AND OTHER ERYTHROCYTE ENZYMES. J CLIN INVEST 56:1164-1169

218. VALENTINE,W.N., PAGLIA,D.E., FINK,K. AND MADOKORO,G., 1976,
      LEAD POISONING. ASSOCIATION WITH HEMOLYTIC ANEMIA, BASOPHILIC
      STIPPLING, ERYTHROCYTE PYRIMIDINE 5'-NUCLEOTIDASE DEFICIENCY,
      AND INTRAERYTHROCYTIC ACCUMULATION OF PYRIMIDINES. J CLIN
      INVEST 58:926-932

219. HAAS,E., 1943, CYTOCHROME OXIDASE. J BIOL CHEM 148:481-493

220. HIRSCHHORN,R., HIRSCHHORN,K. AND WEISSMANN,G., 1967,
      APPEARANCE OF HYDROLASE RICH GRANULES IN HUMAN LYMPHOCYTES
      INDUCED BY PHYTOHEMAGGLUTININ AND ANTIGENS. BLOOD 30:84-
      102

221. WHITE,J.M. AND SELHI,H.S., 1975, LEAD AND THE RED CELL. BR
      J HAEMATOL 30:133-138

222. ODA,S. AND TANAKA,K.R., 1976, ERYTHROCYTE PYRIMIDINE 5'-
      NUCLEOTIDASE DEFICIENCY: METABOLIC STUDIES. 16TH CONGRESS
      INTERNATIONAL SOCIETY OF HEMATOLOGY, KYOTO ABSTRACT 2-69

223. GIBLETT,E.R., ANDERSON,J.E., COHEN,F., POLLARA,B. AND
      MEUWISSEN,H.J., 1972, ADENOSINE DEAMINASE DEFICIENCY IN
      TWO PATIENTS WITH SEVERELY IMPAIRED CELLULAR IMMUNITY.
      LANCET 2:1067-1069

224. VALENTINE,W.N., PAGLIA,D.E., TARTAGLIA,A.P. AND GILSANZ,F.,
      1977, HEREDITARY HEMOLYTIC ANEMIA WITH INCREASED RED CELL
      ADENOSINE DEAMINASE (45-TO 70-FOLD) AND DECREASED ADENOSINE
      TRIPHOSPHATE. SCIENCE 195:783-785

225. ROSA,R., NAJEAN,Y., PREHU,M., BEUZARD,Y. AND ROSA,J., 1977,
      TOTAL DEFICIENCY OF RED CELL DIPHOSPHOGLYCERATE MUTASE
      (DPGM). BLOOD 50: (SUPPL. 1) 84

INDEX